KU-484-363

NORMAN DOIDGE

The Brain's Way of Healing

*Stories of Remarkable Recoveries
and Discoveries*

PENGUIN BOOKS

PENGUIN BOOKS

UK | USA | Canada | Ireland | Australia
India | New Zealand | South Africa

Penguin Books is part of the Penguin Random House group of companies whose addresses can
be found at global.penguinrandomhouse.com.

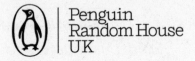

Penguin
Random House
UK

First published in the United States of America by Viking,
an imprint of Penguin Random House LLC, 2015
First published in Great Britain by Allen Lane 2015
Published in Penguin Books 2016
001

Text copyright © Norman Doidge, 2015, 2016

Illustration on page 338 by Laura Hartman Maestro

The moral right of the author has been asserted

Printed in Great Britain by Clays Ltd, St Ives plc

A CIP catalogue record for this book is available from the British Library

ISBN: 978-0-141-98080-5

www.greenpenguin.co.uk

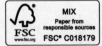

MIX
Paper from
responsible sources
FSC® C018179
www.fsc.org

Penguin Random House is committed to a
sustainable future for our business, our readers
and our planet. This book is made from Forest
Stewardship Council® certified paper.

For Karen, my love

ON DISCOVERIES

Just as the hand, held before the eye, can hide the tallest mountain, so the routine of everyday life can keep us from seeing the vast radiance and the secret wonders that fill the world.

Chasidic saying, eighteenth century

ON RECOVERIES

Life is short, and Art long; opportunity fleeting, experience misleading, and decision difficult. It is the duty of the physician not only to provide what he himself must do, but to enable the patient, the attendants, and the external circumstances to do their part as well.

Hippocrates, father of medicine, 460–375 BC

Contents

Appendix 2

Appendix 3

Note to the Reader

ALL OF THE NAMES OF people who have undergone neuroplastic transformations are real, except in the few places indicated, and in the cases
of children and their families.

The Notes and References section at the end of the book includes
comments on finer points in the chapters.

Preface

THIS BOOK IS ABOUT THE discovery that the human brain has its own unique way of healing, and that when it is understood, many brain problems thought to be incurable or irreversible can be improved, often radically, and in a number of cases, as we shall see, cured. I will show how this process of healing grows out of the highly specialized attributes of the brain—attributes once thought to be so sophisticated that they came at a cost: that the brain, unlike other organs, could not repair itself or restore lost functions. This book will show that the reverse is true: the brain's sophistication provides a way for it to repair itself and to improve its functioning generally.

This book begins where my first book, *The Brain That Changes Itself*, ended. That book described the most important breakthrough in understanding the brain and its relationship to the mind since the beginning of modern science: the discovery that the brain is *neuroplastic*. Neuroplasticity is the property of the brain that enables it to change its own structure and functioning in response to activity and mental experience. That book also described many of the first scientists, doctors, and patients to make use of this discovery to bring about astonishing transformations in the brain. Until then, these transformations had been almost inconceivable, because for four hundred years, the mainstream view of the brain was that it could not change; scientists thought the brain was like a glorious machine, with parts, each of which performed a single mental function, in a single location in the brain. If a location was damaged—by a stroke or an injury or a disease—it could not be fixed because machines cannot repair themselves or grow new parts. Scientists also believed the circuits of the brain were unchangeable or "hardwired," meaning that people born with mental limitations or learning disorders were in all cases destined to remain so. As the machine metaphor evolved, scientists took to describing the brain as a computer and its structure as "hardware" and believed the only change that aging hardware undergoes is that it degenerates with use. A machine wears out: use it, *and* lose it. Thus, attempts by older people to preserve their brains from decline by using mental activity and exercise were seen as a waste of time.

The *neuroplasticians,* as I called the scientists who demonstrated that the brain is plastic, refuted the doctrine of the unchanging brain. Equipped, for the first time, with the tools to observe the *living* brain's microscopic activities, they showed that it changes as it works. In 2000 the Nobel Prize in Physiology or Medicine was awarded for demonstrating that as learning occurs, the connections among nerve cells increase. The scientist behind that discovery, Eric Kandel, also showed that learning can "switch on" genes that change neural structure. Hundreds of studies went on to demonstrate that mental activity is not only the product of the brain but also a shaper of it. Neuroplasticity restored the mind to its rightful place in modern medicine and human life.

THE INTELLECTUAL REVOLUTION DESCRIBED IN *The Brain That Changes Itself* was the beginning. Now, in this book, I tell of the astounding advances of a second generation of neuroplasticians who, because they did not have the burden of proving the existence of plasticity, have been liberated to devote themselves to understanding and using plasticity's extraordinary power. I have traveled to five continents to meet with them—the scientists, clinicians, and their patients—in order to learn their stories. Some of these scientists work in the cutting-edge neuroscience labs of the Western world; others are clinicians who have applied that science; and still others are clinicians and patients who together stumbled upon neuroplasticity and perfected effective treatment techniques, even before plasticity had been demonstrated in the lab.

One patient after another in this book had been told they would never get better. For decades, the term *healing* was seldom used in connection with the brain, as it was with other organ systems, such as the skin or the bones or the digestive tract. While organs such as the skin, liver, and blood could repair themselves by replenishing their lost cells using stem cells to function as "replacement parts," no such cells were found in the brain, despite decades of searching. Once neurons were lost, no evidence could be found that they were ever replaced. Scientists tried to find ways to explain this in evolutionary terms: in the course of evolving into an organ with millions of highly specialized circuits, the brain simply lost the ability to supply those circuits with replacement parts. Even if neuronal stem cells—baby neurons—were to be found, how, it was wondered, would they be of any help? How would they ever integrate into the sophisticated but dizzyingly complex circuits of the brain? Because it wasn't thought possible to heal the brain, most treatments used medication to "prop up the failing system" and decrease symptoms by temporarily changing the chemical balance in the brain. But stop the medication, and the symptoms would return.

It turns out that the brain is not too sophisticated for its own good after all. This book will show that this very sophistication, which involves brain cells being able to constantly communicate electrically with one another, and to form and re-form new connections, moment by moment, is the source of a unique kind of healing. True, in the course of specializing, important reparative abilities, available to other organs, were lost. But some were gained, and they are mostly expressions of the brain's plasticity.

EACH OF THE STORIES IN this book will illustrate a different facet of these neuroplastic ways of healing. The more I immersed myself in these different kinds of healing, the more I began to make distinctions among them and to see that some of the approaches targeted different stages of the healing process. I have proposed (in Chapter 3) a first model of the stages of neuroplastic healing, to help the reader see how they all fit together.

Just as the discoveries of medication and surgery led to therapies to relieve a staggering number of conditions, so does the discovery of neuroplasticity. The reader will find cases, many very detailed, that may be relevant to someone who has, or cares for someone who has experienced, chronic pain, stroke, traumatic brain injury, brain damage, Parkinson's disease, multiple sclerosis, autism, attention deficit disorder, a learning disorder (including dyslexia), a sensory processing disorder, a developmental delay, a part of the brain missing, Down syndrome, or certain kinds of blindness, among others. In some of these conditions, complete cures occur in a majority of patients. In other cases, illnesses that are moderate to severe can sometimes become milder. I shall describe parents who were told that their autistic or brain-damaged children would never complete a normal education, but who saw them do so, graduate, even go to university, become independent, and develop deep friendships. In other situations, an underlying serious illness remains, but its most troubling symptoms are radically reduced. In still others, the risk of getting an illness such as Alzheimer's (in which the brain's plasticity decreases) is significantly reduced (discussed in Chapters 2 and 4), and ways of increasing plasticity are introduced.

MOST OF THE INTERVENTIONS IN this book make use of energy—including light, sound, vibration, electricity, and motion. These forms of energy provide natural, noninvasive avenues into the brain that pass through our senses and our bodies to awaken the brain's own healing capacities. Each of the senses translates one of the many forms of energy around us into the electrical signals that the brain uses to operate. I will show how it is possible to use these different forms of energy to modify the patterns of the brain's electrical signals and then its structure.

In my travels, I saw examples of sounds played into the ear, to treat autism successfully; vibration on the back of the head, to cure attention deficit disorder; gentle electrical stimulators tingling on the tongue, to reverse symptoms of multiple sclerosis and heal stroke; light shone onto the back of the neck to treat brain injury, into the nose to help sleep, or administered intravenously to save a life; and the slow, soft movements of the human hand over the body to cure a girl, born missing a huge section of her brain, of cognitive problems and near paralysis. I will show how all these techniques stimulate and reawaken dormant brain circuits. Among the most effective ways to do so is by using thought itself to stimulate brain circuits, which is why most of the interventions I witnessed paired mental awareness and activity with the use of energy.

The use of energy and the mind together to heal, while novel in the West, has of course been central to traditional Eastern medicine. Only now are scientists beginning to glimpse how these traditional practices may work in terms of Western models, and it is remarkable the extent to which almost all the neuroplasticians I visited were deepening their understanding of how to use neuroplasticity by linking insights from Western neuroscience to insights from Eastern health practices, including traditional Chinese medicine, ancient Buddhist meditation and visualization, martial arts such as tai chi and judo, yoga, and energy medicine. Western medicine has long dismissed Eastern medicine—practiced by billions of people for millennia—and its claims, often because it seemed too far-fetched to accept that the mind can alter the brain. This book will show how neuroplasticity provides a bridge between humanity's two great but hitherto estranged medical traditions.

IT MAY SEEM ODD THAT the ways of healing described in this book so frequently use the body and the senses as primary avenues to pass energy and information into the brain. But these are the avenues the brain uses to connect with the world, and so they provide the most natural and least invasive way to engage it.

One reason clinicians have overlooked using the body to treat the brain is the recent tendency to see the brain as more complex than the body and as the essence of who we are. In this common view, "We are our brains," the brain is the master controller, and the body is its subject, there to follow the master's orders.

This view was accepted because 150 years ago neurologists and neuroscientists, in one of their greatest accomplishments, began to demonstrate the ways in which the brain can control the body. They learned that if a stroke patient couldn't move his foot, the problem wasn't in his foot, as he felt it to be, but in the brain area that controlled the foot. Through the nineteenth and twentieth centuries, neuroscientists mapped where the body was represented in the brain. But the occupational hazard of brain mapping was to begin to believe that the brain was "where *all* the action is"; some neuroscientists began to talk about the brain almost as though it were disembodied, or as though the body were a mere appendage to it, mere infrastructure to support the brain.

But that view of an imperial brain is not accurate. Brains evolved many millions of years *after* bodies did, to support bodies. Once bodies had brains, they changed, so body and brain could interact and adapt to each other. Not only does the brain send signals to the body to influence it; the body sends signals to the brain to affect it as well, and thus there is constant, two-way communication between them. The body abounds with neurons, the gut alone having 100 million. Only in anatomy textbooks is the brain isolated from the body and confined to the head. In terms of the way it functions, the brain is always linked to the body and, through the senses, to the world outside. Neuroplasticians have learned to use these avenues from the body to the brain to facilitate healing. Thus, while a person who has had a stroke may not be able to use his foot because the brain is damaged, moving the foot can, at times, awaken dormant circuits in the injured brain. The body and mind become partners in the healing of the brain, and because these approaches are so noninvasive, side effects are exceedingly rare.

IF THE IDEA OF POWERFUL and yet noninvasive treatments for brain problems seems too good to be true, it is for historical reasons. Modern medicine began with modern science, which was conceived as a technique for the conquest of nature, for—as one of its founders, Francis Bacon, put it—"the relief of man's estate." This idea of conquest gave rise to the many military metaphors that are used in everyday medical practice, as Abraham

Fuks, a former dean of medicine at McGill University, shows. Medicine became a "battle" against disease. Drugs are "magic bullets"; medicine fights
"the war against cancer" and "combats AIDS," with "doctor's orders," from
the "therapeutic armamentarium." This "armamentarium," as physicians
call their bag of therapeutic tricks, honors invasive high-tech treatments as
more scientifically serious than noninvasive ones. There is definitely a time
for a martial attitude in medicine, especially in emergency medicine: if a
blood vessel in the brain bursts, the patient needs invasive surgery and a
neurosurgeon, with nerves of steel, to operate. But the metaphor creates
problems too, and the very idea that it is possible to "conquer" nature is a
fond, naïve hope.

In this metaphor, the patient's body is less an ally than the battle-
field, and the patient is rendered passive, a helpless bystander, as he
watches the confrontation that will determine his fate between the two
great antagonists, the doctor and the disease. The attitude has even
come to influence the ways many physicians now talk to their patients,
interrupting their story as they speak, because often the high-tech physician is less interested in their narrative than in their lab test.

NEUROPLASTIC APPROACHES, ON THE OTHER hand, require the active
involvement of the whole patient in his or her own care: mind, brain,
and body. Such an approach recalls the heritage not only of the East but
of Western medicine itself. The father of scientific medicine, Hippocrates, saw the body as the major healer, and the physician and patient working together *with* nature, to help the body activate its own
healing capacities.

In this approach, the health professional not only focuses on the patient's deficits, important as they may be, but also searches for healthy
brain areas that may be dormant, and for existing capacities that may aid
recovery. This focus doesn't advocate naïvely replacing the neurological nihilism of the past with an equally extreme neurological utopianism—
replacing false pessimism with false hope. To be valuable, discoveries of
new ways of healing the brain do not have to guarantee that all patients
can be helped all the time. And often, we simply don't know what will

happen, until the person, with the guidance of a knowledgeable health professional, gives the new approaches a try.

The word *heal* comes from the Old English *haelan* and means not simply "to cure" but "to make whole." The concept is very far from the idea of "cure" in the military metaphor, with its associated ideas of divide and conquer.

What follow are stories of people who have transformed their brains, recovered lost parts of themselves, or discovered capacities within that they never knew they had. But the true marvel is less the techniques than the way that, through millions of years, the brain has evolved, with sophisticated neuroplastic abilities and a mind that can direct its own unique restorative process of growth.

Chapter 1

Physician Hurt, Then Heal Thyself

*Michael Moskowitz Discovers
That Chronic Pain Can Be Unlearned*

MICHAEL MOSKOWITZ, M.D., IS A psychiatrist-turned-pain-specialist who has often been forced to use himself as a guinea pig.

Burly, buoyant, and six feet tall, Moskowitz looks a decade younger than his sixty-odd years. He wears oval John Lennon glasses; has slightly long, graying curls of hair, a mustache, and a beatnik's soul patch beneath his lower lip. He smiles a lot. I first saw Moskowitz in Hawaii, where he was moderating a serious and sober panel at the American Academy of Pain Medicine. He was in a suit, but he seemed too big a personality, too boyish, to be wearing one. A few hours later, on the beach, he wore shorts and wild colors and was unconstrained, joking, bringing out the boyishness in me. We somehow got into a conversation about how physicians—so often interested in diagnostic categories, which are supposed to be like ideal forms, unvarying from person to person— can easily forget how different people really are. "Like me, for instance," he said.

"How so?" I asked.

"My anatomy." Whereupon he pulled off his Hawaiian shirt to proudly display that his chest bore not two but three male nipples.

"A true freak of nature," I joked. "Does it do you any good?"

Like the medical students we once were, we plunged into a juvenile, jocular debate: because nipples on the male are useless, which of us was more useless, the one with two or the one with three? Thus we got acquainted, and everything about him—his love of singing and playing the guitar, his hugely engaging manner and youthful voice—suggested that he was still very much a creature of the happy-go-lucky world of love, music, and easygoing, carefree abandon of the 1960s in which he came of age.

Not so.

Moskowitz spends most of his time immersed in the chronic pain of others. Their agony is unknown to most people, in part because they are often so drained by their pain that they stop wasting what little energy they have to express distress to those who can't help them. Chronic pain may be invisible on a patient's face, or it can give its victim a drawn, ghostly presence, because it sucks the life out of a person. Moskowitz, on the other hand, gets to share in its full burden. He and another psychiatrist-turned-pain-specialist, his long-standing southern friend Robert "Bobby" Hines, M.D., set up a pain clinic, Bay Area Medical Associates, in Sausalito, California, which treats West Coast patients with "intractable pain": those who have tried all other treatments, including all known drugs, "nerve blocks" (regular anesthetic injections), and acupuncture. The patients who end up there failed to recover in all known mainstream and alternative treatments and have usually been told, "Everything that can be done for you has been done."

"We are the end of the line," Moskowitz says. "We are where people come to die with their pain."

Moskowitz came to pain medicine after working for years as a psychiatrist. He has all the professional and scholarly credentials: he was on the examination council for the American Board of Pain Medicine (setting the exams for doctors in pain medicine); he is a former chairman of the education committee of the American Academy of Pain Medicine; and he has an advanced psychiatric fellowship in psychosomatic medicine. But Moskowitz became a world leader in the use of neuroplasticity for treating pain only after making some discoveries while treating himself.

A Lesson in Pain—The Kill Switch

On June 26, 1999, when he was forty-nine, Moskowitz and a friend snuck into the local San Rafael dump because he had heard that army tanks and other armored vehicles were being stored there for the Fourth of July parade. He couldn't resist the boyish pleasure of climbing up onto a tank turret. When he jumped off, a metal prong for holding gas cans on the tank's side caught his corduroys. As he fell, one leg shot up five feet, and he heard three popping sounds: his femur, the longest bone in the body, was cracking. When he looked down at his leg, he saw it was pointed way to the left, at a ninety-degree angle to the other leg. "I was a bit too old to be on tanks and a jeep. When I spoke afterward to a friend who was a personal injury lawyer, he said, 'You would have a great case if you were seven.'"

As a pain physician, he used the situation to observe a phenomenon that he had taught his students about but had never experienced; it would become central to his neuroplastic research. Immediately after he fell, his pain was a true 10 out of 10—that is, 10/10, as pain physicians measure it. Pain is rated from 0/10 to 10/10 (10 is being dropped into boiling oil). He had never known whether he himself would be able to stand a true 10. He realized he could.

"The first thing I thought was: how will I get to work Monday?" he told me. "The second thing I realized, while lying motionless on the ground waiting for the ambulance, was that once I stopped moving, I had literally no pain at all. I thought, 'Wow, this really does work! My brain simply shut off the pain—something I had been teaching my students for years. I had a firsthand experience that the brain, all on its own, can eliminate pain, just as I, a conventional pain specialist, had tried to do for patients by using drugs, injections, and electrical stimulation. As long as I didn't move, the pain was zero within about a minute.

"When the ambulance came, they gave me six milligrams of IV morphine. I said, 'Give me another eight.' They said, 'We can't,' and I said, 'I'm a pain doctor,' so they did, but when they moved me it was ten out of ten."

The brain can shut pain off because the actual function of acute pain is not to torment us but to alert us to danger. True, the word *pain* comes from the ancient Greek *poine,* which means "penalty," via the Latin *poena*, which means "punishment," but biologically, pain is not punishment for punishment's sake. The pain system is the hurt body's implacable advocate, a reward and penalty signaling system. It penalizes us when we are about to do something that *might* further damage our already injured body, and it rewards us with relief when we stop.

As long as Moskowitz didn't move, he was in no danger, so far as his brain could tell. He also knew that the "pain" was never really in the leg itself. "All my leg did was send signals to my brain. We know from general anesthesia, which puts the higher parts of the brain to sleep, that if the brain doesn't process these signals, there is no pain." But general anesthesia has to render us unconscious to eliminate pain; here he was, lying in agony on the ground, and in one moment, his completely *conscious* brain turned all his pain off. If only he could learn how to flip that switch for his patients!

But it wasn't just movement that posed a danger for Moskowitz. While waiting for the ambulance, he nearly died, because he bled about half of his entire blood volume into his leg, so it ballooned to twice the normal size: "my leg was the size of my waist." With all his blood pooling in his leg for hours, it was a miracle he didn't die from insufficient blood supply to his vital organs. But he made it to the hospital, where "the surgeon put the largest plate they had into my leg and said that if they had needed one more screw, they would have had to amputate."

During the surgery he almost died two more times. First he threw off an embolus—a blood clot—that could have lodged in his lungs or brain. Then the catheter implanted to drain his urine pierced his prostate, and he spiked a high fever and went into septic shock—a life-threatening condition in which the body is overwhelmed by infection. His blood pressure fell to 80/40.

Yet he survived—and learned another pain lesson: the wise use of sufficient morphine during his acute pain prevented his nerves from being chronically stimulated and saved him from developing a chronic pain syndrome. (This was the reason he requested more morphine when his acute pain was not covered.) Despite the severity of the accident, as the years have passed, he has had very little pain in the leg, and he can walk, about a mile and a half, as we did along the beach in Hawaii, without experiencing pain.

The fact that the brain has the ability to turn pain off so suddenly goes against our "commonsense" experience that pain comes from the body. The traditional scientific view of pain, as formulated by the French philosopher René Descartes four hundred years ago, was that when we are hurt, our pain nerves send a one-way signal up to the brain, and the intensity of the pain is proportional to the seriousness of our injury. In other words, pain files an accurate damage report about the extent of the body's injury, and that the role of the brain is to simply accept that report.

But that view was overturned in 1965, when the neuroscientists Ronald Melzack (a Canadian who studied phantom limbs and pain) and Patrick Wall (an Englishman who studied pain and plasticity) published the most important article in the history of pain, "Pain Mechanisms: A New Theory." Wall and Melzack argued that the pain perception system is spread throughout the brain and spinal cord, and that the brain, far from being a passive recipient, controls how much pain we feel. Their "gate control theory of pain" proposed that when pain messages are sent from damaged tissue through the nervous system, they must pass through several controls, or "gates," starting in the spinal cord, before they get to the brain. These messages ascend to the brain only if the brain gives them "permission" to do so, after determining whether they are important enough to be let through. (When President Reagan was shot through the chest in 1981, he initially just stood there, and neither he nor his Secret Service men knew he had been shot. As he later joked, "I had never been shot before, except in the movies. Then you always act as though it hurts. Now I know that does not always happen.") If "permission is granted" for the signal to proceed to the brain, a gate will open and increase our feeling of pain by allowing certain neurons to turn on and transmit their signals. But the brain can also close a gate and block the pain signal by releasing endorphins, the narcotics made by our bodies to quell pain.

Before his accident, Moskowitz taught the latest versions of the gate theory to his residents, and that switches control the gates. But knowing such switches exist is one thing; knowing how to turn them off when you are lying in agony is another.

Another Lesson in Pain—Chronic Pain Is Plasticity Gone Wild

Moskowitz's tank accident wasn't the first time he developed important insights about pain by having it himself. Several years earlier a pain in the neck, caused by a water-skiing accident, taught him another lesson, one that helped him understand the role of neuroplasticity in pain. In 1994, while water-skiing with his daughters, big-kid Moskowitz was speeding, splashing, and pounding at forty miles an hour in an inflated inner tube, when he flipped over and hit the water with his head bent backward. The resulting pain persisted. It was often an 8/10, on many days making it impossible for him to work. It soon dominated his life as no pain ever had. Morphine and other heavy-duty painkillers, and all the known treatments—physical therapy, traction (stretching the neck), massage, self-hypnosis, heat, ice, rest, anti-inflammatory drugs—barely touched it. That pain haunted and tormented him for thirteen years, becoming more severe as time passed.

He was fifty-seven when he hit rock bottom with his neck pain and began researching the discovery that the brain was neuroplastic and relating it to pain. The idea that chronic pain was caused by a neuroplastic event of the brain had been proposed by the German physiologist Manfred Zimmermann in 1978, but as neuroplasticity would remain generally unaccepted for another twenty-five years, Zimmermann's idea was hardly known, and its applications to treat pain unexplored.

Acute pain alerts us to injury or disease by sending a signal to the brain, saying "This is where you are hurt—attend to it." But sometimes an injury affects both our bodily tissues and the neurons in our pain system, including those in the brain and spinal cord, resulting in *neuropathic pain* (sometimes called *central pain* because the brain and spinal cord together make up our central nervous system).

Neuropathic pain occurs because of the behavior of neurons that make up our brain maps for pain. The external areas of our body are represented in our brain, in specific processing areas, called brain maps. Touch a part of the body's surface, and a specific part of the brain map, devoted to that spot, will start to fire. These maps for the body's surface are organized topographically, meaning that areas that are adjacent on the body are generally adjacent on the map. When the neurons in our pain maps get damaged, they fire incessant false alarms, making us believe the problem is in our body when it is mostly in our brain. Long after the body has healed, the pain system is still firing. The acute pain has developed an afterlife: it becomes *chronic pain*.

To understand how chronic pain develops, it's helpful to know about the structure of neurons. Each neuron has three parts: the dendrites, the cell body, and the axon. The dendrites are treelike branches that receive input from other neurons. The dendrites lead into the cell body, which sustains the life of the cell and contains its DNA. Finally, the axon is a living cable of varying lengths (from microscopic ones in the brain to others that run down to the legs and can be three feet long). Axons are often compared to wires because they carry electrical impulses at very high speeds (from 2 to 200 miles per hour) toward the dendrites of neighboring neurons. A neuron can receive two kinds of signals: ones that excite it (excitatory signals) and ones that inhibit it (inhibitory signals). When a neuron receives enough excitatory signals, it will fire off its own signal. When it receives enough inhibitory signals, it becomes less likely to fire.

Axons don't quite touch the neighboring dendrites. They are separated by a microscopic space called a *synapse*. Once an electrical signal gets to the end of the axon, it triggers the release of a chemical messenger, called a *neurotransmitter,* into the synapse. The chemical messenger floats over to the dendrite of the adjacent neuron, exciting or inhibiting it. When we say that neurons "rewire" themselves, we mean that alterations occur at the synapse, strengthening and increasing, or weakening and decreasing, the number of connections between the neurons.

One of the core laws of neuroplasticity is that neurons that fire together wire together, meaning that repeated mental experience leads to structural changes in the brain neurons that process that experience, making the synaptic connections between those neurons stronger.* In practical terms, when a person learns something new, different groups of neurons get wired together. As a child learns the alphabet, the visual shape of the letter A is connected with the sound "ay." Each time the child looks at the letter and repeats the sound, the neurons involved "fire together" at the same time, and then "wire together"; the synaptic connections between them are strengthened. Whenever any activity that links neurons is repeated, those neurons fire faster, stronger, sharper signals together, and the circuit gets more efficient and better at helping to perform the skill.

The converse is also true. When a person stops performing an activity for an extended period, those connections are weakened, and over time many are lost. This is an example of a more general principle of plasticity: that it is a use-it-or-lose-it phenomenon. Thousands of experiments have now demonstrated this fact. Often the neurons that were involved in the skill will be taken over and used for other mental tasks that are now being performed more regularly. Sometimes one can manipulate the use-it-or-lose-it principle to undo brain connections that are not helpful, because neurons that fire apart wire apart. Suppose a person has formed a bad habit of eating whenever he is emotionally upset, associating the pleasure of food with the dulling of emotional pain; breaking the habit will require learning to disassociate the two. He might have to actively forbid himself from going to the kitchen when he is emotionally upset, until he finds a better way to handle his emotions.

Plasticity can be a blessing when the ongoing sensory input we receive is pleasurable, for it allows us to develop a brain that is better able to perceive and to savor pleasant sensations; but that same plasticity can be a curse when the sensory system that is receiving ongoing input is the pain system. That can happen when a person slips a disc, which then presses repeatedly on a nerve root in her spine. Her pain map for the area becomes hypersensitive, and she begins to feel pain not only when the disc hits the nerve when she moves the wrong way, but even

* How this was discovered, and the finer points of how this works, are discussed in detail in Norman Doidge, *The Brain That Changes Itself* (New York: Viking, 2007).

when the disc is not pressing hard. The pain signal reverberates throughout her brain, so that pain persists even after its original stimulus has stopped. (Something similar, and even more drastic, happens in phantom limb pain, when a person who has lost a limb feels it is still attached and hurting. This more complex phenomenon is discussed in *The Brain That Changes Itself*.)

Wall and Melzack showed how a chronic injury not only makes the cells in the pain system fire more easily but can also cause our pain maps to enlarge their "receptive field" (the area of the body's surface that they map for), so that we begin to feel pain over a larger area of our body's surface. This was happening to Moskowitz, whose neck pain was spreading to both sides of his neck.

Wall and Melzack also showed that as maps enlarge, pain signals in one map can "spill" into adjacent pain maps. Then we may develop *referred pain*, when we are hurt in one body part but feel the pain in another, some distance away. Ultimately, the brain maps for pain begin to fire so easily that the person ends up in excruciating, unremitting pain, felt over a large area of the body—all in response to the smallest stimulation of a nerve.

Thus, the more often Moskowitz felt twinges of neck pain, the more easily his brain's neurons recognized it, and the more intense it got. The name for this well-documented neuroplastic process is *wind-up pain*, because the more the receptors in the pain system fire, the more sensitive they become.

Moskowitz realized that he was developing a chronic pain syndrome and was caught in a vicious cycle, a brain trap: each time he had an attack of pain, his plastic brain got more sensitive to it, making it worse, setting him up for a new, still worse attack next time. The intensity of his pain signal, the length of time it lasted, and the amount of space in the body it "occupied" all increased.

It was a case of plasticity gone wild.

IN 1999 MOSKOWITZ BEGAN DRAWING pictures on his computer, demonstrating how chronic pain caused an expansion of the brain's pain maps. At the time, the specialty of pain medicine was often far more focused on how pain is processed in the spinal cord and the body's peripheral nervous system than in the brain. As late as 2006, the major text on pain, *Wall and Melzack's Textbook of Pain,* had a chapter on plasticity and the spinal cord but none on plasticity and the brain. A few years later, in his article titled "Central Influences on Pain," Moskowitz began shifting that emphasis.

Moskowitz defined chronic pain as "learned pain." Chronic pain not only indicates illness; it is itself an illness. The body's alarm system is stuck in the "on" position, because the person has been unable to remedy the cause of an acute pain, and the central nervous system has become damaged. "Once chronicity sets in, the pain is much more difficult to treat."

Moskowitz's thinking was beginning to converge with another Melzack theory, called the neuromatrix theory of pain. Acute pain is a sensation we feel, an "input" that comes into the brain from the bottom up, from our sense receptors. But chronic pain is more complex and more a top-down process. The essence of the neuromatrix theory of pain is that chronic pain is more a perception than a raw sensation, because the brain takes many factors into account to determine the extent of danger to the tissues. Scores of studies have shown that along with assessing damage, the brain, when developing our subjective experience of pain perception, also assesses whether action can be taken to diminish the pain, and it develops expectations as to whether this damage will improve or get worse. The sum total of these assessments determines our expectation as to our future, and these expectations play a major role in the level of pain we will feel. Because the brain can so influence our perception of chronic pain, Melzack conceptualized it as more of "an output of the central nervous system."

Thus, the pain circuit is not a one-way circuit from body to brain; it constantly recycles signals, from the body to the brain and back. The full pain response doesn't stop once the pain signal enters the brain. It begins myriad automatic responses that evolved to avoid further damage and promote healing. We recoil; we guard our damaged limbs so they won't be moved; we groan and cry out for help; we assess and reassess the severity of our wound, if we can; and as studies show, we ride a roller coaster of ups and downs in our distress, based on our latest assessment. If a person develops chest pain behind his breastbone that radiates down the left arm, and thinks these are symptoms of a heart attack, he will experience that pain as more intense than he will if his physician assures him that it's caused by a muscle strain.

"The brain," Moskowitz wrote (using the military metaphor), "mounts a counteroffensive against the incoming activity in an attempt to turn the excessive activity down." He detailed all the pain-modulating pathways that could do so—from the highest ones that originate in the brain's cerebral cortex (where reasoning occurs) to the "lower" input areas in the spinal cord.

A Neuroplastic Competition

Wishing to take charge of his own pain, in 2007 Moskowitz read fifteen thousand pages of neuroscience. He wanted to better understand the laws of neuroplastic change and put them into practice. He learned that not only can one strengthen circuits between brain areas by getting these areas to fire at the same time, but that one can weaken connections because "neurons that fire apart wire apart."

Could he, by fiddling with the timing of input to his brain, start to weaken links that had formed in his pain maps?

He learned that in our use-it-or-lose-it brain there is an ongoing competition for cortical real estate, because the activities the brain performs regularly take up more and more space in the brain by "stealing" resources from other areas. He drew three pictures of the brain that summarized what he had learned. The first was a picture of the brain in acute pain, with sixteen areas showing activity. The second was of the brain in chronic pain, showing those same areas firing but expanded over a larger area of the brain, and the third picture was of the brain when it is not registering pain at all.

As he analyzed the areas that fire in chronic pain, he observed that many of those areas also process thoughts, sensations, images, memories, movements, emotions, and beliefs—when they are not processing pain. That observation explained why, when we are in pain, we can't concentrate or think well; why we have sensory problems and often can't tolerate certain sounds or light; why we can't move more gracefully; and why we can't control our emotions very well and become irritable and have emotional outbursts. The areas that regulate these activities have been hijacked to process the pain signal.

The neuroplastician Michael Merzenich showed the competitive nature of plasticity by first mapping a monkey's brain over time. *Mapping a brain* means finding where in the brain different mental functions occur. For instance, sensations coming from each of the fingers in our right hand are processed in the touch area in our left hemisphere, and each finger has a separate location in the map where its touch sensations are processed. The signals from the neurons that process these sensations can be detected by microelectrodes, pins inserted into individual neurons, or right beside them, to detect when they fire. These electrical signals are passed to an amplifier, then to an oscilloscope with a screen that allows scientists to both see and hear the neuron as it fires. By inserting a microelectrode into the brain's sensory map for the thumb, then touching the actual thumb, a scientist can see "thumb" neurons firing on the screen.

Merzenich mapped a monkey's entire hand map. He began by touching the monkey's first finger and seeing which brain area started to fire. Once he found its brain map and defined its borders, he went on to the next finger. He found five finger areas, side by side for each of the five digits.

Then he amputated the animal's third finger. After a number of months, he remapped the monkey's remaining fingers and found that the brain maps for the second finger and fourth finger had grown into the space he had originally mapped for the third. Because the map was no longer getting input from the third finger, and because the second and fourth fingers were doing more work now that the third was missing, they took over that map space. Here was a very clear demonstration that brain maps are dynamic, that there is competition for cortical real estate, and that brain resources are allocated according to the principle of use it or lose it.

Moskowitz's inspiration was simple: what if he could use competitive plasticity in his favor? What if, when his pain started—instead of allowing those areas to be pirated and "taken over" by pain processing—he "took them back" for their original main activities, by forcing himself to perform those activities, no matter how intense the pain was?

What if, when he was in pain, he could try to override the natural tendency to retreat, lie down, rest, stop thinking, and nurse himself? Moskowitz decided the brain needed a counterstimulation. He would force those brain areas to process anything-but-pain, to weaken his chronic pain circuits.

Years as a pain medicine specialist had fixed in his mind the key brain areas he was targeting. Each of them could process pain and do other mental functions, and he listed what each did other than process pain, so he would be prepared to do those things while he was in pain. For instance, a part of the brain called the somatosensory area (*soma* means "body") processes much of the body's sensory input, including pain, vibration, and touch. What if, while he felt pain, he was to flood himself with vibration and touch sensations? Might those sensations prevent the somatosensory areas from being able to process pain?

He drafted a list of brain areas he would target (Table 1).

Table 1.
Major Brain Areas Where Pain Is Processed

Somatosensory 1 and 2 (the sensory maps for our body parts):
Pain; touch, temperature sense, pressure sense, position sense, vibration sense, sensation of movement

Prefrontal Area:
Pain; executive function, creativity, planning, empathy, action, emotional balance, intuition

Anterior Cingulate:
Pain; emotional self-control, sympathetic control, conflict detection, problem solving

Posterior Parietal Lobe:
*Pain; sensory, visual, auditory perception; mirror neurons
(neurons that fire when we see other people move), internal
location of stimuli, location of external space*

Supplementary Motor Area:
Pain; planned movement, mirror neurons

Amygdala:
*Pain; emotion, emotional memory, emotional response, pleasure,
sight, smell, emotional extremes*

Insula:
*Pain; quiets the amygdala (the brain area just above);
temperature, itch, empathy, emotional self-awareness, sensual
touch, connects emotion with bodily sensation, mirror neurons,
disgust*

Posterior Cingulate:
Pain; visuospatial cognition, autobiographical memory retrieval

Hippocampus:
Helps to store pain memories

Orbital Frontal Cortex:
*Pain; evaluates whether something is pleasant vs. unpleasant,
empathy, understanding, emotional attunement*

Moskowitz knew that when a particular brain area is processing acute pain, only about 5 percent of the neurons in that area are dedicated to processing pain. In chronic pain, the constant firing and wiring lead to an increase, so that 15 to 25 percent of the neurons in the area are now dedicated to pain processing. So about 10 to 20 percent of neurons get pirated to process chronic pain. Those were what he would have to steal back.

In April 2007 he put this theory into practice. He decided that he would first use visual activity to overpower the pain. A huge part of the brain is devoted to visual processing, and it couldn't hurt to have it on his side in this competition. He knew of two brain areas that process visual information and pain, the posterior cingulate (which helps us to visually imagine where things are in space) and the posterior parietal lobe (which also processes visual input).

Each time he got an attack of pain, he immediately began visualizing. But what? He visualized the very brain maps he had drawn, to remind himself that the brain can really change, so he'd stay motivated. First he would visualize his picture of the brain in chronic pain—and observed how much the map in chronic pain had expanded neuroplastically. Then he would imagine the areas of firing shrinking, so that they looked like the brain when there was no pain. "I had to be relentless—even more relentless than the pain signal itself," he said. He greeted every twinge of pain with an image of his pain map shrinking, knowing that he was forcing his posterior cingulate and posterior parietal lobes to process a visual image.

In the first three weeks, he thought he noticed a very small decrease in pain, and he doggedly continued to apply the technique, telling himself to "disconnect the network, shrink the map." After a month he was getting the hang of it and applying the technique so conscientiously that he *never* let a pain spike occur without doing some visualization or other mental activity to oppose it.

It worked. By six weeks, the pain between his shoulders in his back and near his shoulder blades had completely disappeared, never to return. By four months, he was having his first totally pain-free periods throughout his neck. And within a year he was almost always pain free, his average pain 0/10. If he had a brief relapse (usually from his neck being in a weird position, after a long drive, or having the flu), he was able to get his pain down to 0 in a few minutes. His life was totally changed, after thirteen years of chronic pain. During those thirteen years, his average pain had been 5/10, but could range up as high as 8/10 even on medication, and even his best days were 3/10.

The disappearance of the pain reversed the original pattern of its expansion. After his injury, he had acute pain on the left side of his neck, exactly where the injury had occurred. As time passed and the pain became chronic, it had neuroplastically extended to the right side of his neck and down to his midback. Now, with the visualizations, he noticed that the borders of the pain on the right were the first to get smaller. Then the pain on the left side began to retract and went away.

After six weeks of results, he started to share his discovery with his patients.

His First Neuroplastic Patient

Jan Sandin was in her forties, a registered nurse on a cardiac ward at Sequoia Hospital in Redwood City, California. One day when she was working with a 280-pound woman patient, the patient accidentally gashed her own leg and became hysterical. Terrified that she would fall, she reached out her arms and grabbed Jan's neck, hanging on so tightly Jan couldn't breathe: "It felt like a death grip." The woman was screaming, too panicked to put her weight on her injured leg. Jan couldn't dislodge her, so she asked an assistant to maneuver the patient toward the bed and get ready to do a "one, two, three" lift. Jan heaved, but her assistant, in shock from the patient's screaming, didn't put her arms out to help. Suddenly Jan was supporting the full weight of nearly three hundred pounds. "I heard the sound of a rubber band snapping," she recalled, "and felt something inside me break." All five of her lumbar (low-back) discs were damaged, and the bottom one slipped and pressed against a nerve root. She developed sciatica pain down both legs and could not walk. Whenever she moved, her spine made a crunching sound.

In intense pain, Jan was taken to the emergency room. She was diagnosed as having damage to all the discs in her five lumbar vertebrae. After subsequent tests she was told she had so much degeneration of the spine, she would probably need to have those five vertebrae fused with surgery. Over the next few years she was given all the usual treatments for pain, including physiotherapy and heavy-duty opioid medications. Nothing helped, and the pain became chronic. Surgeons told her there was too much damage in her lower back to operate. After several brave attempts to return to work, she was declared disabled. She felt her life was over. "I was depressed and suicidal. And it didn't matter what drugs the doctors gave me—the pain never went away. I couldn't even watch TV or read because, on top of the pain, the drugs I took put me in a gray zone. There was no reason to live." She spent the next decade at home, never going out except to doctors' visits.

By the time she got to Moskowitz, she had been disabled with chronic pain for a decade. The slightest movement would trigger unbearable exacerbations. She spent entire days in her Jacuzzi, on huge doses of heavy-duty painkillers like morphine, which would lower her pain to a 5/10. Often she spent twelve hours a day in a Japanese massage chair but got little relief. Bent over with a cane, she could hardly get herself into Moskowitz's office.

IT'S JULY 2009. THE WOMAN I see before me, Jan, is sixty-two years old, beaming, perky, relaxed, and off all medication. Moskowitz had been working conventionally with her for five years, using heavy-duty painkillers, when, in June 2007, he introduced her to the idea of training herself, using his neuroplastic technique. To motivate her for the neuroplastic challenge ahead—and she would have to counter the pain mentally *every* moment over the next weeks—he decided she would first have to understand plasticity and take inspiration from the successes of others who had been deemed incurable.

"One day, Moskowitz said, 'Okay, I have thought of something new,' and he gave me your book," Jan told me. "And I went right through it, so I could understand how the plasticity of the brain works. The book opened up a way for me to think I might be able to do something. I realized I was stuck in a fixed logic. Reading all the examples of different connections forming in the brain made me think something else might be possible."

Moskowitz showed her his three pictures of the brain and told her that she had to be more relentless than the pain in focusing on them. He asked her first to look at the pictures, then put them down and visualize them, while thinking about transforming her brain into the no-pain version. He urged her to hold on to the thought that if her brain looked like the no-pain picture, she couldn't have any pain.

"I started to take what you were saying in the book," she told me, "and what he was saying and put them into practice. He told me to look at the brain pictures seven times a day. But I sat in the massage chair and I looked at them *all day long*, because I had nothing else to do. I would visualize the pain centers firing, and then I thought about where my pain was coming from in my back. Then I would visualize how it went into the spine and then into my brain—but with no pain centers firing. In those first two weeks, I had moments when there was no pain. . . . It wasn't profound, because I felt, *Oh, it's not going to last.* Then I thought, *Oh, it's back again—don't get your hopes up.*

"By the third week I was starting to have a couple of minutes a day without chronic pain. It just stopped me in my tracks. And then it would come back. By the end of the third week, the time without pain seemed to increase. But it happened for such a short period of time that, honestly, I never really thought it would go away.

"By the fourth week, the pain-free periods were up to fifteen minutes to half an hour. I thought, *This is going to go away.*"

And it did.

Next, she started going off all her medications, terrified the pain would return, but it didn't. "I wondered, *Is it a placebo?* But the pain still hasn't come back. It has never come back."

When I first saw Jan, she had been free of all medication and pain for a year and a half, and life was returning to normal. "It is like I was asleep for a decade. Now I want to stay up twenty-four hours a day and read, and catch up on all that I have missed. I want to be awake all the time."

The MIRROR Acronym

Moskowitz began formulating acronyms, based on neuroplastic principles, to remind patients in chronic pain how to organize their minds (minds that were slightly foggy and disorganized by the pain) as they sought to undermine that pain. One was MIRROR, for Motivation, Intention, Relentlessness, Reliability, Opportunity, and Restoration.

Motivation is the first MIRROR principle. Most chronic pain patients go to their physicians with a passive attitude toward their pain. They have been trained that their role is to take a pill or submit to an injection. Generally they are so sapped by their pain, they assume this passive role easily, living from visit to visit, hoping the physician will find the magical medication to make life more bearable.

Now, in the Moskowitz approach, the patient must become active, must read about how pain develops, must actively visualize (or some equivalent) and take charge of her treatment. Motivation is especially difficult in the early weeks of Moskowitz's technique, when the patient can't be sure it is having any effect and finds that after the first small success, the pain returns. Patients tend to take these setbacks as a reason to feel helpless and hopeless and stop. The trick is to use each attack of pain as a motivator, an opportunity to apply the technique, which will ultimately work.

Intention is a subtle concept. The immediate intention is not to get rid of pain—it is to focus the mind, in order to change the brain. Thinking that the immediate reward will be pain reduction will make it hard to get there, because that reward comes slowly. In the early stages what counts is the mental effort to change. These mental efforts help build new circuits and weaken the pain networks. The initial reward, after an episode, is being able to say, "I got a pain attack and used it as an opportunity to exercise mental effort and develop new connections in my brain, which will help in the long run," rather than "I got a pain attack, I tried to get rid of it, but am still in pain." Moskowitz writes, in his patient handout: "If focus is merely on immediate pain control, positive results will be fleeting and frustrating. Immediate pain control is definitely part of the program, but the real reward is to disconnect excessively wired pain networks and to restore more balanced brain function in these pain processing regions of the brain."

Relentlessness is the simplest concept of all. Pain intruding into consciousness is the signal to push back. What is challenging about relentlessness is that when the pain is just beginning to act up, the patient may think perhaps it will be enough to tolerate the pain or distract himself, hoping it will pass, or that it might be easier to pop a pill and nip it in the bud. But putting up with some pain, while trying to distract oneself with work, is not an intense enough focus to break the strangle-hold of chronic pain. Research on neuroplasticity shows that intense focus is generally required to alter the circuits and make new connections. So casual distraction must be resisted, because it allows the pain to run unopposed. Thus, even if the pain seems mild, letting it go unopposed may mean it gets stronger next time. Relentlessness means: every time pain is detected, push back, with full focus, and with the specific intention of rewiring the brain back to what it was before the chronic pain began. No exceptions. No negotiations with pain.

Reliability is a reminder that the brain is not the enemy, and that the patient can rely upon it to restore and maintain normal function if it has clear and unrelenting directions to do so. For psychological reasons, when in pain, the sufferer feels penalized and tormented by it. But except in the case of certain neurotic psychological conflicts, which generally have to do with unconscious guilt, the brain and nervous system are not "trying to punish" the person in pain. The brain, like all living systems, constantly seeks a stable state. The problem is that at times, it stabilizes in a state of chronic pain. But if the brain is given a way to get back to its previous, pain-free state, before chronic pain set in, it will not generally oppose the change. After all, the pain system evolved to protect. It is an alarm system, not an enemy. "When unconscious systems are not enough to solve a brain/body problem," Moskowitz writes, "we have to bring in conscious control in the form of new learning until the brain and body can carry on without that conscious input. It is a fact that brain and body reliably turn conscious effort into unconscious action that allows us to move from learning to mastery, returning the disease of persistent pain to the fleeting symptom of acute pain."

Opportunity means turning each pain episode into a chance to repair the faulty alarm system. While it's hard to welcome an attack of pain, using it to rally oneself can feel constructive, knowing one is taking charge and is using the pain spike to heal. That attitude by itself can alter the mindset and brain chemistry. "Pain that persists," Moskowitz says, "is terrifying because it sets off the amygdala, before the parts of the brain that modify our emotional responses can be turned on.

"The result is that we reexperience the trauma that caused the pain and this trauma is continuously reinforced by it. The terror demoralizes us, and as pain-processing areas expand in the brain, we lose our full ability to problem-solve, regulate emotions, resolve conflicts, relate to others, distinguish other sensations from pain, effectively plan, and even remember how to apply our past experience to control pain. Every time the pain worsens, it feels like it is here to stay, and we must avoid it at all costs. The amygdala is not a place of moderation. It is a place of extreme emotions, fight-and-flight and post-traumatic stress disorder. Persistent pain demoralizes most people who have it. If, on the other hand, we turn the pain episodes into an opportunity to practice using our brains and bodies differently to gain control of the pain, then pain spiking shifts from an act of terror to a chance to soothe. . . . Essentially we are turning the disease of pain back to a symptom, a signal to rally us to do something to stop it."

Restoration means that the goal isn't to mask pain or take the edge off it, as medication or anesthetics would, but to restore normal brain function.

Once Moskowitz was able to put these six tools in his patients' hands, and motivate them toward the ambitious goal of completely normalizing their brain function, their attitude changed. Now when they had modest improvements, they felt not just temporary feelings of "relief" but a progressive increase in hope, which they then used to energize themselves, to continue applying the technique. A vicious cycle was turned into a virtuous one.

How Visualization Decreases Brain Pain

So far we have explained the cure that Moskowitz achieved as caused by competitive plasticity. For instance, a part of the brain, the posterior parietal lobe, normally processes both pain and visual perception. By visualizing constantly, Jan prevented that lobe from processing pain. Repeated visualization is a very direct way of using thought to stimulate neurons—neurostimulation. On brain scans, we can see signs of the blood rushing to the visual neurons of the brain that are being activated. What we have left out is that she and Moskowitz did a very *specific* form of visualization: they imagined that the area of the brain devoted to processing pain was shrinking.

I was intrigued by the use of visual imagery, which is not entirely new—hypnotists often use it to bring about pain relief, by asking patients to imagine that the area in pain is shrinking, or fading, or farther away. Put in neuroscientific terms, the hypnotists are actually getting their clients to experiment not with their physical bodies but with the subjective image they have of their bodies in their minds, what clinicians call the "body image." The body image was first described in the 1930s by a psychiatrist and student of Freud, Paul Schilder, who pointed out that it is not identical to the physical body.

The body image is formed in the mind *and* is represented in the brain, then is unconsciously projected onto the body. Neuroscientists sometimes call it the "virtual body" to emphasize that it has an existence in the brain and mind that is *independent* of the physical body. This body image is built up with input from multiple brain maps including vision but also touch, pain, and proprioception (where our limbs and bodies are in space)—indeed, from any map that has information, sensory or even emotional, about our bodies. It is thus the sum total of all the different *inputs* to the brain from the different senses, but also includes the person's own emotionally laden ideas about his or her body.

The body image can be quite in sync with the actual body, meaning it can be a fairly accurate representation of it. In those situations, we may even forget that our image of the body is a mental phenomenon that is different from the actual body. But when the body image doesn't match the body, the difference is easy to detect. Many of us have experienced this mismatch without realizing it when the dentist gives a local anesthetic: suddenly the jaw and cheeks feel subjectively much larger than they really are. The mismatch is pronounced when someone with anorexia nervosa looks in the mirror and insists she is fat, when she is actually skin and bones, on the brink of starvation. She has the body image of a fat person, though her physical body is emaciated.

Around the time when Moskowitz was starting to use visualization, having chronic pain patients imagine that areas of their brain were shrinking, scientists in Australia were getting similar results by having patients in the lab "shrink" their body image to rewire their brains. In 2008 G. Lorimer Moseley, an Australian neuroscientist and one of the most creative pain researchers alive, with his colleagues, Timothy Parsons and Charles Spence, conducted an ingenious study of people with chronic hand pain and swelling. He asked them to observe their hands in different conditions. First, in the control situation, they looked at their hands while doing ten hand movements. Then they looked through binoculars without magnification (another control situation, just in case using binoculars had an influence on results) and moved their hands. Third, they watched their hands performing the movements through the binoculars at two times magnification. Finally, they looked through the wrong end of the binoculars, so that their hands looked smaller.

Intriguingly, the researchers found that the pain increased when the image of the hands was magnified, and decreased when it was miniaturized.

A skeptic might question the reliability of patients rating themselves. But these patients did have actual swelling in their hands, and when the researchers measured the circumference of the patients' fingers during the experiment, they observed that the swelling increased when the patients were viewing their hands under magnification.

What this remarkable study shows, once again, is that the experience of pain is not wholly driven by sensory input from pain receptors but is influenced by the body image. When the brain, because of distorted visual input coming from the binoculars, determines that the pain is coming from a smaller area, it concludes, "Less damage." (Moseley proposes that the reason the pain is lessened is that the brain has "visuotactile cells" that simultaneously process both visual and tactile senses, and that magnifying the view of the area being touched increases input into these cells.)

Another breakthrough experiment in pain management involving visualization occurred by accident when academics from the University of Nottingham, England, went to a fair to demonstrate the use of an optical illusion called Mirage. The university's psychology department had developed Mirage in order to distort the body image, as part of a study of how the body map works.

At the fair, the researchers invited children to put their hands inside a box with a camera in it. Mirage then displayed distorted images of their hands on a large screen, where the children could see the distortions—a computerized version of a fun-house mirror.

Encouraged by the researchers, the children tugged gently on their fingers. When they did, on the screen it appeared as though their fingers were being stretched to three or four times their normal size. When they compressed their fingers, they would then appear to shrink on the screen. In other words, the image on the screen was altering their visual body image (leaving their physical body unchanged).

A grandmother of one of the children thought it looked fun and insisted on having a go. But she told the researchers they had better be gentle when they demonstrated the tugging on her hands, because she had arthritis in her fingers.

Dr. Catherine Preston explains, "We were giving her a practical demonstration of an illusory finger stretching when she announced, 'My finger doesn't hurt anymore' and asked whether she could take the machine home with her. We were just stunned—I don't know who was more surprised, her or us."

Preston followed up with a study of twenty volunteers with osteo-arthritis, some of whom had constant pain in their hands, feet, and lower back. That study showed that using the device halved the level of pain in 85 percent of the volunteers. A number of people got the greatest pain reduction when the fingers were shrunk; others got most relief when their fingers were stretched; and some got pain reduction as long as the image of the finger was changed in any way. Many were able to use their fingers more easily while using the device.

It is not clear why "stretching" the imaged fingers would reduce pain; perhaps a stretched finger has different dimensions, and appears slimmer. What does seem clear is that real-time modification of the visual body image can lower the pain experience. It reminds us that the formation of the sense of the body in pain is dynamic—it is being re-made all the time, depending on visual input. It shows that altering the visual imagery of the body can modify pain circuits. This is an important clue as to why Jan Sandin was able to look at imagery of her brain and imagine the pain signal shrinking: she said she strongly identified with those pictures of the brain in chronic pain and then imagined a transition to the picture of the brain out of pain—the signals shrinking away.

Jan hadn't simply been looking at brain pictures; she had also linked them to the pain she felt in her back. Ultimately, she formed a new body image map, which included the brain pictures, and was able to do so because our "master" brain map of our body image is a highly integrated combination of many different maps. It includes the primary biological ones, based on sensory input from our bodies, but also artificial ones, such as our reflection in a mirror, or a favorite photograph of ourselves, or even medical imagery, as when we get an echocardiogram and see our heart contracting, or we are shown an X-ray that displays our insides. Whatever can be defined as representing us can ultimately make its way into our master body image. (The ways the body image can be extended to include artificial images is discussed in detail in Chapter 7 of *The Brain That Changes Itself*.)

Is It a Placebo?

"Is it the placebo effect?" I ask Moskowitz, echoing Jan's question after she got better unexpectedly, fearing it wouldn't last. It's not that I believe it is, but I know that this is the question skeptics will ask him.

The term *placebo* derives from the Latin "I shall please." The placebo effect occurs when a patient with symptoms is given a dummy pill, such as a sugar pill, or injections with no active ingredients, or pseudo-surgery* (when a physician opens a patient's body up but doesn't operate,

---

* In 2002 a study was done of the most commonly performed orthopedic operation conducted in the United States. "Arthroscopic debridement" involves opening the knee joint and surgically removing loose cartilage, inflamed tissue, and bits of bone. About 650,000 such $5,000 operations are conducted each year in the United States. Earlier studies had shown that about half of those who underwent it had some pain relief. In the 2002 study, 180 patients with painful osteoarthritis were assigned to two groups. One group got the usual surgery. The second was given sham surgery, in which an incision was made and the arthroscope was inserted and removed but no surgery was performed. Not only was the sham surgery as effective for pain relief as the actual surgery, but the placebo surgery patients actually functioned better physically. See J. B. Moseley et al., "A Controlled Trial of Arthroscopic Surgery for Osteoarthritis of the Knee," *New England Journal of Medicine* 347, no. 2 (2002): 81–88. While one might argue that perhaps that only means that the usual surgery isn't much good, the point is that the patients got as much relief from the placebo surgery as from the real operation. It also suggests that the same "kill switch" for pain that Moskowitz had learned to master was working in these patients, without their knowledge.

just pretends to, then closes it). The patient is told she is getting effective treatment, and surprisingly, she often gets immediate relief and sometimes as much improvement as might occur with the "real" or "active" treatment. Placebos can be used to treat pain, depression, arthritis, irritable bowel, ulcers, and a wide range of illnesses. But it doesn't work for all illnesses—cancer, or viruses, or schizophrenia, for instance. Most physicians assume that whenever a patient gets better inexplicably, some powerful psychological factor is involved.

So I ask Moskowitz, "Is it the placebo effect?"

"I hope so," he laughs.

He laughs because he knows that if it is placebo, it wouldn't be nearly the problem most skeptics believe it to be. The latest brain scan research shows that when the placebo effect occurs in pain patients, or in patients with depression, the changes in the brain are *almost identical* to those that occur when they get better with medication. Clinicians and scientists who study mind-body medicine argue that if we could develop a way of systematically activating the brain circuitry that underlies the placebo effect, it would represent a huge medical breakthrough.

For pain, the placebo effect generally runs at 30 percent or higher, meaning that if a pain patient is given a sugar pill instead of real medication, or injections that consist only of salt water (saline) instead of anesthetic, at least 30 percent will report significant pain relief. Before the discovery of neuroplasticity, researchers tended to assume that patients who experienced the placebo effect were mostly psychologically unstable, flighty, immature, poor, or female (all of which has since been shown to be untrue). Brain scan studies demonstrate that when the placebo effect occurs, brain structure changes. Placebo cures are not "less real" than cures by medication. They are examples of neuroplasticity in action: mind changing brain structure.

One of the groups pioneering these studies was led by a researcher who had serious doubts. Tor Wager, a Columbia University neuroscientist, was raised as a Christian Scientist and as a boy was taught that all illnesses were products of the mind, requiring prayer not medication. When he developed a severe skin rash that would not disappear through prayer, his mother took him to a doctor, who treated him with medication, success-fully. Wager became skeptical of the idea that the mind could heal, and of the placebo effect, which he began to study, expecting to find it was inef-fective. He gave painful shocks to volunteers, then gave them a placebo cream that he told them would diminish the pain. To his surprise, his studies showed the placebo cream worked. He then used fMRI scans to study what was happening in their brains. When the subjects were given shocks and felt pain, some of the same brain areas that Moskowitz had seen activated by pain lit up. When Wager gave them the placebo, he found reduced activation in the same areas that Moskowitz told his patients could be modified through visualization.

Using PET scans of the brain, Wager has also shown that placebo treatment turns off pain by getting key brain areas to increase the pro-duction of endogenous opioids—the opiumlike substances that the brain produces to erase pain. He showed that the placebo response strengthened the brain's wiring in the opioid-producing areas of the brain's pain system. In other words, the mind can release an internal supply of the natural balm that the brain normally produces. And un-like the opioids in medications like morphine, these opioids are nonad-dictive.

Why It Isn't Just Placebo

"I'm totally open to the idea that this is placebo and suggestion," says Moskowitz, "but I have done this a long time, thirty years, since 1981, and I have never seen placebo or suggestion stick this long. I have never seen the changes for pain based on hypnosis or suggestion last longer than a week or so."

Moskowitz's assertion that placebos generally don't last reflects the consensus based on numerous placebo studies. If a response is very rapid, it is more likely to be a placebo response, but the placebo responders were more likely to suffer a relapse, though some studies show the placebo effect can last for weeks.

However, the exact opposite pattern is seen in Moskowitz's patients using the MIRROR approach and competitive plasticity. His patients often have no response for weeks, then gradually have less and less pain; once they have rewired their brains, they generally have to do the intervention less and less. I have seen the same pattern in people who used neuroplastic techniques to rewire their brains to cure learning disorders and to improve after strokes and traumatic brain injury: the symptoms didn't disappear quickly. Moskowitz's patients' pattern of change is also consistent with what we see when the brain learns a new skill, like playing a musical instrument or learning a language. The time frame is typical of what I have seen in significant neuroplastic change: the change occurred over weeks (often six to eight weeks) and required daily mental practice. It's hard work.

A skeptic, who has difficulty imagining that visualizing a specific brain pain area can diminish pain, might argue that all Moskowitz is doing is finding a way to relax his patients and lower their general level of arousal, so that their pain bothers them less. But one thing that has been learned from studying the placebo effect is that the mind has the ability to target pain with laserlike precision.

The mind-brain-body healing process is *not* merely a general, non-specific process that resets the entire nervous system, the way relaxation does. Mysteriously—because we don't yet know the mechanism—it targets only what the patient believes is the focus. With elegant simplicity, the researcher Guy Montgomery placed weights heavy enough to cause pain on both index fingers of his subjects. He then applied a placebo cream to only one index finger. He found that pain was relieved only in the finger that got the placebo cream. These people were not being relaxed or put in a trance: they were in normal states of conscious arousal, and still their minds could pinpoint the exact spot of acute pain and eliminate it.

What Moskowitz has added to our understanding of this ability of the mind to eliminate a particular pain is that constant mental practice is necessary to strengthen this ability and change the firing of the brain in a way that is sustained.

Unlike medication or placebo, the neuroplastic technique allows patients to reduce its use over time, once their networks have rewired.

The effects last. Moskowitz has patients who have kept their gains for five years. Many of his relatively pain-free patients still have damage in their bodies, which can, on occasion, trigger acute pain. He thinks that once they have learned and practiced the technique over hundreds of hours, their unconscious mind takes over the task of blocking pain by using competitive plasticity. When it doesn't, they can still use the spike of pain as the signal to consciously use competitive plasticity to do more rewiring.

ONE OF MOSKOWITZ'S MOST IMPORTANT insights is that the new opioid narcotics, so popular for pain treatment, have actually made pain problems worse, because neither the drug companies nor most physicians take into account the role of neuroplasticity in pain. Opioid narcotics, the most potent pain medications we have, generally don't work well over long periods of time. Often within days or weeks, patients become "tolerant" to such a drug: the size of the initial dose loses its effect, so they need ever more medication, or they experience "breakthrough pain" while on the drug. But as the dose is increased, so too is the danger of addiction and overdose. To better block pain, drug companies invented "long-acting" opioids, such as OxyContin, a long-acting morphine. People with chronic pain would often be placed on OxyContin-like drugs for life.

As we've seen, the brain makes its own opioidlike substances to block pain, and the manufactured drugs supplement them by attaching to the brain's own opioid receptors. As long as scientists believed that the brain couldn't change, they never anticipated that bombarding the opioid receptors with opioid medications could do harm. However, says Moskowitz, "once we saturate all our God-given receptors, the brain produces new ones." It adapts to being inundated by long-term opioids by becoming less sensitive to them—and thus patients become more sensitive to pain, and more dependent on their drugs, which can make their chronic pain worse. The problem exists, says Moskowitz, with all the pain medicines.

Once he made his discoveries, he slowly began to wean many

patients from their long-term opioids. A key to success was to lower the dose very slowly, thereby giving the neuroplastic brain the time it needed to adapt to being without drugs, so the patient wouldn't experience any "breakthrough pain." Tapering slowly, down to 50 to 80 percent of the original dose, could break the cycle of opioid-induced pain sensitivity.

"I DON'T BELIEVE IN PAIN management anymore," says Moskowitz. "I believe in trying to cure persistent pain."

He has helped patients with a whole range of chronic pain syndromes to diminish their pain, including those with chronic low-back pain from nerve injury and inflammatory damage, diabetic neuropathy, some cancer pain, abdominal pain, neck degeneration pain, amputation, trauma to the brain and spinal cord, pelvic floor pain, inflammatory bowel, irritable bowel, bladder pain, arthritis, lupus, trigeminal neuralgia, multiple sclerosis pain, post-infectious pain, nerve injuries, neuropathic pain, some central pain, phantom limb pain, degenerative disc disease in all regions of the spine, pain from failed back surgery, and pain from nerve root injury, among others. I met many of his patients who had either come off their medications or radically reduced them, so that they have far fewer side effects. Patients have had successes in all these pain syndromes, but only when they were able to do the relentless mental work required.

This burden of work is one of the limits of his approach. Not everyone is like Jan, willing to apply themselves relentlessly, especially in the early weeks, when nothing appears to be changing, even if they have a physician as inspiring as Michael Moskowitz. He's observed that when patients have not benefited, they have seemed unable, for whatever reason, to mobilize themselves mentally for the challenge. Many, perhaps most, need positive reinforcement.

Jan, Moskowitz, and others were restored by understanding how to use competitive plasticity. Pleasure returned. Many clinicians would, at that point, have focused the rest of their career on teaching visualization, because so many patients responded to it. But not all had responded, and that left Moskowitz dissatisfied. Perhaps some needed approaches other than visualization to compete with pain. Moskowitz wondered: in addition to helping his patients to slowly unwire their brain's pain circuitry, could he make use of the body's own pleasure chemistry to alleviate pain more rapidly? And what if the idea of truly restoring patients meant not only achieving the absence of pain but nothing less than bringing them back to a fuller life?

In studying these questions, he would be helped by Marla Golden, a physician who specializes in chronic pain, whom he met in 2008. Golden, an emergency physician, also trained in osteopathy, a hands-on practice. She has profoundly deepened Moskowitz's understanding of how to use touch, sound, and vibration, each in a unique way, to flood the brain and to competitively counter pain. (In Chapter 8 we shall see how sound, vibration, and touch can heal many kinds of serious brain problems.) She has achieved remarkable results by using her hands, approaching pain through the body.

"I had always thought the body was a bag for the brain," Moskowitz said to Golden when they met, on the assumption that what a patient feels in his body is the product of brain activity. But Golden was able to show Moskowitz that the body is as much an avenue into the brain as is the mind. "She's the yin to my yang," he says, and he has totally internalized her approach. Now, they collaborate and have pioneered a true brain-body approach to chronic pain, in which patients receive simultaneous neuroplastic input from the mind and body to influence the brain. Golden's hands are so sensitive, Moskowitz says, she sometimes seems to "see" with them, finding problem areas and rapid ways to ease chronic pain. I have seen Moskowitz and Golden work together, in demonstrations, on the same patient at once. Moskowitz talks to the patient, helping her to use her mind to alter brain circuits neuroplastically, while Golden works on the patient's body, stimulating touch and vibration sense at the same time. I have followed a number of their patients and seen remarkable progress.

As for Jan Sandin, who was cured in 2009, I returned to visit her in

2011. Her chronic pain syndrome had not returned, and she actually looked younger than she had in 2009. Today, in 2014, she continues to be pain free, knowing that her relentless application of her mind in those days—when she was confined to a chair, immobilized, depressed and suicidal from her pain—was the best investment of mental energy she ever made.

Chapter 2

A Man Walks Off
His Parkinsonian Symptoms

*How Exercise Helps Fend Off Degenerative Disorders
and Can Defer Dementia*

MY WALKING COMPANION, JOHN PEPPER, was diagnosed with Parkinson's disease, a movement disorder, over two decades ago. He first started getting symptoms nearly fifty years ago. But unless you are a perceptive and well-trained observer, you would never know it. Pepper moves too quickly for a Parkinson's patient. He doesn't appear to have the classic symptoms: no shuffling gait; no visible tremor when he pauses or when he moves; he does not appear especially rigid, and seems able to initiate new movements fairly quickly; he has a good sense of balance. He even swings his arms as he walks. He shows none of the slowed movements that are the hallmark of Parkinson's. He hasn't been on anti-Parkinson's medication for nine years, since he was sixty-eight years old, yet appears to walk perfectly normally.

In fact, when he gets going at his normal walking speed, I can't keep up with him. He's now going on seventy-seven and has had this illness, which is defined as an incurable, chronic, progressive neurodegenerative disorder, since his thirties. But instead of degenerating, John Pepper has been able to reverse the major symptoms, the ones that Parkinson's patients dread most, those that lead to immobility. He's done so with an exercise program he devised and with a special kind of concentration.

The beach we are on is called Boulders because of the huge, round rocks that ring it, lined up like adjacent marbles. It is just off the southern tip of Africa, where the Indian and Atlantic Oceans meet, and we have come to observe an African penguin colony. Slightly off the beaten path, we are in search of jackass penguins, so known because of their braying mating calls. We see our first penguin as it rockets out of the Indian Ocean with optimistic grace. It's called porpoising. But when the penguin comes ashore, he has an ungainly waddle.

We have been told that in the next little stretch of sand, which is surrounded by the huge ten-foot-tall boulders, we will find a group of penguins and their babies. But I don't see how we will reach them through the wall of rock because the cracks between the boulders are so narrow and low. Still, Pepper urges me to go through one of the gaps. I manage to contort myself, crouching on my hands and knees, in a claustrophobic passage only a couple of feet high, crawling and twisting my spine under the low ceiling over the water-lapped sand, and barely get through. Then I look back. He follows.

My initial thought is that this is not a good idea. Pepper is six feet tall, 212 pounds and muscular, thick limbed, with a huge chest, much bigger than mine, and I just made it with barely an inch to spare. In Parkinson's, rigidity is a central feature, and I imagine him getting stuck in that hole because his body will be too stiff to do the necessary contortions. Another feature of Parkinson's is "freezing," due to difficulty initiating new movements, which is why, when walking, Parkinson's patients, on encountering the smallest obstacle, even at a line drawn on the path, can suddenly freeze in their tracks. If Pepper should freeze in that hole, it might be impossible to get him out.

But I have seen him move so well in the last few days, I have no reason to play the Nervous Nellie. He scrambles through.

Now we can hear but not see the penguins, and to get to them, we will have to climb up over a huge rock. Pepper leaps ahead of me, scurrying up and over the top of the boulder, sure-footed. Another symptom of Parkinson's is absent or slowed movement, called akinesia or bradykinesia respectively. He displays neither.

I struggle up, my limbs splayed out on the rock, trying to get a good grip, but I'm having difficulties. This rock is unexpectedly moist. Not just glistening, it has a slimy surface, and I keep slipping.

"I thought the soles of these shoes were stickier, but I keep sliding back," I say, blaming my sneakers, as I finally make it over.

He laughs. "It's the guano."

"Guano?"

"Penguin poop. And seabird dung. It's thick on these rocks and on the cliffs, too many centuries' worth. In days gone by, ships would moor off the coast and send in small boats to dig the guano off these rocks. It's magnificent fertilizer." His face is Anglo-Saxon, he has cropped gray hair, and his voice is like Alec Guinness's with a South African accent.

I rub my hands clean on the sides of my pants and discover we are standing in a small waddle of penguins. They are adorable and are not bothered by our presence.

We spent that morning in Cape Town, where Pepper was teaching a woman at the Parkinson's support group there, as he's taught hundreds, to overcome her shuffling gait and to move more freely and effectively. Now at Boulder Beach, I see that penguins have much the same shuffling gait as the patients we spent the morning with. Penguins' feet are set so far back on their bodies—to reduce drag when they swim—that they look stooped when they walk, like people with Parkinson's. Penguin bodies appear stiff, and when they turn, they do so *en bloc,* without fluidity, again like people with Parkinson's. Penguins' legs look stiff too (because they are so very short), and their feet seem to stick briefly to the ground between steps, so that they too "shuffle" along.

Patients with Parkinson's shuffle because their legs have begun to rigidify, and they lose normal postural reflexes that would allow them to change their muscle tone as they change the position of their limbs and joints. Their movements slow, and their steps shorten. They shuffle because these uncertain, stiff-legged steps can cause the toes or even the whole foot to drag, and they barely pick up their feet, so their soles hardly clear the ground. Thus they never get a spring in their step. Nor do they swing their arms. The Parkinson's stoop and the shuffling gait are the features physicians can most easily pick out at a distance. It was that gait that one of Pepper's physicians thought he noticed one day, many years before, when he asked what seemed to Pepper a bizarre question:

"Would you mind leaving the room, then coming back in again?"

Pepper went out and came back, and the physician examined him in more detail. At the end of the visit, the physician identified the shuffling gait that goes with Parkinson's disease, called PD for short.

A Letter from Africa

In September 2008 I received an e-mail letter from John Pepper:

I live in South Africa and have had Parkinson's disease since 1968. I do a lot of exercise and have learned to use my conscious brain to control the movements, which are normally controlled by the subconscious brain. I wrote a book about my experience, but it has been rejected by the medical profession without looking into my case, because I no longer look like a PD sufferer. I no longer take PD medication, although I still have most of the symptoms. I walk fifteen miles per week, in three sessions of five miles. The glial-derived neurotrophic factor produced in the brain appears to have restored the damaged cells. However, they do not cure the cause of PD, and if I stop exercising, I go backward. . . . I am sure that I can help many newly diagnosed patients, if I can encourage them to do serious regular exercise. Please let me know your thoughts on this matter.

My thought was that, as far-fetched as it might seem, Pepper, by battling aspects of Parkinson's with the low-tech approach of walking, might indeed be triggering neuroplastic change in his brain. The glial-derived neurotrophic factor (GDNF) that he referred to is a brain growth factor. It functions like a growth-promoting fertilizer in the brain. GDNF is made by glial cells, one of the major types of cells in the brain. Fifteen percent of our brain cells are neurons; the other 85 percent are glial cells. For a long time, scientists hardly discussed glial cells because they believed they were merely the "packing material" of the brain, that they simply surrounded and supported our far more active neurons. Now we know that glial cells are constantly communicating with one another, interacting with neurons and modifying their electrical signals. They are also "neuroprotective" of neurons, helping them to wire and rewire the brain. Frank Collins and his colleagues discovered GDNF in 1993 and found that it contributes to plastic change in the brain by promoting the development and survival of dopamine-producing neurons (the cells that die off in Parkinson's). Collins immediately wondered if it might be useful in the treatment of Parkinson's. GDNF also helps the nervous system recover from injury.

Pepper was aware of the recent discovery by Michael Zigmond and others that exercise in lab animals had been found to increase GDNF. I wrote him back:

> I'm not an expert in Parkinson's, but I'm in touch with people who are making significant progress that we didn't think possible on neurological illnesses, such as progressive MS, so I'm fascinated by your story, and do know—from other sources—that exercise has been helpful in PD and have spoken with people who are experts in this and neuronal stem cells, and intensive walking like you are doing sounded to them like the kind of dose that would be necessary.

As we corresponded, it became clear that his claim was not that he had completely cured himself of the disease; rather, as long as he kept up his walking, he could reverse the main *movement* symptoms of Parkinson's. The changes had so helped him that he was no longer suffering from the main disabilities of PD and was living a full life. "I will be ashamed to die with all this information," he wrote, "and not be able to do something for Parkinson's patients."

His claim seemed remarkable; only a few have ever professed to reverse the main symptoms of Parkinson's without medication. Some people experience a mild version of the illness, but without medication, most lose the ability to walk within eight to ten years of diagnosis. Typically, Parkinson's movement problems begin on one side, in an upper or lower limb; over time they progress, in most cases, to both sides of the body. Those on medication find that their drug's effects begin to wane after about five years.

Physical disability is not the only worry. Parkinson's can also give rise to cognitive deficits. As in any neurological condition that restricts mobility, the effects of the illness (as opposed to the illness itself) can weaken the brain in a secondary way. The neuroplastic brain evolved in ambulatory beings who ranged around the world, always having to explore unknown territories. In other words, the brain evolved to learn. As people become immobile, they see less, hear less, and process less new information, and their brains begin to atrophy from the lack of stimulation (unless they are fundamentally thinkers, and even then the neuroplastic systems require physical movement to generate new cells and nerve growth factor). Whether the cause of the atrophy is Parkinson's or the lack of stimulation, Parkinson's patients develop cognitive deficits at rates higher than does the normal population. The cognitive problems can progress to dementia in advanced cases: Parkinson's patients have a six-times-normal risk of dementia.

Finally, they risk premature death. Margaret Hoehn and Melvin Yahr conclude at the end of their scientific study that "the state of Parkinsonism severely limits life expectancy." Pneumonia is the most common cause of death, along with falls and choking as a result of difficulty swallowing.

Today's medications can dramatically improve the ability to move, especially early in the illness, but they don't stop the progression of the disease, which begins to affect more and more of the body and slowly overwhelms a medication's ability to deal with it. Mainstream thinking has been that the illness is caused by the increasing inability of part of the brain, called the substantia nigra, to produce the brain chemical dopamine, which is necessary for normal movement. The substantia nigra is called "nigra" because it has a rich dark pigment. As its neurons are lost, so too is the pigment—a loss that can be seen with the naked eye on autopsy.

In 1957 the Swedish Nobel laureate Arvid Carlsson, an extraordinary scientist and physician, discovered that dopamine was one of the brain chemicals used to send signals between neurons. He then discovered that about 80 percent of our brain's dopamine is concentrated in the part of the brain that contains the substantia nigra, the basal ganglia. Dopamine does many things, including—as we now know, years after Carlsson's discovery—helping to consolidate neuroplastic change. The researcher Oleh Hornykiewicz showed that low dopamine gives rise to Parkinson's symptoms, and that giving dopamine boosters like levodopa (a chemical that the body can easily transform into dopamine) relieves symptoms. Levodopa is a substance the body normally produces, and in the brain, the neurons can convert it to dopamine to replace what is missing. Ultimately studies in humans showed that dopamine levels can fall by 70 percent without appearing to affect a person, but when they fall by 80 percent, Parkinsonian symptoms develop.

Levodopa, still the commonest drug used to treat Parkinson's, can give dramatic relief for some time. It is most effective for countering the rigidity and slow movements but less effective with the tremor and balance problems.

These discoveries led many physicians and scientists to conclude that Parkinson's is *caused* by the loss of dopamine. But while dopamine loss may be the immediate cause, it would be more precise to say that loss of dopamine describes a crucial aspect of the disease. But what causes the substantia nigra to lose dopamine in the first place? And how do we account for the fact that other brain areas also stop functioning? Is it because they are not getting proper signals from the substantia nigra, or is there a deeper process affecting the brain that causes all these symptoms? We don't know.

This is why Parkinson's disease is called idiopathic—meaning we don't know the ultimate cause for certain. We know what its *symptoms* are, and we know about some of the major brain areas that are damaged, the *pathology*. But we have only limited knowledge of the *pathogenesis*, the underlying processes that cause the pathology.* As we shall see, one of the causes appears to be certain toxins, such as pesticides, but the matter is not settled. Current medications relieve the symptoms to an extent,

---

* Recent discoveries by Heiko Braak give intriguing clues to the pathogenesis and have set the field ablaze. There are suggestions that the disease may begin in the gastrointestinal tract, then affect the part of the brain closest to the spine, and then move upward, finally affecting the substantia nigra. This would explain why Parkinson's patients often have many symptoms related to brain stem functions. This will be discussed in more detail in Chapter 7.

but they do not correct the underlying pathology or influence the pathogenesis.

There is another problem: the mainstream dopamine medications have side effects. Levodopa has lots of them. Though not every patient gets them, they are among the most challenging in all of medicine. Between 30 and 50 percent of patients on these medications (after two to five years of treatment) develop a new movement disorder from their medication, called dyskinesia, which often causes them to writhe in an unsightly way. Doctors adjust the dose, hoping to find a small window through which to escape dyskinesia, without allowing a reemergence of the Parkinson's symptoms. Animal experiments show that these medication-induced dyskinesias are a result of undesirable neuroplastic changes brought about in the brain's synapses.

In addition, psychiatric problems can develop in patients on levodopa, including psychotic hallucinations caused by the higher amount of dopamine it creates. (Arvid Carlsson showed that excess dopamine can produce symptoms that mimic paranoid schizophrenia, which helped us better understand that psychotic illness and develop drugs for it.)

Patients may escape many or most of these symptoms, especially if they get Parkinson's late in life and die from some other ailment before the worst of the Parkinson's sets in. But even when levodopa significantly improves patients' quality of life, after four to six years its good effects tend to wear off more and more quickly, so that patients need to take more, increasing the risk of the dyskinesias. For levodopa is only a symptomatic treatment, and behind the scenes, the disease is worsening. As Werner Poewe, who has studied the natural history of the illness, wrote, "Although Parkinson's disease . . . is the only chronic neurodegenerative disorder for which there are effective symptomatic therapies no treatment has yet been identified that would significantly slow its natural progression."

Most neurologists know this to be the case. So do drug companies, which claim, each time a new drug comes along, that it has greater benefits and fewer side effects than the last. This deficiency is why scientists are looking at nondrug ways to treat PD.

Deep brain stimulation is one such treatment, used for patients who don't respond to medication. It involves implanting electrodes in brain areas that govern movement, which can improve symptoms. It was thought that the stimulation "jams" the abnormally firing circuits, but additional research indicates that the electrical stimulation changes synapses and alters axonal branches, through neuroplastic mechanisms. But brain surgery has risks.

Given the lack of ideal clinical options, John Pepper's claim to have reversed the worst symptoms and to have built up his health to the point where he could go off the medication would, if true, be of breathtaking importance to millions of people.

Exercise and Neurodegenerative Disease

Pepper offered to come to Toronto, but I wanted to visit South Africa to meet him and his doctors and to watch him be physically examined and to understand how the diagnosis was made. I wanted to meet with those who had known him before he was ill, who watched him decline, and who saw him get better. And I wanted to meet with the people he had claimed to help.

As it happened, a staggering series of neuroplastic breakthroughs had just occurred in Melbourne, Australia, that were of immediate relevance. The neuroscientist Anthony Hannan, head of the Neural Plasticity Laboratory at the Florey Institute of Neuroscience and Mental Health, working with T. Y. C. Pang and others, had done a series of experiments that would change our understanding of the role of the environment and exercise in altering the course of catastrophic neurodegenerative disorders that were believed to have a genetic basis.

Huntington's disease is a more horrifying neurodegenerative movement disorder than Parkinson's. It is a genetic disorder: if a parent has it, a child has a 50 percent chance of getting it too, usually between the ages of thirty and forty-five. It is currently thought to be incurable. Its victims progressively lose the ability to move normally; they develop severe jerking movements, become depressed, then demented, and die a premature death. It enfeebles the part of the brain called the striatum, which is dysfunctional in Parkinson's disease.

Hannan and his team used young mice that had had the human Huntington's disease gene transplanted into them. Over time such mice developed the disease. The team studied the effects of providing the mice with running wheels. A mouse on a running wheel is not really "running," though it looks as if it is. Because there is no resistance on a running wheel, what the mouse is really doing is more like "fast walking." A second group of the mice were raised under normal lab conditions, without the running wheels. Those raised under normal lab conditions, without much exercise, developed Huntington's disease, as expected. Those that got a lot of fast walking and stimulation got the disease too, but onset was significantly delayed. It is always problematic to extrapolate literally from an animal lifetime to a human one. But for very rough purposes, the average mouse lifetime is two years. The exercise delayed the onset of the illness by approximately a decade in human years. Here was perhaps the first instance of a terrifying genetic neurodegenerative disorder being affected by, of all things, walking.

BEFORE I LEFT FOR SOUTH AFRICA, Pepper's small self-published book, *There Is Life After Being Diagnosed with Parkinson's Disease,* arrived in the mail. It was a combination of personal memoir and self-help book for Parkinson's; he led off by pointing out that he had had little formal education and no science background. When he wrote me in his original e-mail that the "medical profession" had been put off, he was not completely accurate, though close. His own physician, Dr. Colin Kahanovitz, had written the preface and testified to Pepper's Parkinson's diagnosis and to witnessing his progress, innovations, integrity, and rare determination.

One of the book's purposes was to lift up the sagging spirits of Parkinson's patients, so many of whom are depressed—not just because they have Parkinson's but because one of the disease's direct effects on the brain is to alter the mood centers. At times, the book seemed quite different from the succinct e-mails he had written me. It contained phrases that authors often put in self-help books, such as "I still believe in miracles, and that nothing is impossible"—the kind of cheerleading that might well have put off some physicians who deal with end-stage Parkinson's every day. It also told stories of neurologists who had told their patients their illness was incurable.

Cheerleading aside, the book made quite clear that Pepper was not claiming to have cured his Parkinson's, only to have turned back the most dreaded symptoms, through daily exercise of a very specific kind. The book's title means, as he explains, that the diagnosis does not have to be taken as a death sentence, that there are ways to manage with the disease better than most have thought. Chapter 3 is called "My Symptoms," and in an appendix he lists more than a dozen Parkinson's symptoms that he still has. He makes clear his claim is only that there are new neuroplastic ways to manage the symptoms, stop their progress, and in some cases reverse them.

Though he himself is now off medication, he is far from being dogmatically antimedication. The book mentions medication more than fifty times, making clear that he is not counseling others to go off it. He describes how his medications improved him initially. Early in his illness he stopped his medication three times (twice naïvely, because he felt so much better, and once because it drove his blood pressure dangerously high), but when he got worse, he went back on it.

While he feels all patients should exercise if they can, he explicitly writes, in bold letters, "Do not even contemplate going off medication, unless you have consulted your doctor first" (page 69), and later, "I do not recommend that patients stop taking their medication" (page 73). He stresses that only after he had done fast walking for a number of years was he able to wean himself off his drugs, and that that course might not be best for everyone.

The overall message is sober, and the author's unpretentious authenticity, vulnerability, and friendly charm are unmistakable. More important, some of the innovations he made were uncannily consistent with the latest discoveries of neuroplasticity. And reading it made clear to me why it was John Pepper who was able to make his breakthrough.

A Dickensian Childhood During the Blitz

John Pepper was born on October 27, 1934, in London, into a Dickensian childhood—which he turned into a series of lessons in resourceful living, while under constant threat. In 1932 his father became an economic casualty of the Great Depression and had to borrow money to stave off starvation in those hard times. He spent the rest of his life conscientiously paying off his debt to those who had helped him. One consequence of his honesty was that the Pepper family was impoverished throughout John's childhood in wartime England. The family couldn't buy clothing, food was unobtainable much of the time, and John never had a single toy throughout his childhood.

When the Second World War began, the family began a life on the run, fleeing from house to house. John was almost six when the Nazis began dropping bombs on London in the Blitz. Because there was no shelter near where they lived, John and his brothers hid under the stairs, while their parents, somewhat pathetically, took shelter under the kitchen table. In those early days of the war, the Nazis so dominated English skies that they could fly daytime raids with impunity. When the British mounted some defenses, the Nazis switched to nighttime bombings, and the Pepper family moved to another house for protection. The Blitz went on for eight months. London was bombed on fifty-seven consecutive nights, destroying about a million houses.

"One day," Pepper says, "a bomber was being chased by one of our fighters, and he came very low over the houses, straight down our street, where he hurriedly off-loaded his incendiary bombs as he flew past. One of these bombs hit the house to the left of ours and the next one hit the house to the right."

While his father worked in an aircraft factory, John, his mother, and his two brothers carried their rubber gas masks wherever they went, or raced to hide in bomb shelters. Throughout much of the war, the family was sent to live with other families, who were not grateful to have them. Typically the three boys slept in one bed—two lying in one direction, and the third the opposite way so they could all fit in—listening to the bombs dropping. John went to nine different schools before he got to high school. In one case his class met in an outdoor ditch that had been turned into an air raid shelter. After two of John's schools were bombed out, the family was evacuated to a series of small villages outside London, where they lived without water or lights.

Despite moving around so much, at the age of ten, John won a scholarship to an English public school in Winchester and was placed with older boys, giving him his first exposure to a better-educated class. But "I never overcame the enormous emotional and developmental gap between myself and my classmates," he says. "Consequently, I became a loner." These older boys, with their money and breeding, had a superior attitude and took to ostracizing and bullying him. As a scholarship student he was never able to afford a school uniform, and the older, bigger, pubescent boys would strip ten-year-old John of his ragged trousers so that he was completely exposed, ridiculing him, mocking his endowment, and chasing him around the playing field in front of the school. In sports, little John Pepper almost always came in last.

In impoverished circumstances, one can't always choose one's own career. When he was sixteen, in 1951, "my father came in and said you start work Monday at Barclays Bank." He started at the bottom, as the lowly office boy, changing nibs in pens and filling inkwells, establishing himself as a hard worker.

One morning he came to work on time as usual and saw that the boss, who kept banker's hours and never arrived early, happened to be there. John, alone with him, said what came naturally to this man in his gray pinstripe suit: "Good morning, Mr. Challen."

"Don't you call me Mr. Challen. You call me 'Sir.' Now get out" was the cold reply.

This reproach was the first time the banker had spoken to his office boy in John's ten months of working at the bank. There and then John decided he was so sick of the class system that he wrote a letter to Barclays Bank saying "I am willing to take a job with the bank anywhere in the world, as long as it is abroad." A week later, to his surprise, he got a reply. There was a job in South Africa. "Any place that has food and a job, and I am good," he thought.

Within three weeks, the seventeen-year-old was aboard a mail boat on his way to South Africa. It was 1952. He soon rose from the lowliest job at the bank up to the level of accountant, then got a better position at Burroughs Machines as a sales representative and serviceman. He offered to go to a mining town where no one else wanted to go and opened up a branch office. He went from success to success wherever he worked, and when South Africa changed to the decimal system, he started selling accounting machines. He lived as though the Depression were still on, never buying snacks, going to the movies, or taking the bus to work if he could walk. In that way he was able, by 1963, to save enough money to buy a printing press and open his own small printing business. In 1987 it went public and became the largest form-printing company in South Africa and one of the largest in the southern hemisphere. His life was full; he was a self-made success, happily married to Shirley Hitchcock, with two children, and performing in plays regularly, singing.

But all this came at an extraordinary cost. He achieved his success through a remarkable determination and through, in his own words, his "compulsive workaholia." He was unable to delegate work in what had become a large company. Driven, he would go to bed at eleven p.m. and find himself awake at three a.m., so he would write and update complex computer programs he felt were urgently needed to run his business. For eighteen years he was unable to sleep more than four hours a night and assumed he had insomnia because of stress. He would work six or seven hours, then bring Shirley some coffee to wake her. Then he would commute thirty miles to his factory, putting in eighty-hour weeks. Being so preoccupied, he ignored a staggering number of symptoms. "I was too busy to be sick," he told me. "I am the type of person who does not know when he is beaten."

Illness and Diagnosis

By his midthirties, Pepper was showing many signs of becoming ill, though he never dreamed that his troubles, including his insomnia, might have been driven not simply by his workaholia but by an illness such as Parkinson's. Long before Parkinson's fully declares itself, there is often a "premotor period," with mild symptoms that may have little to do with movement difficulties. Sometimes called the prodrome, this phase represents the earliest sign of the illness, when it is still difficult to detect.

By the time PD is fully expressed, a person will have several of the four cardinal symptoms of PD, all in some way connected with movement. These symptoms are also often called "the Parkinsonian features," because they are so characteristic. They include rigidity, slow movements, tremor, and unsteady postural and related balance problems. Together they give rise to the famous shuffling gait. There are two groups of people who get Parkinsonian syndromes: those with Parkinson's disease proper (which is the most common group), and those who have an atypical Parkinsonian disorder.

But the cardinal symptoms are only the best-known symptoms. Some people have only two of them yet still receive the PD diagnosis. PD is, at this point in conventional neurology, a clinical diagnosis based on the extent to which the patient exhibits symptoms, not on a brain scan or blood test; one very expensive brain test for it, which is rarely done, will be discussed later in this chapter.

In fact, Parkinson's has so many different symptoms, some affecting movement, some not, that no two people have quite the same experience, and depending upon how the symptoms unfold, a patient can go for decades, as Pepper did, with the nonmotor prodrome symptoms before the full-blown illness becomes apparent.

Until about a decade ago, physicians paid little attention to the prodrome symptoms. Pepper's earliest symptoms, dating all the way back to the early to mid-1960s, were a mix of nonmotor and motor. Parkinson's usually strikes people in their fifties and sixties, but 5 percent can get it before they are forty, and Pepper, like Michael J. Fox, showed his first signs when he was about thirty.

Pepper noticed that when he tried to throw a ball, he was unable to let go of it at just the right moment—a sign of rigidity and perhaps the first indication his brain was having difficulty coordinating a seamless switch from one movement (propulsion) to the next (the release of the ball). He also developed constipation, often an early symptom that is easily overlooked because it is so common. In 1968, in his midthirties, he developed a peculiar problem with his handwriting: it was becoming hard to decipher and, mysteriously to him, smaller. (Because Parkinson's slows movement, his hand made smaller excursions on the page; hence the micrographia.) Eventually he became unable to sign his own name. By the mid-1970s, when he was around forty, he was occasionally unable to move his feet after standing still for a while (freezing) and having trouble walking on uneven surfaces (a coordination problem). Then he developed depression and an inability to clear his throat. These symptoms seemed unconnected, and he was still such a comparatively young man that he never dreamed they might be signs of early Parkinson's, which seemed to him a disease of the elderly—in part because as a person gets it, he begins to look much older, stiffer, and less animated.

His daughter, Diane Wray, told me that in the late 1970s her father "underwent a huge personality change. We [the family] were overseas in 1977, and he got really angry about an ice cream that I wanted and he would not let me have. I was sixteen at the time. He jumped up and down like a child and shouted at a robot—the traffic lights—in the street. This was the first time that I noticed something was different about my dad. . . . We also noted that his face had changed. He had been a very animated person and was onstage in plays and was always singing and dancing. We all noticed at the dinner table his face drooped and sagged and became very deadpan. A very different look. And at that stage he did a self-portrait, which you can see in his house, and you can see the difference." Pepper lost the ability to smile normally, and his face became increasingly frozen and masklike.

By the mid-1980s he was having significant trouble controlling his emotions, controlling his finger movements, and multitasking (doing more than one mental task at once). He had become clumsy, regularly knocking over glasses at dinner. By the late 1980s, when he was in his fifties, he developed a tremor that was so bad he could no longer depress the keys of his computer keyboard—a real problem because his work involved writing computer programs. Then a torrent of symptoms afflicted him: on occasions his body perspired intensely when he was under the slightest pressure, his eyes watered when he read, he fell asleep while at work or driving (some Parkinson's patients begin to sleep in the day and wake at night), and he had trouble finding words, remembering names, and concentrating at work. He garbled his words when he spoke, choked on certain foods, started to make involuntary arm movements, and developed restless legs at night. He struggled to dress himself in the morning and frequently lost his balance. He noticed that his body was becoming very rigid.

Yet he still didn't dream he had a movement disorder. And being fiercely independent, with a high pain threshold, not wanting to burden others, and willing to go to the doctor only if his symptoms completely stopped him from working, he kept many of his difficulties to himself and rarely saw a physician.

Nevertheless, in 1991, he went to see Dr. Colin Kahanovitz, his family doctor, for fatigue. Now, finally, he was feeling very tired. In May 1992 he complained of depression. Then in October of that year, Dr. Kahanovitz noticed that Pepper had a hand tremor. He suspected early Parkinson's and referred him to a well-thought-of neurologist whom I'll call "Dr. A."

Dr. A wrote detailed notes each time he saw him and sent eleven medical notes back to Dr. Kahanovitz, who kept all of them and, in fact, every doctor's consult note he ever ordered on Pepper.

According to the notes, when Dr. A examined him physically on November 18, 1992, he found that Pepper had a classic physical sign of Parkinson's, called cogwheel rigidity, in his left wrist and neck. If you move the limbs of Parkinson's patients, they have a ratchety or jerky feel. He also had the famous masklike face, and his gait was abnormal too. He had a *festinating* gait: the small hurried steps that many Parkinson's patients sometimes take to avoid falling over. He didn't swing one of his arms when walking, another sign. He also had "a positive glabellar tap." When you tap someone who doesn't have Parkinson's on the forehead between the eyes, the person initially blinks reflexively, but as you keep tapping, the blinking stops. Not so with many Parkinson's patients and people with other neurodegenerative disorders; they just keep on blinking.

Dr. A put those findings together with Pepper's tremor at rest or holding a cup, the personality change (Pepper had become short-tempered and hyperemotional), his lost libido, poor concentration, and depression. Dr. A wrote, "I agree entirely with your assessment that he has mild early Parkinson's disease, and I think he will benefit greatly from medication." Dr. A started him on the main drug for Parkinson's, Sinemet (which has levodopa in it), as well as Symmetrel.* He saw him two weeks later, after which he wrote, "There does seem to be an improvement." Dr. A saw him again a month later, in January 1993, and noted "a tremendous improvement." Neurologists often take a response to levodopa as a strong indication that the person has Parkinson's disease. Dr. A also told him, at that visit, to add another medication, called Eldepryl. When Pepper complained of confusion and memory problems the next year, Dr. A did an MRI to see whether Pepper had a brain disease other than Parkinson's and didn't detect one.

While skiing in Switzerland, in January 1994, Pepper showed a marked deterioration in his motor skills, which he reported to Dr. A. The Sinemet was stopped in March 1994. By January 1995, Dr. A noted that Pepper was now starting to limp, to fall on uneven surfaces, and to drag his legs: the shuffling gait was beginning.

At this point, Dr. A emigrated from South Africa. A third doctor, a neurologist whom I'll call "Dr. B," took over his care next and, in his consult note of April 1997, wrote that he had examined Pepper and found the physical signs of Parkinson's that Dr. A had found. He too wrote he found the "cogwheeling," "a tremor," "diminished arm swing," "masked faces," and an abnormal response to the glabellar tap. His speech was "monotone." Dr. B wrote, "He has, I think, deteriorated slightly . . . being a little more bradykinetic [slow-moving] and slightly more rigid than he was six months ago." He also observed that when Pepper changed his position, his blood pressure dropped, "in keeping

---

* Interestingly, when Pepper wrote his book, he did not remember trying Sinemet during this period, which partially coincided with the period when he had memory problems. But the Sinemet, and his initial positive response, are meticulously documented in his neurologist's notes for all the sessions, from after it was started, November 18, 1992, until March 18, 1994, when it was stopped because he seemed to be doing better on another medication, Eldepryl, begun in the middle of that period on January 9, 1993. Perhaps this lapse was caused by the fact that this first neurologist tried him on seven different medications for his many symptoms: Sinemet, Symmetrel, Tryptanol, Inderal, Eldepryl, Lexotan, and Imovane. The Sinemet was stopped before he began his walking program in earnest in 1994.

with the mild autonomic neuropathy not uncommonly associated with Parkinson's disease." (An autonomic neuropathy involves a disorder of the autonomic nervous system, which regulates bodily functions.) Dr. B thus documented the same physical signs as Dr. A. He continued Pepper's anti-Parkinson's medication and did not alter the diagnosis. With Pepper's encouragement, I contacted Dr. B when I visited, to see whether he had any other documentation on his former patient to share, but he said he did not have access to Pepper's chart, and he wasn't prepared to speak on the record about Pepper's case.

Thus the three doctors who had seen Pepper toward the beginning of the illness had diagnosed John Pepper with Parkinson's disease. "The family was hugely shocked at the time," his daughter, Diane, recalled, because "in essence the doctors said it is a degenerative disease, and you should take this medication, and 'there is no hope.' And then in his usual way, he didn't take no for an answer."

Walking Among Snakes and Birds

John Pepper was convinced his doctors had made a mistake. What followed were two years in which he moved from denial to mourning. His ready-for-action character was not ready for something that would make action itself difficult. He was stunned that he had pushed aside discomfort for so long. He decided to quit work, which had been immensely stressful, to live more modestly and to turn his attention to his health. But his usual ability to engage now seemed unavailable to him; he spent much of two years in a chair, thinking, reading, listening to music, and more than anything else, "feeling sorry for myself."

After grieving and moping, he realized, "I had allowed myself to become a victim, when I always thought of myself as a winner." As a self-reliant person, he was most terrified of making himself a burden on his wife, Shirley. Because of his rigidity and tremors, he was dependent on her to help button and unbutton his shirts and put on his shoes and socks. He made a pledge to alter his attitude fundamentally, based on what might be thought of as a naïve approach to his degenerative illness. "I decided to start doing anything I could that might stave off the inevitable progression of PD. Because PD is a movement disorder, I assumed that the more I moved, the slower the PD would be able to take over my life."

As a youth, Pepper had never enjoyed working out because of his poor coordination. But when he was thirty-six years old, because of a back condition that ultimately required two surgeries and a disc removal, he took up regular exercise to build a stronger back and also some jogging for general fitness. By the time he was diagnosed with Parkinson's, he was already in the gym for ninety minutes, six days a week. He did cardio for an hour: twenty minutes on the treadmill walking six kilometers per hour, twenty minutes of cycling at fifteen kilometers per hour, and twenty minutes on a step-climber at two steps a second. After that he would do another thirty minutes of six different muscle-building exercises on weightlifting machines.

But in the days leading up to his diagnosis, all this exercise was failing him. He noticed that he had been accomplishing about 20 percent less per workout than he had in the previous six months, and that he was having to lower the amount of work he was doing on each of the machines. He was lifting less and couldn't understand why. He noticed that he was, for the first time, exhausted long before he had finished his workout; it was this very exhaustion that had brought him to Dr. Kahanovitz in the first place and set in motion the recognition he had Parkinson's.

His gym work, despite his pledge to get over his movement disorder by moving more, was proving a fantastic failure.

WHEN PEPPER AND I FINISH speaking to a Parkinson's group at a church in a small city in the Eastern Cape province, we go for another walk together in a huge field at the edge of a huge pond, at sunset. He is teaching me to look out for the rich variety of African snakes in the low bush—grass snakes, rinkals, black and green mambas, and pythons. As we approach the pond, Pepper, a bird-watcher, points out some Egyptian geese landing on the water, to join some coots and a great heron. He points out blacksmith plovers, crowned plovers, hadadas, and cattle egrets.

At one point we have to go over a small fence, the kind of obstacle that would be impossible for most Parkinson's patients, but Pepper doesn't hesitate as he lifts one leg, then another, over it. As we cross a field, we see a sign that says, "Run/Walk for Life" and posts some meeting times.

It's a coincidence, because Run/Walk for Life, an organization with branches throughout much of South Africa, was key to his breaking out of his exercise disaster.

Shirley had joined it a year before Pepper's diagnosis, to lose some weight and get fit. It seemed to Pepper a slack program, invented to help sedentary people with no fitness whatsoever to develop some. All it involved, as far as Pepper could see, was walking. In 1994, seeing him faltering, Shirley urged him to join, and he impatiently told her, "I already walk twenty minutes a day."

Moderation may not have been Pepper's strong suit, but moderation is the essence of Run/Walk for Life, even though it was designed for people of all ages, races, and backgrounds. The point is to avoid injury and start very slowly, then, with great patience, work up to significant walks—in some cases, even marathons—making sure to give the muscles time to rest between sessions.

After ten minutes of stretching to fend off injuries, beginners were permitted to walk for only ten minutes around a school playing field, three times a week. Every two weeks they would increase their walking time by five minutes. To increase their strength, they had to increase the distance they covered in that time. After they could do four kilometers, they were allowed to try to improve their time. When they could walk four kilometers, or two and a half miles, they could switch to walking on the road. At the end of every second week, the distance would be raised one kilometer, if the participant was ready for that. Once the person reached eight kilometers, the goal became to decrease the time. After a walk, there was a cool-down lap. The goal was to get to eight kilometers a session. Once a month each person was timed doing four kilometers. The program helped South Africans all over the country to lose massive amounts of weight and reduce their blood pressure, cholesterol, insulin dependence, and even need for medication. Instructors

watched to make sure that people walked properly and to stifle the over-
enthusiasm that leads to injury and burnout.

No sooner had Pepper started the program than he was frustrated
that he was allowed to walk only ten minutes! So the instructor let him
walk twenty minutes, but no more. He was never allowed to skip a level
of exercise. He had to spend at least two weeks walking a given distance
before she would permit him to add a kilometer more. She noticed that
he was walking with a stoop, with his head facing downward, and perhaps not knowing that this was typical of Parkinson's, she started shout-
ing at him, "Stand up straight, and look ahead!" She was the first person
to begin the long process of reeducating him to pull his shoulders back
and keep himself upright. He noticed that walking on a field was difficult for him, because it was uneven. But to his surprise, by using the
take-it-slow approach and exercising only every other day so he could
rest between sessions, he began to improve his times significantly.

This was the turning point—the first time, in years of decline, that
he had shown the slightest improvement in any kind of movement.
Within several months, he was walking eight kilometers, at about eight
and a half minutes per kilometer, then got down to six and three-quarter
minutes a kilometer. He allowed himself to exercise only every other
day, for an hour, but when he did, he always broke a sweat. His goal was
to get his pulse racing at over 100 beats per minute and keep it there for
an hour, three times a week. His biggest obstacle was his own tendency,
time and again, to increase his rate of walking too quickly, causing unnecessary injury.

Still, his walking appeared somewhat odd. He walked very quickly.
Indeed, the first time I went walking with him, early one morning, when
he usually walks the tree-lined streets of Johannesburg, I said, "Let's
go," and started walking, but he pulled away from me so fast, I thought
he might be running—but he wasn't. In those early years, when he began his fast walking, his fellow walkers often accused him of running,
not understanding he had Parkinson's and couldn't get his legs to move
properly.

With change happening so gradually, only in retrospect did Pepper
begin to realize that one or another of his Parkinsonian symptoms had

either improved or disappeared. Family pictures from the period before Pepper started fast walking, in which his relatives were all smiling, show Pepper with an unexpressive Parkinsonian mask (even though he thought himself smiling when the photo was taken). Now when he visited his factories, people began to comment on how well he looked. He had spent a decade appearing to others to be an "invalid" and living with the belief that "I could never get better . . . because everybody knows that Parkinson's is incurable." Now he was feeling "perky" and realizing that perhaps by exercising every other day, and giving his body time to rest, he had found the formula. He began concentrating on getting as much rest as possible and on avoiding stress as much as he could—which, given his constitutional tendency to act, required a lot of effort.

During this entire period, while Pepper was trying to eliminate the stress from his life and heal, South Africa was undergoing remarkable change as apartheid was ending. While political violence was contained, a period of increased crime ensued that has never totally abated.

Pepper's daughter, Diane, was swarmed when she stopped her car at an intersection and was robbed at gunpoint. Her car was stolen. Others were murdered in their cars. John and Shirley's car was stolen. By 1998 Shirley became frightened of being mugged, and decided to stop walking on the roads. So John agreed to walk with her, which meant he had to walk much more slowly. This gave him an opportunity to begin thinking about how he was walking. The secret was that instead of saying to himself "I shall walk now and watch myself," he broke down the normally complex automated activity of walking into parts and meticulously analyzed each and every muscle contraction, movement, shift of weight, placement of his arms, legs, feet, and so on.

Walking slowly, he discovered his major problems—problems typical of almost all Parkinson's patients. Understand that typical modern walking is a kind of controlled fall forward. What keeps us from falling over is that our feet normally support our weight, first on one side and then on the other. But Pepper observed that when he walked, his weight was never well supported on the ball of his left foot, so he didn't dare lift his right leg enough, and that he tended to drag his right foot. He observed that his left foot had no spring to it, and he was not pushing up and forward on it. His left heel was still touching the ground when his right touched down. His right foot didn't always clear the ground as it passed his left leg, giving rise to his shuffle. If the right foot did clear the ground, he could never straighten his rigid right knee fast enough, so that his right foot landed heavily because his body weight wasn't sufficiently supported by his left foot. These were just the most obvious of many subtle observations he made as to why he could not experience the controlled fall that his walking should have been.

It took him three months to get his left foot to support his body weight. If he concentrated on supporting his body weight on the left foot, he was no longer in an uncontrolled fall, and his right knee had the time to straighten out before the heel touched the ground. Such attention required an extremely focused, almost meditative concentration, as when a child learns to walk for the first time, or when a student does the slow-motion walking of tai chi, which teaches more perfect movement by slowing things down.

His close observations exposed all the other problems of his gait. He saw that his steps were too short; that he wasn't swinging his arms; that he was stooping forward from the hips; and that his head was hanging down to the left. He lengthened his stride with mental effort and some stretching. He also began to carry a one-kilogram weight to force himself to swing his arms. He corrected the Parkinsonian stoop by forcing himself to stand straight, shoulders back, chest out, whenever he noticed he was slouching. It took him over a year of practice to internalize all these changes.

His walking normalized—as long as he paid attention and concentrated on each action. Even today he doesn't just tell himself to "take one step at a time." Rather, he observes himself in far more detail. He senses how he is lifting his back left leg, bending his knee, launching from his toe, swinging his leg forward, making sure his foot is weight-bearing long enough, clearing the ground with a straight right foot, and planting his right heel, while swinging his opposite arm, fighting the tendency to stoop.

We might think that this level of proficiency in walking would be impossible for a person who had illnesses in addition to Parkinson's and thus would be useful for only the healthiest Parkinson's patients. But at the time of his diagnosis, Pepper had dangerously high blood pressure; high cholesterol; an ear disorder called Ménière's disease with hearing loss, balance problems, vertigo, and ringing in the ears; osteoarthritis in his shoulders and knees; and an irregular heartbeat. And still he walked.

Conscious Control

When I walk with Pepper, I marvel that he can hold all these movements in his head. He insists he can, and because neither of us can bear to walk in silence, we talk as we go, and I observe that he can do two things at once; he can keep up the motor movements that the rest of us perform automatically, by using his conscious mind, and still have "mental space" left over for conversation. But as the conversation deepens—when I ask him about something that intrigues him, or that stumps him, or when he sees a bird he can't identify, I can hear a foot drag, reminding us both that he still has Parkinson's; it's just that he's found a way to overcome it.

Pepper describes this conscious control over walking as "the final piece of the puzzle" that he needed to take on other motor symptoms.

After mastering walking, he began to take conscious control of his tremor. Parkinson's patients usually have an "involuntary tremor at rest," meaning it occurs when the body part is not being consciously moved; but they can also have "action tremors" when they consciously reach for something. Formerly, when Pepper held a glass, his hand shook. But he started playing with how he held the glass and found that if he held it very firmly, the tremor disappeared. He understood that the brain knits together actions and turns them into complex "automated" sequences, so that one no longer has to use a lot of mental energy to put multiple movements together. It is this unconscious ability to automate and link all these movements that is lost in PD. All Pepper's new techniques, he realized, involved "using a different part of my brain to control an action, which was normally controlled by my unconscious." In practice, this meant consciously performing tasks in slightly different ways than he had originally learned them. Likely this approach helped because it did not engage the brain areas that processed his existing unconscious programs, which seemed to be the source of the trouble. It worked to control his tremors, as long as he wasn't too stressed.

The smallest actions once stymied him, but soon he no longer needed Shirley to help him button and unbutton his shirts because he was becoming less rigid and inflexible and regaining control of his fine motor movements. After he was diagnosed with PD, he took up painting, but his lines were always shaky. As he perfected his conscious movement technique, his painting instructor marveled at the loss of his tremor when holding the brush, so that his once-shaky lines became smooth and straight. To deal with the shrinking handwriting of Parkinson's, he switched from cursive writing (which he could no longer read) to printing capitals.

In his work for a Parkinson's support group, he helped a woman who had a terrible tremor when she brought a glass to her lips to approach the glass from behind consciously, instead of automatically from the side, as she normally did. This forced her to use consciousness to bypass the unconscious processing of her already-automated Parkinson's movements, and her tremor disappeared. Pepper took to holding his own fork at forty-five degrees toward himself and to grasping his spoon very loosely instead of tightly like his glass. Eating with Pepper, you would never recognize he had Parkinson's, except that his hands take odd paths to bring food to his mouth, and he occasionally knocks something over when the conversation becomes animated.

Over lunch in the Cape, I heard Shirley cry, "John, watch it."

"It's okay, luv," he told her. "Shirley is always moving things out of my reach," he said to me, "because when I reach subconsciously, I'll knock a glass of wine with my hand. It goes on mostly when I should be concentrating. If I'm not, I'm always pulling wine back on to me because I don't let go of it"—one of his original Parkinson's symptoms.

But then I heard a loud "ow" as he was explaining this very point. "I just bit into my cheek." He explained that it happens all the time, particularly if he doesn't concentrate on chewing and swallowing.

The Science Behind the Conscious Technique

When we walked together, Pepper always had the same burning question. Was it possible that he had found, through conscious walking, a way of using a different part of his brain to walk?

He had done so, I believe, by "unmasking" existing brain circuits that had fallen into disuse. He has been able to teach others to walk faster, more freely, to swing their arms, and to shed their shuffle and stoop, often in a matter of minutes, as I saw on several occasions. As far as we know, change that happens so quickly can happen only in one way in the brain. Preexisting circuits are unmasked, or uninhibited. Then over time, these circuits can be strengthened neuroplastically.

There is a logical explanation for why conscious walking works, rooted in the anatomy and function of the substantia nigra (the section of the brain where the loss of dopamine is most profound) and the basal ganglia of which it is part.

The basal ganglia are a clump of neurons deep in the brain, and they light up on brain scans when a person learns to knit together complex sequences of movements and thoughts. Numerous studies have shown that the basal ganglia help us to form automatic programs for the complex actions of everyday life, then to select and initiate these complex actions. Many of these we take for granted—getting out of bed, washing, dressing, writing, cooking, and so on—but we learned each one step by step, until it became habitual and automatic. When the dopamine system in the basal ganglia doesn't work, it becomes difficult for people to perform such complex motor sequences or learn new automatic sequences. It also becomes difficult to learn new cognitive sequences of thought, and so great patience is required in teaching Parkinson's patients both to move and to acquire complex cognitive skills.

There are advantages to "automating" sequences of thoughts and movements. If an action is automatic, a person doesn't have to concentrate on it consciously and so can use his conscious mind for other purposes. From an evolutionary perspective, a hunter can pace through the forest while concentrating on his prey. This "threaded cognition," in which he moves, observes his prey, and moves again, allows him to do two or more things at once, and at least one of them can be a complex activity. More mundanely, healthy people can dress while listening to the radio or eat automatically and sustain a high-level conversation at the same time. But people with basal ganglia damage, like Pepper, can't do both well—he bites his cheek. He can drive well if he concentrates— but occasionally he misses a turn if a pesky visitor from overseas is plying him with questions.

We accomplish complex automatic actions—even those as "natural" as walking—in two steps. First, we learn them, by paying close attention to each and every detail. (Think of a child learning to play a piece on the piano.) This conscious learning phase is preautomatic and requires focused mental effort. It involves prefrontal brain circuits (behind the forehead) and subcortical circuits (deep inside the brain). Only after the child has learned all the details do the basal ganglia come into play and allow him to put the details together into an automatic sequence. (The cerebellum is also involved.)

Because Pepper's basal ganglia are not functioning, he had to learn to pay close *conscious* attention to each movement *by activating* the prefrontal and other subcortical circuits, as a child would when first learning to walk. He appears to be bypassing his basal ganglia.

One of the greatest difficulties Parkinson's patients have is initiating new movements. For instance, if you put a small elevated obstacle in the way of a person with Parkinson's, she will stop walking before it as she prepares to step over it. But she may find that having stopped walking, she can't start again and will remain at a standstill, because the substantia nigra—that part of the basal ganglia that is especially lacking dopamine—is not working well, and it is responsible for initiating automated sequences of behaviors.

Though the patient is at a standstill and seems frozen, as the neurologist Oliver Sacks points out, she is very easily helped, when stimulated by others, to initiate a new sequence of movements. Sacks reports a famous case of an English footballer with Parkinson's who sat frozen and immobile all day; yet when thrown a ball, he reacted by catching it, leaping to his feet, and running and dribbling it. Sometimes the rhythm of music is enough to initiate movement in a Parkinson's patient at a standstill. Sacks also points out that Parkinson's patients may appear mute unless they are spoken to, or motionless unless they are motioned to, whereupon they can respond quite well. They require another person to initiate the conversation, because they can't themselves.

"The central problem in all Parkinsonian disorders," Sacks has written,

> is *passivity* . . . as the central cure for them all is *activity* (of the right kind). The essence of this passivity lies in peculiar difficulties of self-stimulation, and initiation, not in the capacity to respond to stimulation. This means, in the severest cases, that the patient is totally unable to help himself, although he can be very easily helped by other people. . . . [I]n less severe cases . . . the Parkinsonian patient *can* help himself in a limited fashion, by using his normal and active powers to regulate his pathological or "de-activated" ones. . . . The problem, then, is to provide a continual stimulus of the appropriate kind.

Sacks, in explaining that lending a hand can help a person with severe Parkinson's initiate an ongoing movement, is describing a helpful short-term intervention, but not a recovery the likes of which Pepper has shown. Pepper doesn't need another person to "lend a hand" to his brain—because he has found a way to use a healthy part of his brain to take over for the damaged basal ganglia and substantia nigra and to initiate a flow of movement. He has found a way not only to initiate movement but to keep the stream of movement flowing, and to improve his brain circuitry by constantly stimulating growth factors because he walks so much. Pepper has solved the problem Sacks described, having found a way to provide himself "a continual stimulus of the appropriate kind" with his conscious walking technique.

Helping Others

Watching Pepper walk, I wondered whether others could show the kind of *sustained* mental control he did. His conscious walking was certainly a marvelous neuroplastic exercise, exactly the kind of concentration required to preserve existing neurons in the brain. It reminded me of the kind of *attention* a rock climber must pay to each and every move; or of how the student of tai chi must concentrate his or her full attention on each joint movement, breath, and muscle contraction. But at times I feared Pepper was a man caught in some Dantesque level of hell. He had longed so much to return to movement; now his wish was granted, but only if he concentrated on each and every muscle fiber as it twitched. He might be walking, but was it at the cost of losing the free flow of spontaneous thought?

So I asked him my burning question: "How is it possible for you to hold all these sensory observations and movements in your head, and still walk, and talk, and appear to enjoy it? Does it burden you, or can you enjoy these walks?" Silently, I was wondering: Would others without his grit be able to do it?

"I don't resent having to concentrate on my movements," he said. "It's been a big challenge, and I'm often amused by what happens when I'm not concentrating on what I'm doing. It certainly isn't a burden, as it helps me so much." It did, though, take some getting used to and at the beginning was very tiring.

Though he insisted he had to concentrate on each and every movement, I began to suspect that his brain was sometimes beginning to automatize the new way of walking, releasing his conscious mind for other activities. Though at times in our animated conversations a foot might drag, at other times, it seemed to me, he could be deep in thought and the foot was fine. Was the substantia nigra beginning some self-repair, with the release of neurotrophic growth factors such as GDNF?

With the success of Pepper's conscious movement technique, his physician, his wife, and his children all began to notice improvement. Pepper began studying how his progress might have been possible. He started reading about neuroplasticity and other research describing how exercise can promote brain growth factors. He dug up important studies by Dr. Michael Zigmond's group from the University of Pittsburgh, showing that animals whose dopamine neurons had been chemically destroyed had less likelihood of getting Parkinson's symptoms if they exercised.

Pepper disseminated this information on neuroplasticity to others with PD, threw himself into the local Parkinson's support group, and rose to become the head of it. He was, as in all things, relentless, maintaining that exercise was not optional for Parkinson's—it was mandatory. But he was always surprised when other patients didn't follow his advice. The ability to walk is a natural resource we all have, but most people, he found, would rather ride in a car than walk. Now that exercise is no longer forced on us by necessity, only the most motivated patients get enough of it. Pepper often failed to understand why others with the illness were not as motivated as he was.

He began to believe that the emphasis on medication in treating Parkinson's had the psychological side effect of rendering patients more passive in dealing with an illness that can itself promote passivity. In the common medical model, patients take their medicine and wait until a better one comes along. Visits to the doctor consist of checking the progression of the disease and examining for medication side effects. Treatment becomes a race between patients' deterioration (over which they have no control) and pharmacological research (over which they also have no control). Responsibility for patients' well-being is shifted to others. Pepper worried that reliance on medication alone might hasten a person's deterioration.

Pepper went to a dozen different support groups throughout South Africa, and found that over time he was able to help every patient he worked with to improve his or her walking, if they could stick with it. One of them was Wilna Jeffrey.

Wilna has had Parkinson's for fourteen years, but she has a normal-looking, assertive gait. She is seventy-three years old, has blond hair, and is stylishly dressed; she moves quickly and indeed more gracefully than most people her age, but also more deliberately, revealing that she's using Pepper's conscious walking. When she and I sit down in the café of the Sunninghill Hospital in Johannesburg, I see she has only the mildest tremor, a barely perceptible twitch of her wrist, and one slightly restless leg.

Widowed in 1995, Wilna had two children, but her son was killed in a motor vehicle accident. Her daughter lives in Newcastle, Australia. "In

1997 I suddenly noticed I couldn't sign my name," she told me. She saw several physicians, including the head of the Parkinson's division of the General Hospital in Johannesburg, and in 1998 they diagnosed her with Parkinson's. Without family nearby, she couldn't be dependent on others, as most Parkinson's patients become.

"When I was diagnosed, I didn't want to hear about it. I said I will bring this right. I denied the diagnosis. But then the tremor started. My doctor put me on Sinemet, then Azilect, Stalevo, Pexola." Her hand improved a bit, but her leg "got the shakes," and she developed a shuffling gait.

She heard from a mutual acquaintance that John Pepper worked with Parkinson's patients as a public service, and telephoned him. When he first met her, she was stooped, physically crestfallen, and so demoralized she didn't see herself as having any future.

In three sessions with him, "my whole attitude toward PD changed into something positive." He gave her the courage to aim for a normal life, despite the Parkinson's. He visited her at home, analyzed her gait, her dragging right foot, and other symptoms. He got her to join Run/Walk for Life and to continue stretching and physiotherapy. She now does eighteen kilometers a week of Pepper-style fast walking, using her conscious mind for each step. He also taught her his conscious movement technique so she could hold a glass without spilling it, and he taught her to correct her voice (which can go faint in Parkinson's patients) with exercises. She also swims in a pool three times a week. "I don't swim lengths. I do sit-ups and stretching of the leg and pulling up the legs. I also stretch a lot before I get up in the morning, and I do a lot of core exercise." Her friends all noticed the improvement. "It has made all the difference," she says. Wilna has remained on medication, showing that the exercise can be of use to those taking Parkinson's drugs.

Wilna grew up on a farm, rode horses as a child, and was always physically active, which may be why she could begin serious exercise later in life. Now her gait is normal, but she still has Parkinson's.

"When I see other Parkinson's patients, I see that I haven't deteriorated like they have. In my daily life, I can do everything I wish: drive, play golf, play tennis if I have to."

"What happens to you when you can't exercise?" I ask.

"If I don't do the exercise, I know all about it. I go very stiff, I get cramps, I just don't feel well."

"Does your doctor know you are exercising?"

"Yes. David Anderson is my neurologist, and he gets very cross with you if you don't exercise. He emphasizes exercise and biokinetics and walking."

"In what ways does the Parkinson's limit your life now?"

"I can't multitask. If we go out to a cocktail party, and I stand with a drink and then take something to eat, I will shake or spill the drink. And I fumble quite a bit opening my bag, especially when I'm rushed. Dressing, I battle sometimes with tiny buttons. I must never hurry because the minute I hurry, I can't cope. If I don't take my medicine, I start shaking. If I send an e-mail, and I am battling with it, I will knock the wrong key. Then I get frustrated and abandon it."

Wilna says that though she is not deteriorating at nearly the rate of those who were diagnosed when she was, she thinks the disease is progressing, "very, very slightly, and slowly, because I didn't have it in the leg, and do now."

She draws inspiration from Pepper. "He's got energy for Africa," she says. "That's a South African expression. It means he's got a tremendous amount of energy. When we walk together, I can't keep up with him." But that agility, she adds, has made a lot of trouble for him, and some neurologists have been talking about John Pepper. "You know, in the neurological world, people say he doesn't have Parkinson's."

The Controversy

From his attempts to help others, the Parkinson's community thought extremely well of John Pepper. In 1998 he became the chair of a Parkinson's organization in South Africa, a volunteer position, and he was re-elected five years in a row. Under his leadership, the group provided support to sufferers, helped set up new support groups, distributed information about new research and medications, and represented PD sufferers at meetings with pharmaceutical and medical aid companies.

Pepper made it his goal to persuade Parkinson's sufferers that the illness was not a death sentence but a manageable condition.

In August 2003, at the group's annual general meeting, the vice-chair argued that it was not good for any organization to have the same person serve as chair for too many years. Pepper, having been chair for five, thought this reasonable and fair and agreed not to run for another term. The then vice-chair was elected chair, and Pepper was elected vice-chair.

In the meantime, he was about to self-publish his book *There Is Life After Being Diagnosed with Parkinson's Disease*. To let others know about it, he took a proof copy around. He showed it to a neurologist I'll call "Dr. O." He met with her to get feedback about his book and to spread the word about his walking technique. He was not trying to establish a doctor-patient relationship, and she did not ask him to see his past medical chart; nor did she do a physical exam. "I asked her [Dr. O] for her reaction to the book. She was very noncommittal," says Pepper. "She did not touch me or ask me any questions about my condition. She did not come around from her side of her desk at any time."

In addition to Dr. O, Pepper sought comments to improve his book from a second neurologist who was the group's medical adviser at the time, whom I'll call "Dr. P." (Together with a third neurologist mentioned below, "Dr. Q," I will refer to all three as the "outside neurologists" because they did not treat Pepper.) Dr. P read it, and on July 2, 2004, he sent an e-mail to Pepper and to the group's director.

Dr. P said that while he was "very impressed" with Pepper's book, especially his ideas about using his frontal lobes for his conscious walking technique, "what is problematic is that by everyone's definition you don't have typical Parkinson's as we know it. . . . [F]or the vast majority of patients, your approach is going to HAVE to be there to supplement medication. . . . [P]eople with Parkinson's need medication and we would do them a grave disservice by denying them that." If Pepper failed to acknowledge the primary importance of medication, Dr. P said he feared Pepper would end up like South Africa's AIDS-deniers who promoted "garlic and African potatoes" over lifesaving AIDS medications. He added that probably Pepper had something called Parkinsonism, which is not the same as Parkinson's disease, and that Parkinsonism can be caused by encephalitis (a viral infection of the brain) from which people can recover.

The e-mail was gentlemanly and respectful and in some respects admiring. The problem for Pepper was the statement that by everyone's definition he didn't have typical Parkinson's. It contradicted Pepper's own physician, Dr. Kahanovitz, who had known him the longest, had actually examined him physically, and had extensive documentation on Pepper's chart, including all the neurologists' notes that he ever received on Pepper, documenting his many physical exams, signs, and symptoms, and which stated that the diagnosis was Parkinson's disease, without any suggestion his case was atypical.

In addition, Dr. Kahanovitz saw Pepper in the early prodrome years, when the Parkinson's symptoms developed; he then saw those symptoms emerge full force, before he began his exercise program; and finally he watched him laboriously put his method into effect and slowly get control of many of his symptoms. Dr. P overlooked the fact that Dr. Kahanovitz had written the preface to Pepper's book, affirming Pepper's PD diagnosis and saying that in his observation Pepper was "able to circumvent the standard treatment through his perseverance and original thinking." Clearly, not everyone agreed that Pepper's diagnosis was atypical. For Dr. Kahanovitz, what was atypical was not the diagnosis but what Pepper did about his diagnosis.

Dr. P had not done a physical exam on Pepper or reviewed his complete chart. The reasoning seemed to Pepper to be that typical Parkinson's is progressive, and Pepper had not gotten worse. And he seemed to assume that Parkinson's couldn't be helped significantly, except through medication.

On August 17, 2004, the Parkinson's group wrote Pepper a letter, citing Dr. P's comments about his book, and asked Pepper to resign immediately. (He was serving as vice-chair.) The letter also said, "We agree with our medical advisor, that your book will give people with Parkinson's false hope and therefore cannot endorse your book any longer." The chair wrote again on August 25, stating: "You attribute your recovery to exercise and positive thought, to the exclusion of medication, which is in conflict with the opinions of the neurologists associated with the association."

At a meeting of the group on September 14, 2004, organized by one of Pepper's supporters to clarify the situation, Dr. O, who by then had been appointed as a second medical adviser to the group, asked the director why Pepper had been asked to resign. As stated in the minutes of the meeting, the director said that earlier in September at a Parkinson's information day in Durban, a third neurologist, Dr. Q, "told Mr. Pepper that he does not have Idiopathic Parkinson's* . . . [because Pepper] shows no progression of illness and does not take any anti-Parkinson medication." Again, the reasoning was that because *only* medication could stop progression of the illness, if Pepper wasn't taking medication, his diagnosis must be wrong. Pepper, to his knowledge, had never met or talked to Dr. Q. "Dr. Q never came anywhere near me," he said, "nor did he examine me at any other time. His opinion was based on what he saw of me at the meeting. His statement was made in front of everybody." Once again an outside neurologist was challenging Pepper's diagnosis—in public—because he appeared, from across the room, to be moving well.

According to the minutes, when asked about Pepper's book, "Dr. O replied that the book is harmful." The minutes reflect that Pepper then asked Dr. O to assist him in revising parts of the book that she thought were harmful, and she declined. Finally, Dr. O said that if Pepper were to continue in an official role in the organization, he "must be monitored at meetings" lest his statements be taken for official policy. After a few days, he agreed to step down. At a subsequent meeting, despite the fact he had already stepped down, Pepper was publicly denounced by the new leadership, in front of all the members, for misleading patients.

According to Pepper, Dr. O "said that my book gave the impression to readers that I claimed to be cured without the use of medication! When I asked her, 'Where in my book do I say this?' she answered, 'You don't say it, but that is the impression the reader is left with, after reading your book.'"

---

* *Idiopathic Parkinson's,* as we have seen, is another term for typical Parkinson's disease, sometimes used to emphasize that it is degenerative and that we do not yet understand what drives the degeneration.

Why, a bewildered Pepper wondered, were the three outside neurologists and the chair so passionately defending the role of medication in treating Parkinson's, when he too saw it as having a role and said so repeatedly in his book? What harm could be done by encouraging more physical activity? Why wouldn't curious scientists and clinicians be trying to understand the case of a man who had learned to control his symptoms—regardless of the kind of Parkinson's they thought he might have—given that medications wane, or can cause hallucinations or new movement disorders?

Parkinson's Disease and Parkinsonian Symptoms

"He is a very gentle man," says Dr. Colin Kahanovitz, remembering the painful years Pepper experienced. "He is a man of great integrity, and they have put him through a hard time here. He was ostracized. He was devastated. Very hurt. He is not a man of many words; he says what has to be said. But being the type of person he is, and having felt he helped himself so much, he wrote the book for others. But the neurologists were saying 'You're talking rubbish.'"

Among questions raised, the one that was worth serious thought was the medical adviser's claim that Pepper didn't have typical Parkinson's disease but rather some variant. It would have been more helpful had he raised this as a possibility, rather than asserting it as a probability, especially because he supported this idea by writing erroneously that "by everyone's definition" Pepper had atypical Parkinson's disease. But the medical adviser's letter, unlike the use to which it was put by others, was attempting to come to grips with the fact that Pepper displayed symptoms that appeared to be a variant of Parkinson's and he nonetheless got control of them. He also conceded Pepper's approach had some merit.

As I said earlier, Parkinson's disease is called idiopathic when we don't know the cause and when it appears in a form assumed to be degenerative, progressive, and incurable.

The medical adviser, Dr. P, used the term *Parkinsonism* to describe Pepper's symptoms, in contrast to idiopathic Parkinson's disease.

Parkinsonism and *Parkinsonian symptoms* (the terms are often used in-terchangeably) are not always progressive. Often the term *Parkinsonian features* is used to describe the cluster of motor symptoms—the tremor, the rigidity, the lack of movement, and the postural instability. There can be no dispute whatsoever that John Pepper has shown these to multiple physicians.

As we've said, Parkinson's disease is the most common cause of Parkinsonian symptoms. But there are other causes of Parkinsonian symptoms, and the terms *Parkinsonian symptoms, Parkinsonism,* and *atypical Parkinson's* are often used *when we know the cause* of these motor symptoms. In some cases where we know the cause, we can elimi-nate that cause, or it passes and the symptoms go away. (Dr. P referred to one such case in his letter, when he described a patient who had enceph-alitis and "Parkinsonism" and who then got better.) Interestingly, in many cases, atypical Parkinson's has a far worse prognosis than Parkin-son's disease, and leads to earlier loss of life.

But raising the possibility that John Pepper merely had "Parkinson-ism" or was "Parkinsonian" opened the door to the possibility that he had once had symptoms that looked like those of idiopathic Parkinson's disease but were not. The implication was that his symptoms disap-peared when the cause was removed, and thus he mistakenly thought he had cured himself of Parkinson's disease. (Of course, Pepper never claimed to have been cured, and he still has multiple nonmotor Parkinson's-type symptoms. His claim was only that the movement symptoms were now under his control.)

There are two well-known causes of atypical Parkinsonian symp-toms. The first is a form of encephalitis, an infectious disease of the brain. Just after the First World War, this disease caused its victims to succumb to what was popularly called sleeping sickness but was really a Parkinsonian state of corpselike immobility, in which they remained for decades. These are the patients Oliver Sacks described in *Awaken-ings;* they were "awakened" from their states by the levodopa he gave them—until its effects waned. Clearly, that couldn't apply to John Pep-per: he had never had sleeping sickness or a case of encephalitis or as extreme an impairment.

A second cause of atypical Parkinsonian symptoms is seen in patients who are prescribed one of several medications known to cause the symptoms as a side effect, most commonly antipsychotic medications that lower brain dopamine. Usually these Parkinsonian symptoms are reversed when the patient goes off these drugs. In the few cases where they are not reversed, it is often thought that these patients probably already had, or were going to develop, idiopathic Parkinson's disease. So it is important to ask whether Pepper had been exposed to any medication known to cause Parkinsonism.

The only drug Pepper had ever been on that might cause Parkinsonian symptoms is Sibelium, which he used for his Ménière's disease, an ear disorder that can affect balance and hearing and cause ringing in the ears. Sibelium is not an antipsychotic, so it is far less likely than that class of drugs to cause Parkinsonism. Rather, it is a calcium channel–blocking agent and only rarely gives rise to Parkinsonian symptoms, the overwhelming majority of which are reversible. Parkinsonian side effects usually occur in people over sixty-five. But Pepper's Parkinsonian symptoms began in the early to mid-1960s, when he was in his thirties. Pepper began to take Sibelium only in 1972, almost a decade *after* he had shown signs of a movement disorder. That chronology alone would disqualify Sibelium as the cause of his illness, though he took it for several years.

Drug-induced Parkinsonism is more likely to occur on both sides of the body, and Pepper had symptoms on one side at the time. Drug-induced symptoms often come on quickly and dramatically, but neither Pepper nor his physician noticed a dramatic change when he was on Sibelium. Though drug-induced Parkinsonian symptoms tend to remain static, Pepper's disease was progressing in a way that is typical of idiopathic Parkinson's disease—in the years before, during, and after he took Sibelium.

Finally, most people recover when those drugs are stopped—usually within two months, though some take up to two years. When Pepper went off Sibelium, he didn't notice an improvement in his symptoms. He has now been off that medication for thirty-five years and still has many movement disorder symptoms. All these reasons make it *highly* unlikely that his Parkinson's symptoms were Sibelium-induced. There are other causes of Parkinsonism—for instance, very rare strokes, boxing injuries, and significant head trauma, and some rare diseases—but so far there is no evidence that Pepper has any of these.

The fact that Pepper also has many signs of Parkinson's disease outside the usual Parkinsonian symptoms—sensory problems (which make it difficult for him to know where his limbs are in space), intermittent memory loss, and nervous system problems typical of Parkinson's disease, such as trouble regulating his blood pressure, telling if it is cold or hot, profuse sweating, and urinary difficulties—also suggests that he certainly has a widespread, serious disease. Finally, to argue that the fact that he was able to reverse some of his symptoms proves he doesn't have the disease, is a stretch. When medication or brain stimulation reverses symptoms, practitioners don't say that proves the person never had an illness in the first place.

So the case that Pepper does not have Parkinson's disease comes down to, as Dr. P says in his letter, the belief that Parkinson's disease is "progressive," that "people with Parkinson's need medication," and the fact that Pepper was now *improving* by his specific kind of walking, *without medication.* This argument rejects the possibility that conscious walking might be a neuroplastic form of treatment.

Those who doubted that Pepper had Parkinson's disease emphasized that PD is progressive; indeed, we often assume that "incurability" and "progression" are *central* to the definition and diagnosis of Parkinson's disease, which is "degenerative." But this assumption creates a problem. Whether an illness is "incurable" or "curable" or "progressive" or "stable" or "degenerative" is a decisive observation but is a better criterion of *prognosis* than of *diagnosis.* Prognosis describes a disease's likely outcome, a forecast based on what we have seen in the past. Pepper's critics were arguing that because he was doing better than they expected, he couldn't have had the diagnosis in the first place. They were confusing diagnosis with prognosis and overlooking the fact that he was treating himself very intensively.

Those who said that Pepper was raising false hope were no doubt trying to protect patients. There is a long, noble tradition in medicine that when physicians have knowledge that their patient will deteriorate or die, they take upon themselves the extremely unpleasant, thankless task of protecting the patient from wishful thinking and telling it like it is. That way the patient can make a sound judgment about how best to handle the remainder of his life: to do things now that he soon will not be able to do, or even say his good-byes and set his affairs in order.

But there is a catch. If a physician is going to pronounce a person incurable for his own good, the physician had better be correct, especially if the illness is one in which neuroplasticity—which requires that the patient mobilize himself for mental and physical exercise—can play a role in the recovery. We know, from the placebo effect, that when a physician delivers a prognosis and says, with confidence, "This pill will help you," even if it is a sugar pill, the symptoms will often improve, triggered by the patient's positive expectations. We also know that the placebo response has an evil twin, the "nocebo" response: if you lower a patient's expectations of a treatment, the symptoms often worsen, regardless of what is in the pill. Delivering a prognosis is not just passing on information; telling someone how you believe he will do becomes a part (even if a modest part) of the treatment itself.

False hope and false despair are worthy rivals in doing inadvertent harm. To navigate between them, a physician cannot simply rely on knowledge of how an illness unfolds in most people, or of what happened with the last patient he or she saw with that diagnosis, or make a diagnosis based on how the patient looks from the other side of the room. It is important to gather as much current information as possible about the individual with the illness. That was why it was essential to see Pepper's neurologist.

A Visit to His Neurologist

The energetic Dr. Jody C. Pearl is doing a physical exam on Pepper, holding his limbs out and letting me move them, demonstrating some of his Parkinson's disease symptoms. His right hand is cogwheeling as I move it. I get a ratchety feeling. She goes through the normal neurological exam and shows me that Pepper has cogwheel rigidity in all four of his limbs, and I feel it.

Dr. Pearl is a busy young neurologist at the Sunninghill Hospital. Dr. Kahanovitz began referring patients to her and found her "incredibly competent." She is warm with her patients, very alert, direct, and up to date on much of the latest research—with an interest in the latest medications but also in stem cells and other kinds of interventions. She's the editor in chief of *Neuron SA,* a South African neuroscience newsletter. She has followed Pepper for six years and has also read his book.

"He's got this unique way he's approached everything, in terms of the way he's managed to stay off medication," she says, conveying a sense of appreciation for what he's done. "He was very proactive in the way he handled his disease. He didn't sit back and allow the disease to handle him. And you know, John is quite controversial in terms of the way he has approached things locally with the local organizations here. But be that as it may, he certainly has overcome many challenges with regard to his Parkinson's, and he remains extremely well in certain aspects of his condition."

I ask Dr. Pearl to clarify one thing. "When you say Parkinson's, do you mean Parkinson's disease?"

"Parkinson's disease. Absolutely," she says.

Dr. Pearl knows that our brains are neuroplastic and that each of us wires up somewhat differently, and she therefore knows that each patient requires a different approach, because a brain illness will have a different expression in each person. "Patients don't read textbooks, and every patient is different," she says. "All patients progress differently, and there is a spectrum of disorders. We cannot therefore say that all patients need x medication for x condition. The only reason that he and I managed to have this relationship is because I was willing to accept what his needs were. It wasn't because I was able to do something amazingly different for him. And now we've shown that if Parkinson's patients exercise and walk, they seem to release the neurotrophic growth factor—which obviously he knew before all of us did."

Though Pepper's face can be emotionally expressive when he uses his conscious technique, she points out that when she gets him to tap his index finger and thumb together, a typical Parkinson's masklike face emerges. It's a subtle, quick demonstration that Pepper doesn't even notice, but she explains out of his earshot: "When I distract him, by getting him to do two things at once, or concentrate on another task, his Parkinson's symptoms come up." She explains she has to use these "tricks" to see the symptoms and signs, "because he has trained himself to use his conscious movement technique."

She also points out that as he taps his thumb against each of the different fingers on the same hand repeatedly, the movements become slower and smaller because his motor pathways are not working properly—another sign of the bradykinesia typical of Parkinson's disease. She has continued to see these kinds of subtle findings in Pepper's physical examination since she took over his care in 2005.

Her earliest notes documented the same physical signs that Dr. A, his first neurologist, recorded twenty years before. When she first saw Pepper, she noted that he displayed cogwheel rigidity on his right side, had a tremor, dragged his right leg if he didn't use his conscious walking technique, and had decreased arm swinging if he didn't consciously focus on it. He had signs and symptoms that would be almost impossible to fake. Physicians know the kinds of tremors Parkinson's patients have, right down to the number of times they shake per second—4 to 6 Hz (vibrations per second). When she first examined him, she did a well-known, widely respected assessment test, the Hoehn and Yahr Scale rating. The scale grades Parkinson's disease in terms of severity, for clinical and research purposes; Pepper had 2.5/5 in terms of severity.

"John also had an abnormal response on the 'pull test,' which is a sign of postural instability," Dr. Pearl says. He didn't have the abnormal response initially but developed it over time, a sign that the underlying PD had progressed. In the test, the patient stands with his feet slightly apart, and the physician stands behind him. She explains that she will pull the patient gently, while he tries to keep his balance. If the patient has to take three or more steps back, or falls without taking a step, this represents a positive pull test.

She has carefully documented Pepper's many PD symptoms. "When he originally saw me," she says, "he complained of difficulty walking"—which occurred if he didn't use his conscious technique—"and constipation, fatigue, frequent nighttime urination, irritability, conflict, lack of concentration, sleeping during the day, swallowing difficulties, memory loss, and depression.

"Parkinson's disease is a clinical diagnosis," she explained, meaning that the diagnosis is made by a clinician based on the history and the physical exam. She would do an MRI brain scan, she explained; though it can't demonstrate Parkinson's, it can rule out stroke, dementia, and other problems that might mimic Parkinson's. A new, expensive test, not yet available in Johannesburg, called a DAT scan, scans the brain looking for dopamine depletion but is used only in the rarest situations, "in a patient who presents with Parkinson's disease where you are reticent about making a diagnosis," she explains. "It is not something you do on a routine basis because at the end of the day Parkinson's is a clinical diagnosis. I got one done when I had a patient who was thirty-five years old, and I was uncomfortable telling a patient that age he had Parkinson's."

"Is there a standard recommendation for rehabilitation in South Africa?" I ask.

"There is no standard recommendation," she says. She recommends that her patients go to a biokineticist for evaluation of posture, stretching, strength training, and heart fitness. For the last eight years, Pepper has also attended a one-hour exercise program for seniors twice a week that involves stretching and loosening up movements and light strength training with one-kilogram weights or flexi-bands.

Not Walking

The therapeutic power of Pepper's walking is most clearly revealed when he can't do his fast walking.

Parkinson's patients are prone to chest infections because they often have an impaired cough reflex and stiff chests. On several occasions Pepper developed a tenacious chest infection that required five courses of antibiotics, and he had to stop walking. He also had back surgery in 1999 and was unable to exercise. Both times his Parkinson's symptoms emerged full force. Typically, the first symptom to reemerge was clumsiness: he knocked things over on a table, bumped into objects, spilled food while bringing it to his mouth, dragged his feet, limped. His speech deteriorated quickly, becoming garbled. His voice would get very faint when he was tired, and his sleep pattern became irregular. In less than six weeks, he had almost all the symptoms that he had had just before he was diagnosed. It took Pepper six weeks of exercise to reverse the symptoms that had returned.

In 2008 he tore a ligament in his left foot that took four months to heal, so he couldn't walk. Once again the Parkinson's symptoms that his walking had controlled reemerged full force. Eager to get rid of them, and prone to behaving like a shot out of a cannon, he restarted walking too intensively and reinjured himself. "I had to get into my thick skull that I had to start at the beginning, at a slow speed, walking for ten minutes, three times a week, then build up by five minutes every two weeks." That took him six months of work, but he got back up to seven kilometers in just over an hour, where he is now, just shy of his best, which was eight kilometers in just under an hour.

In other words, the neuroplastic "miracle" of his improvement required constant tending and application because he still had a serious movement disorder. What his walking was doing, by triggering neurotrophic growth factors, was giving support to a system that was still under duress. As we shall see, patients who do not have an ongoing disease process, but experience a onetime loss of brain tissue, as might occur in a stroke, do not need to apply neuroplastic interventions constantly to maintain their gains. That said, what Pepper has shown is the extent to which walking benefits brain health in general, and that exercise must be part of any brain health routine.

FOR MANY YEARS, EXERCISE WAS not recommended for people with Parkinson's disease. Following diagnosis, PD patients tend to reduce their physical activity, and only 12 to 15 percent are referred to physiotherapy. While some studies in those years showed benefits, others reported no measurable effect, and some argued that the exercise might actually worsen the underlying pathology, raising the question: Could a dopamine system that seemed to be wearing out be strained by too much demand?

The general rule, we now know, is that our brains are more likely to waste away from underuse than to wear away from overuse—as long as one builds up to exercise slowly and rests between sessions, ideally starting before the disease has progressed too far. (One study shows that amyotrophic lateral sclerosis, or ALS, may be an exception to this general rule. Female mice with the human ALS gene, raised in stimulating, environmentally enriched environments, got worse faster than those in normal environments.)

Today some physicians seem caught between those old fears and the more recent evidence that exercise is helpful. Most commonly physicians use visits to evaluate disease symptoms and drug side effects, as they should, and only pay lip service to the need for physical activity. They encourage their patients to keep active without telling them how. That advice is rarely sufficient. Since there is nothing Parkinson's disease patients want more than to stay active, the key is to teach them how to do so despite an illness that progressively robs them of that ability. Ironically, neurologists often refer patients to speech therapy for their voice problems, which involves doing exercises; but referring patients for intensive walking seldom happens.

The Science Behind the Walking

What science validates Pepper's walking therapy?

Walking, so natural, so "pedestrian" (in the sense of ordinary), may not be a high-tech neuroplastic technique, but it is one of the most powerful neuroplastic interventions. When we walk fast, regardless of our age, we produce new cells in the hippocampus, the brain area that plays a key role in turning short-term memories into long. For a hundred years, neuroanatomists searched for signs that the adult brain could form new cells to replace those that died, as the liver, skin, blood, and other organs do. None could be found. Then in 1998, two researchers, Frederick "Rusty" Gage, an American, and Peter Eriksson, of Sweden, discovered such new cells in the human hippocampus. (This discovery is described in detail in Chapter 10 of *The Brain That Changes Itself*.)

A host of discoveries followed, which found that placing animals in enriched environments led to neuroplastic change. The first modern use of enriched environments occurred when the Canadian psychologist Donald Hebb, instead of keeping rats in laboratory cages, brought them home and let them roam freely around his living room as pets. He showed that they performed better on problem-solving tests than those raised in cages. The psychologist Mark Rosenzweig was able to show that the animals raised in enriched environments developed more neuroplastic changes in their brains and produced more neurotransmitters, compared with those raised in typical rat or mouse cages. Their brains were heavier, having a larger volume.

Frederick Gage's lab, working with mice, made two other important discoveries. The first was that for mice, the *cognitive stimulation* provided by exposure to an enriched environment of toys, such as balls or tubes, for only forty-five days, preserved neurons (i.e., kept them from dying) in the hippocampus. The second discovery, made by Gage's colleague Henriette van Praag, showed that when mice were put in enriched environments, the most effective contributor to an increased proliferation of neurons (i.e., the "birth" of new neurons) was use of a running wheel. As I said earlier, animals don't really "run" on running wheels, because there is no resistance; what they do is more like fast walking. After a month of fast walking on the wheel, the mice doubled the number of new neurons in the hippocampus. Gage theorizes that this growth happens because in a natural setting, extensive fast walking occurs when an animal is venturing into a new, different environment requiring exploration and new learning, sparking what he calls "anticipatory proliferation."

In response to this discovery, the neuroscientific community exploded with activity. Could fast walking and enrichment increase brain power and preserve it in other parts of the brain? What was the relationship between cognitive activity and physical activity? What other neuroplastic processes, if any, were triggered by fast walking? Could brains with neurodegenerative disorders—such as Parkinson's, Alzheimer's, Huntington's, or even multiple sclerosis—be healed or helped by this activity?

When the young Australian neuroscientist Anthony Hannan was at Oxford, he had a daring idea about Huntington's disease, which causes dementia, a severe movement disorder, and depression. Until that point, Huntington's had been seen as the "epitome of genetic determinism"— so powerfully and exclusively driven by genetics that the environment couldn't possibly affect its outcome. A genetic "stutter" (the mistaken repetition of part of the genetic code) leads the brain to produce too much of a chemical, glutamine, which eventually poisons the victim's brain. Most scientists assumed that overcoming this internal, microscopic process was virtually impossible without a breakthrough in genetic engineering.

But Dr. Hannan thought that the merciless decay seen in Huntington's disease might *in part* be neuroplastic. Aware of Gage's and other neuroplastic breakthroughs, he wondered whether the actual "poisoning" might be causing a neuroplastic dysfunction, affecting how new connections—synapses—were formed between neurons.

"It appeared," Hannan told me, "that in brain diseases like Huntington's and Alzheimer's, the synapses start to malfunction due to a change in the molecules that form their building blocks, and thus don't transmit information accurately between the neurons. This change impairs brain function. In some cases, synapses are completely lost, which also disrupts brain functions such as learning and memory. I wanted to see what happened when we stimulated more synapses to grow and 'drove the synapses harder,' by enhancing sensory, cognitive, and physical activity levels."

Working with a graduate student, Dr. Anton van Dellen, Hannan conducted a breakthrough experiment, demonstrating that mice that had the human Huntington's gene transplanted into their DNA could, through the cognitive stimulation provided by an enriched environment of objects for the mice to explore, significantly delay the onset of the illness. This was the first demonstration ever of the beneficial effects of an environmental stimulation on a genetic model of neurodegenerative disorder.

A second study by Hannan's group showed that spending time on the running wheel contributed to the delay of Huntington's onset in mice, though both cognitive and sensory stimulation were also important. Of course these are the two tasks that John Pepper performs: he walks fast, but he also provides himself with constant cognitive stimulation: the superconcentration he uses to sense and monitor exactly how he places each foot and performs each movement engages his sensory and cognitive capacities. Since his diagnosis, he has also stimulated his mind by doing crosswords and Sudoku; playing bridge, chess, poker, and dominoes; by recording CDs of himself singing, by learning French, and by doing a brain program by Posit Science.

Now he's inventing a computer program that he hopes will pick a winning Lotto number, not just to win the lottery but to challenge his brain. He also travels, a wonderful thing, because the novelty of new countries and cultures forces him to learn and turns on dopamine and norepinephrine (a brain chemical that, as the neuroscientist Elkhonon Goldberg points out, appears more prevalent in the right hemisphere— the hemisphere that is "particularly adept at processing novel information"). Travel also stirs one to voluntary walking. (He's been on more than seventy-five international trips, to areas as diverse as Turkey, Iceland, Lebanon, Egypt, all over Europe, twenty-eight states of the United States including Alaska, and also China, Argentina, Chile and Cape Horn, Malaysia, Australia, and throughout Africa.)

Hannan (head of the Neural Plasticity Laboratory at the Florey Institute of Neuroscience and Mental Health in Melbourne) and his colleagues were able to show that they could use neuroplastic interventions to affect Huntington's motor deficits, cognitive deficits, mood, brain size, and molecular mechanisms in the brains of mice. His lab, his immediate colleagues, and other members of the neuroscience community have now assembled evidence that environmental enrichment and enhanced physical activity can delay onset, or result in milder progression, or produce overall better disease outcomes, in animal models of Parkinson's, Alzheimer's, epilepsy, stroke, and traumatic brain injury. Hannan's lab has been able to show that exercise is as effective as fluoxetine (Prozac) in mice with depressive symptoms from Huntington's, and has demonstrated the beneficial effects of environmental enrichment in mouse models of an autistic spectrum disorder called Rett's syndrome and schizophrenia. Dr. Emma Burrows, Hannan's young colleague, working on mice that have been genetically modified to have mental processes similar to schizophrenia, has shown that schizophrenic-like mice raised in enriched environments—with all sorts of novelties and opportunities for exploration—normalize their cognitive responses to stresses, and the effect is as great as seen with the antipsychotic medication. But only a voluntary running wheel exercise will delay neurodegeneration. "If you force them to run," she says, "it is stressful and cancels the effects."

Almost all the studies done at the Neural Plasticity Lab on neurodegenerative disorders have shown that a combination of physical exercise and mental stimulation (through environmental enrichment) is key to a good outcome. The hope for these experiments is that they will show that mice with the genetic predisposition to these disorders can, with proper exercise and cognitive stimulation through their life cycle, develop a cognitive reserve—extra "backup" brain connections—that protects against their developing the disorder, or helps to compensate for whatever damage is triggered by an animal's, or a person's, genetic predisposition to a neurodegenerative illness.

Scientists began to study the effects of exercise on Parkinson's in the 1950s, in response to clinical reports and small studies that showed that some people with PD seemed to benefit from it. They studied the effects of exercise by using the same animal models they used to test the new medications.

In 1982 it was discovered that two chemicals, MPTP and 6-OHDA, could cause a Parkinson's-like illness in humans. MPTP is a neurotoxin that destroys the dopaminergic neurons in the substantia nigra—causing the same damage as in Parkinson's. When scientists gave MPTP to mice, they became permanently Parkinson's-like, so now researchers had a "mouse model" of Parkinson's upon which they could try new drugs and treatments to see whether they were effective and safe. A second chemical, 6-OHDA, injected into a rat's brain, also led to loss of dopamine and a Parkinson's-like syndrome. Since then 6-OHDA has been found to be present in human beings with Parkinson's disease.

A crucial study by Jennifer Tillerson and her colleagues at the Institute of Neuroscience at the University of Texas at Austin, using both the MPTP and the 6-OHDA animal models, shows that a moderate amount of daily treadmill running—if it is initiated the very day that the chemicals deplete the dopamine in the basal ganglia—protects those basal ganglia dopamine systems from deteriorating. These Parkinson's disease–like animals did moderate treadmill exercise for nine days after being given the chemicals. They were able to preserve their ability to move and have complete recoveries if they exercised twice a day. In addition, the benefits persisted for four weeks, nineteen days after the exercise stopped. At that point, the animals' brains were examined. It was found that the dopamine-producing system in the substantia nigra had been better preserved in the animals that exercised, compared with those that didn't. This experiment is a stunning confirmation, in animals, of what John Pepper was experiencing in himself: that exercise, if it is started early enough in the disease process and is continuous, preserves movement. (The fact that the animals' brains no longer looked as Parkinson's-like should make Pepper cautious in assuming that after his death, a postmortem brain scan could prove to the skeptics he had Parkinson's. It's possible that the neuroplastic exercise he has done will, as in the animals, show some preservation of his dopamine system.)

ANOTHER MAJOR BREAKTHROUGH HAS BEEN the finding that when Parkinson's-like animals exercise, they produce two kinds of growth factors: GDNF (glial-derived neurotrophic factor) and BDNF (brain-derived neurotrophic factor) in their brains that permit them to form new connections between brain cells.

Michael Zigmond and his team at the Pittsburgh Institute for Neuro-degenerative Diseases, a world leader in the study of Parkinson's disease and exercise, writes, "Our own results—both published and unpublished—are unambiguous: increased running as well as environmental enrichment greatly reduces the loss of DA [dopamine] cells in both rats treated with 6-OHDA and in mice and monkeys treated with MPTP, and comparable results have been reported by others."

Dr. Zigmond has shown, using rats, mice, and monkeys on treadmills, that exercise can trigger the production of nerve growth factors, which protect the brain in animals with Parkinson's. He and his colleagues began exercising the animals three months before injecting them with either MPTP or 6-OHDA, and they continued the exercise for two months after the injection. Exercise both reduced the movement problems and increased the amount of the nerve growth factor, GDNF. Since GDNF is lowered in the substantia nigra in human Parkinson's disease, this is a welcome result. Brain scans and chemical analysis of the animals' brains showed that the dopamine-producing cells were preserved in the animals that exercised.

Zigmond's group has also found that inflicting a little bit of stress on an animal, for short periods, can actually increase dopamine availability. Zigmond speculates that a small stressor might be protective, preparing an animal for greater stress. John Pepper has always maintained that he has to walk fast enough to stress himself a bit and break a sweat. The same group also found that continuous stress leads to cell loss. Pepper quit work as part of his approach to handling his illness because it had been so major a stressor in his life.

We also know that exercise increases the number of connections between neurons. BDNF, also triggered by exercise, very likely plays a major role here. When we perform an activity that requires specific neurons to fire together, our brain releases BDNF. This growth factor consolidates the connections between those neurons and helps to wire them together so they fire together reliably in the future. (When BDNF is sprinkled on neurons in a petri dish, they grow branches that connect them. The growth around the neurons of the thin fatty coat that speeds up the transmission of electrical signals also accelerates.) BDNF also protects neurons from degenerating. Rats unable to run produce less BDNF. BDNF is also low in the substantia nigra of Parkinson's patients.

The neuroscience and plasticity researchers Carl Cotman, Heather Oliff, and their colleagues have shown that mice that exercise voluntarily on a running wheel increase their BDNF. The longer the distance, the more the BDNF increases. The increase in BDNF occurs in the hippocampus, which as we've seen turns short-term memories into long-term ones, a task essential for learning. (Short-term memory starts to fail in Alzheimer's,* also a neurodegenerative illness, but Parkinson's patients have memory problems, too.) BDNF can also protect neurons and lead to neuronal growth, in part of the basal ganglia called the striatum, and it has been shown in a few studies to increase with exercise.

Numerous studies now show that exercise can enhance an animal's ability to learn, proportional to a rise in BDNF. People may well do better on a cognitive test if they exercise and stay physically fit during exam time. Cotman and his colleague Nicole Berchtold argue that research on human beings now suggests that a combination of learning and exercise can help maintain brain plasticity and even increase it, because learning turns on genes that express more BDNF, and BDNF facilitates learning. Thus the more people learn, the better they become at learning and at making the brain changes that occur with it.

Learning and exercise together seem to be a good combination. As people reach middle age, and the brain begins to degenerate, exercise is more, not less, important, and one of the few ways to offset this process. Understanding this is more crucial than ever, because so many people live sedentary lives, in front of computer screens, sitting most of the day. Numerous studies show that a sedentary lifestyle is a significant risk factor not only for heart disease but also for cancer, diabetes, and neurodegenerative illness. If there's a panacea in medicine, it's walking.

Learned Nonuse

Parkinson's disease patients are caught in a tightening noose. They may be helped with fast walking, but fast walking is precisely what they cannot

---

* Recent studies show that high BDNF in later life protects against Alzheimer's.

easily do. And the Parkinson's patient who cannot walk does not "stay still"—his disease gets worse. The reasons are several. First, the illness is progressive. Second, the brain is a use-it-or-lose-it organ, and when walking becomes more difficult, slacking off will cause whatever walking circuits the patient still has to wither from disuse. Once they have withered, if he tries to use them again, he may fail, and the brain as a pattern detector will "learn" that he can't walk because of "learned nonuse."

Learned nonuse was first seen in human beings who have suffered a stroke. It has been known for over a hundred years that after a stroke, the brain enters a state of shock, called diaschisis, which means "shocked throughout." The "shock" occurs because in a stroke, after neurons die, chemicals leak out of some cells, harming others, inflammation is very active, and interruptions in blood flow occur around the dead tissue. All these events disrupt functioning not just where the stroke occurred but throughout the brain. In addition, immediately after an injury the brain undergoes an "energy crisis" because it has to consume so much glucose to deal with the injury. (Even when healthy, the brain has a huge energy requirement. Though it accounts for only 2 percent of the weight of the body, it consumes 20 percent of its energy.) The period of diaschisis typically lasts about six weeks, during which an injured brain is especially vulnerable because its energy to deal with additional harm is so low.*

In the years before we realized that the brain is plastic, physicians would examine their stroke patients at six weeks to see what mental functions they still had. Since it was believed that the brain couldn't "rewire" itself or develop new connections, all the physicians could do was wait and see which cognitive abilities remained after the shock wore off. They assumed that this represented 95 percent of the patient's eventual recovery. Perhaps the patient would make minor additional progress over the course of the next six months or year. The rehabilitation the patient underwent merely attempted to reawaken whatever circuits had been spared, like priming a pump that hasn't been used for some time. Such pump priming doesn't take long, so rehab was brief—a few hours a week for six weeks; it

---

* This is one reason why after people have a concussion or brain injury, they should not put themselves at risk for a second one until completely healed.

was certainly not seen as exercise that could develop *new* connections or teach healthy areas of the brain to learn, from scratch, the functions it had lost. (Unfortunately, even today, most patients receive very limited rehab.)

One of the most important neuroplasticians, Edward Taub, discovered, through a series of experiments, that neither animals nor people who have had strokes were necessarily condemned to live with only the level of function they had at the end of six weeks. He demonstrated that when stroke patients tried to use a paralyzed arm during their brain shock, or diaschisis, and found they couldn't, they "learned" not to use it and so relied on their functioning arm instead. Not being used at all, the circuits in the brain that governed the paralyzed arm wasted away. Taub showed that a person with a paralyzed arm can learn to use that arm. He put the patient's good arm in a cast, then trained the paralyzed or partially paralyzed arm. The cast on the good arm functioned as a constraint, so the patient couldn't rely on it. Then the patient incrementally trained the paralyzed arm. This technique works even years after the original stroke occurred.

Taub originally applied his new therapy, called Constraint-Induced Therapy, with success to stroke patients who had lost use of their arms; he then applied it to paralyzed legs. Brain scan studies show that when patients recover with Taub's treatment, neurons adjacent to the injury begin to take over from the damaged or dead neurons. (The details of his work are discussed in *The Brain That Changes Itself,* Chapter 5.)

Experiments by Tillerson, G. W. Miller, Zigmond, and others on animals with Parkinson's-like syndromes show that learned nonuse plays a major role in Parkinson's and that it can be overcome by using Taub's technique to achieve a staggering degree of improvement.

Injecting 6-OHDA into a rat can create severe Parkinson's on one side of the animal's body because the drug causes a 90 percent depletion of dopamine. Some of these animals had their good limbs put in casts for the first seven days after the injection, so they were forced to use their affected limbs. By the time the cast was removed, the affected limbs showed no movement difficulties. This was another stunning result. Somehow exercise stopped a newly injured system from going down—even one with 90 percent of its dopamine absent. Next, the scientists put the cast on the Parkinson's limb for seven days, so that the animals could not use it. Its movement gains were all lost. (Recall that when Pepper was incapacitated by chest infections, or surgery, and he could not exercise, all his symptoms returned.)

Tillerson and Miller were able to show that animals forced to use the affected limb showed no movement problems and their dopamine was preserved. If the scientists delayed putting on the cast for three days, they found that there were partial movement impairments, and that only some dopamine was preserved. If they delayed for fourteen days, dopamine levels were not preserved at all.

This research means that the effects of a serious, life-altering disease, in its advanced state, may at times be prevented—as long as the animal can stay active. If extrapolated to human beings, it implies that exercise should be one of the first recommendations for someone with early signs of Parkinson's. Tillerson, Miller, and Zigmond have shown that animals with only a 20 percent loss of dopamine will soon lose 60 percent if their movements are restricted: "These results suggest decreased physical activity not only is a symptom of PD but also may act to potentiate the underlying degeneration." Perhaps the worst thing a patient can do, on getting the diagnosis, is to decrease her activity.

As I think of Pepper and these experiments, I find myself hoping that in the future Parkinson's patients will not merely be diagnosed and sent home but will instead be enrolled in a "PD boot camp" together with their closest caregivers. There experts will explain that exercise and activity are essential to their dealing with the illness, elaborate the neuroplastic science behind it, analyze their gait, teach them conscious walking and movement, and start them on a walking program like Run/Walk for Life, so they don't injure or exhaust themselves. The goal, as soon as the diagnosis is made, will be to get them moving while they still can, to trigger neurotrophic factors. As members of a group, they will also deal with the psychological trauma of the diagnosis and learn to help one another summon their wills. Though Parkinson's patients often seem passive, that is not quite correct; many have trouble initiating activities, which is precisely why a boot camp is needed, for most, to get them going as co-contributors to the management of their disease, and to get them out of the trap of thinking that the treatment involves only taking their pill.

Walking would not be the only kind of exercise, either. (Recall that Pepper also does stretching, movement, coordination, and strength training for seniors.) Increasingly, movement therapists (see Janet Hamburg's *Motivating Moves* DVD), Pilates teachers, and others recommend exercise for Parkinson's patients, and while nonaerobic exercises may not trigger neurotrophic factors in the way walking does, they may have other advantages in fighting rigidity, overcoming balance problems, and decreasing the loss of facial movement. Taub's Constraint-Induced Therapy should also be taught at the boot camp.

And tricks, other than Pepper's conscious walking technique, might be used. Oliver Sacks described an immobilized Parkinsonian patient who leaped from his wheelchair to save a drowning man. While Parkinson's patients can't *voluntarily* do this, in emergency situations alternative brain pathways can be fired up involuntarily, allowing them to initiate movement. This unexpected movement is called kinesia paradoxa. A neurologist in the Netherlands, Dr. Bastiaan Bloem, was surprised to discover that a patient with very advanced Parkinson's, who could barely walk and often "froze," was able to stay in shape by riding a normal bicycle (not a stationary bike) for miles each day, getting all the exercise benefits from riding. On a bike, he appears to be perfectly normal, with excellent balance and fluid motion. As soon as he gets off, he freezes. Presumably, once the wheels are turning, the problem of initiating movement is overcome. Dr. Bloem is currently conducting a clinical trial of six hundred patients with PD to see if intensive bike riding might also slow the progression of their disease. Since many PD patients have trouble walking because of balance problems, an exercise bike is an excellent alternative. Exercises for balance are also crucial.

NEW BREAKTHROUGHS SHOW THAT THE relationship between motivation and the motor-movement system, dopamine, and neuroplasticity is far more subtle than ever imagined. The conventional view is that dopamine is essential for movement, and because people with PD have too little in the substantia nigra and the striatum, they can't move. But it turns out that dopamine is also essential to "feel" that it is worth making a movement—that is, people need dopamine to feel motivated to move in the first place, particularly for habitual, automatic forms of movement.

Dopamine has another extremely well-known purpose. It is often called the "reward neurotransmitter" because as people progress toward accomplishing any goal, it is released in the brain's reward system, in the expectation of a good outcome. The greater the value of that outcome, the faster people move to bring the outcome about and the more dopamine is released. Dopamine secretion gives a person a sense of rewarding pleasure as well as an energy boost. Also, the dopamine release reinforces the connections among the neurons in the very networks that helped us to perform the rewarding activity.

Thus dopamine has at least three characteristics relevant to PD: first, it enhances motivation to move; then it facilitates and quickens that movement; and finally it neuroplastically strengthens the circuits involved in the movement, so that movement will be easier next time. But if there is no motivation, no movement will occur.

A recent study shows that the "motivation to move" goes awry in PD, and that PD patients, if they are motivated, can often move. A control study by Pietro Mazzoni and his colleagues from the Motor Performance Laboratory at Columbia University has shown that Parkinson's patients (as John Pepper also demonstrated) can make normal movements. Their study compares Parkinson's patients with normal subjects on a variety of movement tasks and shows that the Parkinson's patients are capable of making motor movements as accurate and fast as normal subjects but need more practice to do so.

Mazzoni and his colleagues explain their remarkable finding in this way. Whenever a person is about to move, the brain first estimates and weighs how much *effort* that move will require compared with the *reward* it estimates will be obtained from the movement. In normal circumstances, the dopamine system is necessary for us to perform this "weighing" function. When dopamine is low and the person moves, he does not experience the pleasure of reward. As the neuroscientists Yael Niv and Michal Rivlin-Etzion point out, the system simply "assumes" that the benefit will be negligible and that the "opportunity cost" of the movement will not be worth the effort. Since the speed with which the PD patient performs a movement is in part related to how much reward is anticipated versus the energy cost of the movement, the result of low dopamine is very slow movement: in other words, bradykinesia. This is exactly what Mazzoni found. In more difficult movement tasks, requiring more effort, the PD patients were "more likely than controls to move slowly when the energetic demands of a movement task increase." It is significant that this occurred while the patients performed quite ordinary movements, and not in emergency situations, such as when a patient sees a man drowning and somehow leaps from the wheelchair to rescue him.

It may seem remarkable that few if any neuroscientists or physicians have intuited that much of the PD problem has to do with the chemistry of movement *motivation,* particularly because scientists have known for decades that dopamine is an essential part of the reward chemistry. But the oversight is understandable because this "weighing" function operates outside awareness and is largely unconscious.

The importance of the findings of Mazzoni and his colleagues for understanding Parkinson's cannot be underestimated: it is *not* simply that PD patients have an inherent inability to move normally and at a normal speed; the motivational component of their motor system is also fundamentally compromised. Niv and Peter Dayan have proposed that dopamine "energizes" and gives "vigor" to a habitual action. And Mazzoni and colleagues write, "The motor system has its own motivation circuit. . . . We propose that striatal dopamine also energizes action in a more literal sense, namely by assigning a value to the energetic cost of moving." Parkinson's disease appears in its symptoms as a physical movement disorder, but it has roots that are "cognitive" or "mental," and is thus as much a mental as a physical disorder.

Which is precisely why it is problematic to teach Parkinson's patients that the loss of dopamine prevents them from moving! This instruction will only reinforce passive resignation, at the very moment when that attitude needs to be undermined. And because it is a use-it-or-lose-it brain, the less PD patients move, the faster their neuronal circuits for movement and their muscles will weaken, hastening their decline. Telling PD patients they have a movement disorder and leaving it at that is a self-fulfilling prophecy. It would be better to tell them, "You have a disorder in which the motivation for movement is significantly impaired, along with movement. But by knowing that, and using conscious mental effort, you may be able to override the impairment to a significant degree."

A Parkinson's boot camp would be the ideal place to explain these subtleties, then to show the patients as a group that they can move by bringing in people like John Pepper to demonstrate. Parkinson's patients have a problem *initiating movement*. They can be taught that this may have to do with a problem *initiating motivation*.* This motivational lack is not a product of laziness or apathy or weakness of will. Rather, the brain's dopamine-based motivation circuit for movement often cannot energize particular movements, even when desired, and this appears as weariness or lassitude. This statement is not to reduce the will-to-move to being *merely* a physical-chemical phenomenon, but to emphasize that mind and body evolved together and attempts to understand one without the other are futile.

That John Pepper was able to motivate himself to move, despite limited dopamine, attests to the vital force of his mind and will. But to translate that motivation into movement still required a "neurological" discovery on his part. He still couldn't do normal, everyday walking, which is automatic, and habitual (and thus relies on dopamine circuits in the lateral striatum, which is part of the basal ganglia), until his conscious walking technique got around this circuit and allowed him to use other circuits (in the frontal lobes and likely more medial parts of the striatum).

---

* See also the wide-ranging behavioral neuroscientist Patrick McNamara's subtle discussion of how PD affects the self's sense of agency. P. McNamara, *The Cognitive Neuropsychiatry of Parkinson's Disease* (Cambridge, MA: MIT Press, 2011).

The Double-Sided Parkinsonian Character

Pepper often wonders why more people have not followed his example. At support groups, only 25 percent of PD sufferers did so. All those who did, he says, benefited. But some, he felt, were perhaps too ashamed of their disease to go out walking; some were just unwilling. And perhaps there are exercise-resistant variants of PD that simply don't respond, so they broke it off. I've also wondered whether Pepper's rare determination might be an expression of his Parkinson's—which may sound odd, because Parkinson's is usually seen as a physical, not a mental, disease. But Oliver Sacks points out that James Parkinson, who first described the physical illness in detail, also described its psychological effects, which can include states that appear passive as well as others that appear more willful, speeded up, and urgent. The physical speeding up can be seen in the small hurried steps some Parkinson's patients take. This "festination" has, as Sacks describes it, a mental counterpart as well: "Festination consists of an acceleration (and with this, an abbreviation) of steps, movements, words, or even thoughts—it conveys a sense of impatience, impetuosity, and alacrity, as if the patient were very pressed for time; and in some patients it goes along with a *feeling* of urgency and impatience, although others, as it were, find themselves hurried against their will."

John Pepper does leap into the fray very quickly sometimes. I once wrote him a letter expressing a wish to meet some people he had worked with, expecting to receive a letter with his thoughts on the idea, and instead, within a few days, he had arranged large group meetings in three African cities for me to speak at. When I hesitated (briefly), he wrote back, with great and unmistakable remorse, "You must forgive me for running away with things, without adequate consultation, but that is my way." I wondered whether this urgency was what allowed Pepper to exercise, whereas other patients, who were more slowed down physically and possibly mentally, might not be able to.

Did those with slowed movements have a slowing that would lead to a kind of paralysis of will? Such a physical and mental slowing, as Sacks points out, "is exactly antithetical to hurry or pulsion" and gives rise to an "active *retardation* or *resistance* which impedes movement, speech, and even thought, and may arrest it completely. Such people find themselves embattled, and even immobilized, in a form of physiological conflict—force against counter-force, will against counter-will, command against countermand." Yet John Pepper certainly knew what it was to freeze and become rigid and immobile, and as Sacks has emphasized, people with Parkinson's have tendencies both to slow and to speed up.

THE WORLD OF SCIENCE IS finally catching up to John Pepper. In 2011 a multistudy review was published in one of the most important mainstream medical journals, *Neurology.* Mayo Clinic neurologist J. E. Ahlskog looked at most of the available evidence for exercise and Parkinson's, in animals and humans; it was titled, "Does Vigorous Exercise Have a Neuroprotective Effect in Parkinson's?" Vigorous exercise included walking, swimming, and basically "physical activity sufficient to increase heart rate and the need for oxygen" and that was sustained and repeated. On the basis of examining many hundreds of patients, it concluded, "This overall body of evidence suggests that vigorous exercise should be accorded a central place in our treatment of PD."

And a recent controlled study by Dr. Lisa Shulman and her colleagues from the University of Maryland compared low-intensity treadmill walking with higher-intensity treadmill walking in PD patients. They found that the lower-intensity exercise, at a walking pace chosen by the patients themselves, actually worked better than exercise at a very high intensity and led, ultimately, to an increased walking speed when they were tested off the treadmill. Remember, Pepper started his Run/Walk for Life program at very slow speeds; it was only with long practice that he got to high speeds. This has been replicated by an important 2014 randomized study of PD patients from the department of neurology at the University of Iowa, led by the researcher Ergun Uc. The study found that walking, three times a week for forty-five minutes, for six months, led to improvements in the patients' Parkinsonian movement symptoms, mood, and decreased fatigue. Though the patients were on anti-Parkinson's medication, the authors noted that the improvements could not be attributed to medication.

What this emerging evidence tells us is that even if one wishes to still remain skeptical about John Pepper, whether he has "typical" or "atypical" Parkinson's is beside the point. There is no disputing he *at least* had a severe Parkinson's-like movement disorder, extremely hard to distinguish from Parkinson's disease on close examination; indeed close enough that his neurologists documented it as PD; that it responded, at one point, to levodopa; that his disease has, in ways, been progressive; that it is not confined to Parkinsonian symptoms; that, lasting almost fifty years, and relapsing *severely* when he doesn't walk, it is not a "minor" movement disorder. His triumph has been that whatever variant he has—if it is a variant—it has been something he has been able to learn from, and then help others who have PD. Only now is the science showing that his claims apply to many more people than himself, and that exercise is extremely powerful medicine. Only time will tell whether some others, who have exercised as many years as he has, can make as much progress.

Deferring Dementia

The question inevitably arises: If walking can turn back Parkinson's symptoms, and can delay the onset of Huntington's, both degenerative diseases, might it have a role to play in the commonest degenerative disease of the brain—Alzheimer's disease?

The question is especially important because there are no effective medications for Alzheimer's. Yet Alzheimer's and Parkinson's have similarities. Dr. Mark P. Mattson, chief of the National Neurosciences Laboratory at the National Institute on Aging, National Institutes of Health, has shown that many of the cellular processes that cause problems in Parkinson's also occur in Alzheimer's but in different brain areas. In Parkinson's, the substantia nigra begins to malfunction first. In Alzheimer's, degenerative changes begin in the hippocampus (which turns short-term memories into long), which starts to shrink, so that its victims lose short-term memory. In Alzheimer's disease, the brain literally loses its plasticity, and its ability to make connections between neurons, many of which die.

In 2013 that pressing question about walking and Alzheimer's was answered. Walking was a key contributor to a very simple program that reduced the risk of dementia by a staggering 60 percent. If any drug could do that, it would be the most popular, talked-about treatment in medicine.

The breakthrough study was done by Dr. Peter Elwood and a team from the Cochrane Institute of Primary Care and Public Health, Cardiff University, United Kingdom, and released in December 2013. For thirty years, these researchers followed 2,235 men living in Caerphilly, Wales, aged 45 to 59, and observed the impact of five activities on their health and on whether they developed dementia or cognitive decline, heart disease, cancer, or early death. The Cardiff study was meticulous, examining the men at intervals over the thirty years, and if they showed signs of cognitive decline or dementia, they were sent for detailed clinical assessments of high quality. It overcame study design problems from eleven previous studies (discussed in the endnotes).

Results showed that if the men did four or five of the following behaviors, their risk for cognitive (mental) decline and dementia (including Alzheimer's) fell by 60 percent:

1. Exercise (defined as vigorous exercise, or walking at least two miles a day, or biking ten miles a day). Exercise was the most powerful contributor to decreased risk of both general cognitive decline and dementia.
2. Healthy diet (as measured by eating at least three to four servings of fruits and vegetables a day).*
3. Normal weight (as measured by having a body mass index between 18 and 25).

---

* We know much more about diet and the brain since that study was initiated thirty years ago. For an up-to-date discussion of how diet, food sensitivities, glucose, insulin, and obesity affect brain health, and the relationship between exercise and insulin, see the neurologist David Perlmutter's *Grain Brain* (New York: Little, Brown, 2013).

4. Low alcohol intake (alcohol is often a neurotoxin).

5. No smoking (also a case of avoiding a toxin).

All five factors promote the general cellular health of neurons and glia. All factors require that a person live closer to the ways our hunter-gatherer ancestors lived and thus use the body as it evolved to be used. All these behaviors are basically subtractive: don't do things we didn't evolve to do, such as sit all day, and travel sitting in cars; don't eat processed food, inhale smoke, or drink too much.

One of the reasons this work hasn't received more attention is that the scientific community has been so focused upon "curing" Alzheimer's by coming up with a drug for it, or thinking of it in terms of genetics. Of course, if "it is all in your genes," most people assume there is nothing they can do about it, except pray for "genetic breakthroughs." But as the Alzheimer's researcher and neurologist Tiffany Chow points out, "Only a very small percentage of people in the world carry an indelible familial pattern of inheritance of Alzheimer's." In addition, there are many known environmental causes of Alzheimer's and other forms of dementia: head injuries and exposure to certain toxins, like the pesticide DDT, increase the risk, while a high education level decreases the risk. As Chow puts it, environmental factors "interact with . . . genetic makeup to eventually allow or deny dementia a foothold." People who have genetic risk factors commonly associated with Alzheimer's don't necessarily get it,* and even having multiple copies of the genetic materials associated with risk "is not sufficient to produce Alzheimer's Disease." So while having a first-degree relative with Alzheimer's increases one's genetic risk, that increased risk doesn't mean that protective techniques, like exercise, won't help. On the contrary, it probably makes them especially relevant for self-protection.

As for those without dementia, it is now crystal clear that physical exercise helps preserve brain functioning. Another crucial review, in 2011, shed important light on the cognitive effects of exercise. J. Eric

---

* The most commonly cited genetic risk factors are certain variations of the Apolipoprotein E gene on chromosome 19.

Ahlskog, of the department of neurology at the Mayo Clinic, and his team reviewed all 1,603 studies to date of exercise and cognitive impairment with a focus on dementia. Ahlskog did what is called a meta-analysis, examining all studies of high quality and selecting out the best, including randomized, controlled trials. The twenty-nine randomized, controlled studies that were selected documented that exercise—mostly aerobic—was helpful in improving cognitive functioning in adults without dementia, in terms of memory, attention, processing speed, and ability to form and act on plans. Typical doses in most studies are 2.5 hours of aerobic exercise a week. A recent randomized, controlled trial led by Kirk Erickson shows that those (without dementia) who did aerobic exercise for a year showed significant hippocampal enlargement, compared with sedentary adults. These changes last, too. Another study showed that adults who walked had hippocampal enlargement nine years after they began their exercise program. Ahlskog also found that even those with dementia made some modest improvements with exercise.

Will incorporating these behaviors defer dementia indefinitely? We don't yet know. Right now, 15 percent of people over seventy have some dementia, and that number radically increases by age eighty-five. But it isn't inevitable in a long life: some people live to very advanced years without Alzheimer's. Only now that people are living longer are we able to study people over ninety—the "oldest old"—in significant numbers. These "nonagenarians" are the fastest-growing age group in North America: they number 2 million in the United States now and will number 10 million at midcentury. Though dementia increases with age, the University of California at Irvine's excellent "Ninety Plus" study of sixteen hundred nonagenarians has found that the majority do not have dementia. Studying that group as they age will tell us what characterizes the remarkable brains that don't radically degenerate even after a century of activity.

Cape of Good Hope

We climb up the rocky ascent to the lighthouse at the Cape of Good Hope. It is hard to hear Pepper because the wind today is at gale force,

40 miles per hour. I hadn't quite realized how hard the wind was blowing because as I look at him, he stands bolt upright throughout the climb. The southeasterly has been coming at us as we mount the final steps to the lighthouse, and it will be at our backs as we descend. We are totally exposed. I am reminded how vulnerable Parkinson's patients are to losing their balance, and I remember Pepper taking the retropulsion test in Dr. Pearl's office—how she pulled him to see if he could keep his balance.

This is not your normal Parkinson's walking weather, even for John Pepper. But today his posture is very stable. That is because he's using his conscious technique to balance himself, actively shifting his weight forward, into the wind. He is fit for his age, has no difficulty lifting his feet, and keeps up a strong pace, even though he's in sandals, not proper walking shoes for a climb that is the equivalent of many flights of stairs.

At the top, we look out to where the two great aquamarine oceans meet, the warmer Indian Ocean and the colder Atlantic. We turn and begin to descend the stone steps to the nature reserve.

"Did you notice," he says, "as we've been going down, that we both accelerated just now?" referring to the wind. I nod yes and note that he has now passed nature's retropulsion test from behind.

"This could be Scotland, only it would be colder," he says, as we travel farther down, looking out at the fynbos—the South African name for the fine bush—which covers this nature reserve. "Except it would be a yellow gorse, a prickly bush, and heather, not fynbos."

Enraptured by the view, he gets distracted, stops using his conscious thought technique, and drags his foot. A reminder of his disease returns.

"I just caught my toes, from not lifting my foot high enough. These are not the right shoes for this," he says of his sandals, mad at himself.

Then he turns back to look at the fynbos and flowers. Suddenly, strangely, his face is expressive, nostalgic, but also curious about the wildlife and beauty around him. There is no mask.

ON JULY 13, 2011, FIVE months after I returned home, I wrote Pepper to see how he was doing. I knew he and Shirley had intended to travel through South Africa that summer.

He wrote me right back.

I am currently mourning the death of Shirley, which happened yesterday morning. . . . She had a massive heart attack, and died without gaining consciousness. . . . My family has taken me under their wing. . . . I am surrounded by love from my family, and an incredible number of PD patients who have bombarded me with their thoughts and best wishes. I am truly blessed.

Kindest regards,
John

A few months later I called and learned that just before Shirley died, John developed sores in his mouth and was given another diagnosis. A surgeon, working with a lab, diagnosed pemphigus, an autoimmune disorder, and told Pepper he had a 30 percent chance of survival, and he'd probably be dead in three years. The surgeon referred him to an oncologist, who gave him a medicine that shot his blood pressure up to 190/110, so he couldn't tolerate it. He then wrote me, "My family and I are convinced that Shirley was absolutely shattered by the diagnosis of Pemphigus, as it is a terminal illness. . . . She has gone through so much in the past with my health problems, that she just could not face losing me. . . . The loss of Shirley caused me to just give up everything." That included his exercise, of course. Under the stress of losing her, the sores worsened.

Months pass. In March 2012 a new doctor reevaluates his condition. He's told, if it is truly pemphigus, he would not still be alive and functioning as well as he seems to be. The surgeon now concurs. Instead, he has something more benign that only looks like pemphigus—"pemphigoid." He writes me, "Shirley died before the news came of the mistaken diagnosis. We are all shattered by this revelation."

Many more months pass, and I call him to see how he is doing.

I learn that John Pepper is on his feet, back out on the roads of Johannesburg, walking.

Chapter 3

The Stages of Neuroplastic Healing

How and Why It Works

THE CHAPTERS YOU HAVE JUST read focused on two very different kinds of healing. The work of Michael Moskowitz focused on *specific neuronal functioning issues,* and on using the fact that plasticity is competitive, to rewire the brain by weakening a pathological pain circuit through the use of the mind. John Pepper's radical self-improvement involved using the mind to strengthen *specific neuronal* circuits in parts of his brain not normally involved in walking. But his exercise also helped improve the *general cellular functions* of his neurons and glia, by triggering neuronal and glial growth factors and the development of new cells, and by improving brain circulation.

In the chapters that follow, I will focus on the role of energy, in one form or another, to awaken and assist a brain that is not functioning well. In this chapter, I lay out my understanding of the stages of neuroplastic healing. These stages are to be seen as a flexible framework, not as a rigid scheme. But to understand them, it is first necessary to understand three general processes that frequently occur in the brain when it has problems.

The Pervasiveness of Learned Nonuse

Since I wrote *The Brain That Changes Itself,* three things have become apparent to me.

The first is that learned nonuse applies not only to stroke. As discussed in the previous chapter, people who have had a stroke go through a crisis—diaschisis—in which the brain, immediately after the injury, goes into shock for about six weeks and functions poorly. Edward Taub showed that when a stroke patient tries repeatedly, during this period, to move the paralyzed arm, and cannot, he "learns" it doesn't work and so starts using only his nonaffected limb. In the use-it-or-lose-it brain, the already-damaged circuitry for the paralyzed arm withers further. Taub proved that if the good arm was put in a cast or sling, so that it couldn't be used, then extremely intensive, incremental training of the paralyzed arm could often restore function, even decades later.

By 2007 Taub had shown that brain injuries caused by radiation treatments also lead to learned nonuse. He has since found that it can occur in a partial spinal cord injury, cerebral palsy, aphasia (loss of speech from a stroke), multiple sclerosis, traumatic brain injuries, and people who have had brain surgery for epilepsy, and that these conditions can respond to his therapy.* I began to see that learned nonuse could occur in other brain problems, such as Parkinson's, and even, at times, it seemed, in some psychiatric problems. Indeed, in any situation where brain function is lost or on the wane, a person may be understandably tempted to find ways to work around the deficit—and thereby unintentionally exacerbate the loss of this circuitry. The widespread if not universal existence of learned nonuse means that often we cannot judge the level of a person's deficit, or potential to recover, until we first try to train the individual vigorously.

---

* Taub's many published works show great success in using Constraint-Induced Therapy to help patients deal with lost *movement* from stroke, traumatic brain injury, and multiple sclerosis and should, to my mind, always be considered for movement-related problems caused by brain injury or disease, including Parkinson's disease (with which he has also had anecdotal success). Studies of modified forms of Constraint-Induced Therapy have proven them effective in helping stroke victims with aphasia to regain speech, and they probably can help some vision problems, such as amblyopia, where the circuitry for vision in one eye "turns off." See V. W. Mark et al., "Constraint-Induced Movement Therapy for the Lower Extremities in Multiple Sclerosis: Case Series with 4-Year Follow-up," *Archives of Physical Medicine and Rehabilitation* 94 (2013): 753–60.

I have come to suspect that learned nonuse is such a common phenomenon in the brain because "going dormant" is a common strategy when a cell, or a more complex organ or organism, finds itself in a situation in which its normal ways of adapting to the environment fail.*

The Noisy Brain and Brain Dysrhythmias

The second concept that is applicable to many different brain problems is that of the "noisy brain" that has problems firing in rhythm. I was originally exposed to the idea of the noisy brain in the lab of Paul Bach-y-Rita, where he was working with Cheryl Schiltz (discussed in Chapter 7). Schiltz's balance system was injured by a medication, and she could no longer determine where she was in space. She said that her mind felt very "noisy." The scientists believed her subjective sense of "noise" mirrored what was happening in her neuronal circuits: her neurons couldn't generate enough strong, sharp signals in the balance system to stand out against the background noise of all the other neuronal signals being fired in her brain. *Noise* is a term from engineering, to describe what happens in a system when that system cannot recognize

---

* The temporary shifting into dormant states is a strategy seen in different kinds of organisms. In the plant kingdom, seeds can go into a dormant state if the external environment becomes too hot or too cold for them to control their internal cellular environment, and can survive without water, sun, or nutrients for centuries. The great physiologist who coined the term and concept "homeostasis," Claude Bernard, pointed to many cases of "latent life," wherein animals oscillate between fully active living states and dormant ones. The dormant ones occur when the animal can no longer maintain "homeostasis"—that is, it can no longer control its internal environment, because external conditions are not compatible with normal life. The wormlike tardigrade, which has a nervous system and muscles, can, in drought, completely dry up and remain dormant in an inactive state for extended periods, only to come to life when exposed to moisture. Some of these animals have been kept inert for as long as twenty-seven years. In these protected states of "suspended animation," energy consumption drops radically, until the animal can be revived. The revival often requires an input from the outside. I have discussed these examples of biological dormancy as a possible template for learned nonuse with Taub. He thinks that learning is sufficient to explain what we observe and thinks it is an open question as to whether other factors might contribute. But I would add, it might be both learned and instinctual. There are a number of instinctual capacities that require some "priming" by the environment—which involves learning—to be triggered. See C. Bernard, *Lectures on the Phenomena of Life Common to Animals and Plants*, trans. H. E. Hoff, R. Guillemin, and L. Guillemin (1878; reprinted Springfield, IL: Charles C. Thomas, 1974), pp. 1:49–50, 56.

normal signals because they are too weak compared with the background "noise." Hence the "noisy brain."

I would put it this way. In a brain injury, from whatever cause (toxins, stroke, infection, radiation therapy, blow to the head, degenerative disease), some neurons die and cease to give off signals. Others are damaged, but—and this is key—they don't necessarily "fall silent." Living brain tissue is, by nature, excitable. Even when a brain circuit is "off," it continues to fire some electrical signals, although at a different, often slower rate than when it is activated and "on." In this view, the brain is like the heart. At rest, it doesn't stop; rather, it shifts into a resting rate. When the heart's electrical system is damaged, it loses the ability to regulate its firing rate and gives off aberrant signals of various kinds: its natural pacemakers may run too slowly, or race at dangerous speeds, or lead to chaotic irregular beats called either arrhythmias or dysrhythmias.

In the brain, these irregular signals have an effect on all the networks they are connected to, "messing up" their functioning as well—unless the brain can shut down its damaged neurons. In many brain problems, we now know, neurons are firing at the wrong or unusual rates. This problem occurs in epilepsy, Alzheimer's, Parkinson's, many sleep problems, and brain injuries, among others: they create a noisy brain because so many of the signals are out of sync.* Something similar is seen in the aging brain, in the brains of children with learning disorders, and in sensory problems when neurons can't fire sharp, clear signals.

When sick neurons render the healthy ones that receive their irregular signals ineffective, they may become dormant. A recent important study by Taub's group, using brain scans, has shown that when a stroke kills neurons in what is called the "infarct" area, other neurons, still living but far from the dead cells, can show signs of atrophy or wasting away.

---

* A number of neuroscientists, among them Rodolfo Llinás, Barry Sterman, and Paul E. Rapp, an expert in traumatic brain injury, have documented brain dysrhythmias in a variety of neurological and psychiatric disorders. Support for the idea that "sick" neurons fire improper signals comes from neurofeedback (see Appendix 3). Special EEGs show that in brain injuries, patients often have areas of the brain that fire inappropriate "slow wave" activity. When patients are trained, with neurofeedback, to make slow waves to fire at a more normal rate, their brain injury symptoms can often decrease.

The extent of this atrophy correlates with the patient's difficulties and how well he or she will do in Constraint-Induced Therapy. (Taub thinks, as do I, that this wasting away of neurons most likely occurs because these areas are not getting proper signals from sick neurons, according to the use-it-or-lose-it principle, or because they are exhibiting the poor brain health that predisposed the person to the stroke, or both.) Thus, when patients try to perform an activity that requires all this circuitry, they fail and, at this point, I believe, develop learned nonuse. Worse, not only do they lack access to skills they once had, they have trouble learning new ones because the noisy brain cannot make fine distinctions or differentiations.

In summary, though such patients cannot perform certain tasks, only some of the neurons that normally process those tasks are dead; others are alive but distressed and firing irregular, noisy signals, and others are merely dormant because they are getting bad signals. The approaches I describe in the chapters to come can often foster improved health in the sick, noise-generating neurons and use energy and neuroplastic approaches to retrain the surviving neurons to fire in sync and reawaken dormant abilities.

The Rapid Ongoing Formation of Neuronal Assemblies

The third major factor that allows neuroplastic healing derives from the uniqueness of neurons, compared with other cells. Neurons usually work in large groups, communicating electrically through widely distributed networks throughout the brain. These networks are constantly reforming themselves into new "neuronal assemblies," as the neuroscientists Susan Greenfield, Gerald Edelman, and others have emphasized. This appears to be especially true for conscious activities. Since no conscious mental act is entirely the same as another, in each mental act slightly different combinations of neurons communicate with one another. Thus, as a person goes through the day, her brain is forming, unforming, and reforming new neuronal networks as part of its basic operating procedure. In this respect, the organic living brain is quite the opposite of an engineered machine with hardwired circuits that can perform only the limited number of actions that it has been designed to do. Machines generally perform an action the same way every time.

A neuron, or group of neurons, however, will be used for different purposes, at different times—a sign of how flexible neuronal networks are. In 1923 the neuroscientist Karl Lashley exposed a monkey's motor cortex and stimulated it with an electrode in a particular place. He observed the resulting movement, then sewed the monkey back up. After some time he repeated the experiment, stimulating the monkey in that same spot, only to find that the resulting movement often changed. As Harvard's great historian of psychology of the time, Edwin G. Boring, put it, "One day's mapping would no longer be valid on the morrow."

Lashley's work also raised the hope that if one neuronal network was damaged, perhaps another could form to replace it.

Scientists once imagined that memories, or skills, were processed in discrete, small locations in the brain. But Lashley showed that this was often not the case. His most famous experiments involved teaching an animal, such as a rat, to perform a complex activity to get a reward. Then he would damage brain tissue in the part of the cortex thought to process that skill. Surprisingly, the animal could still perform the activity, though it might take longer or be less precise. Why this result occurs is open to interpretation, but from Lashley's work, scientists learned that many skills involve much more widely distributed neural networks than had been believed. It also showed that these networks have a lot of redundancy, because parts can be removed, and still the animal can perform the task.*

---

* It is possible to integrate the best of Lashley's findings with studies of brain locations, which I do in *The Brain That Changes Itself*, especially in Chapter 11. There is something to finding specific locations for certain mental activities in the brain, or "localizing them," but some forms of localizationism are "immature" and overly rigid, while more mature forms take into account brain plasticity. Just because the brain *tends* to process certain mental activities in certain areas doesn't mean it always must. Immature localizationism doesn't recognize this fact. As the reader can already appreciate, I frequently talk of certain brain areas as being "involved in" processing specific mental functions. What I mean by "involved in" is that these areas tend to participate in these mental functions and may even be necessary for those functions, but the circuit is usually much broader than the named area, involving many other brain areas, and for many functions the brain works more holistically than immature localizationism implies. Saying that "the hippocampus is involved in processing short-term memory" is more accurate than saying "short-term memory is processed in the hippocampus." *The Brain That Changes Itself* gives numerous

It is important for laypeople to remember the following, perhaps shocking, point. It is well established that mental activity correlates with neuronal activity, and that as learning occurs, new connections are formed between neurons. But when neuroscientists sometimes say, using shorthand, that "our thoughts are in our neurons," they are radically overstating what the science has shown. To say that when thoughts occur, neurons fire and form links with one another is to describe two things happening at once. But neuroscientists really do not know where "in" the neurons thoughts are encoded. Nor do they know if they are "in" individual neurons (highly unlikely), or in the connections between the neurons, or distributed throughout the brain. This mystery of the mind remains unsolved.*

Lashley appears to have been the first neuroscientist to propose an interesting alternative: that learning and skills are encoded not "in" specific neurons, or even "in" the connections between neurons, but "in" the *cumulative electrical wave patterns* that are the result of all the neurons firing together. (This important hypothesis was taken up by the neurosurgeon and neuroscientist Karl Pribram, who developed a brilliant theory of how the brain encodes experience.)

Let us imagine that brain functions—such as thoughts, memories, perceptions, and skills—are encoded not in individual neurons but in the patterns that can be generated by different coalitions of neurons. (To use an analogy, the patterns are like a musical piece, and the neurons are the orchestral musicians that play the piece.) Loss of some individual neurons, from neuronal death or disease, would not necessarily lead to the loss of a mental function, as long as enough of the brain's neurons

---

examples of how, when large parts of the brain are damaged or absent, other brain areas can take over their mental functions. Taub's group has shown that there is very little correlation between where a stroke lesion occurs, and its size, and how well patients do in Constraint-Induced Therapy, with the exception of a stroke in an area called the corona radiata. See L. V. Gauthier et al., "Improvement After Constraint-Induced Movement Therapy Is Independent of Infarct Location in Chronic Stroke Patients," *Stroke* 40, no. 7 (2009): 2468–72; V. W. Mark et al., "MRI Infarction Load and CI Therapy Outcomes for Chronic Post-Stroke Hemiparesis," *Restorative Neurology and Neuroscience* 26 (2008): 13–33.

* How neuroscientists overstate our knowledge about "where" mental activity is localized in the brain, and confuse the mind with the material brain, is described in neuroscientist Raymond Tallis's extremely thought-provoking book *Aping Mankind: Neuromania, Darwinitis and the Misrepresentation of Humanity* (Durham, UK: Acumen, 2011).

remained and were able to generate these patterns. (To continue the music analogy: if one member of the string section is sick, the show can still go on, if his replacement has access to the musical score.)

Much of what we consider to be our essence is not in our individual neurons, anyway, all of which are quite similar. So much of the specifics of "who we are" is related to our encoded experience, which is carried in the patterns of energy that our brain generates. The coded patterns of experience can often survive structural damage to the brain.*

The Stages of Healing

I have observed the following stages in neuroplastic healing. Often they occur in the order presented here, but that need not always be so; some patients need to go through only some of these stages to heal, while others must pass through all of them.

Correction of general cellular functions of the neurons and glia. This is the only stage that does not directly address "wiring issues"—that very specialized ability of neurons to connect to and communicate with each other—but instead focuses on the general health of the neurons, and the cell functions they have in common with other cells. In many brain problems, the brain becomes "miswired" because the neurons and the glia have been disturbed by an external source (such as an infection, a heavy metal toxin, a pesticide, a drug, or food sensitivity), or they have been undersupplied with resources, such as certain minerals. These

---

* The biological thinker Ludwig von Bertalanffy reminds us that the sharp separation between structure and function really best applies to machines, which can only be on or off and are made of inanimate matter. In organisms, it is better to think of processes. "The antithesis between *structure* and *function* . . . is based upon a static conception of the organism. In a machine there is a fixed arrangement that can be set in motion but can also be at rest. In a similar way the pre-established structure of, say, the heart is distinguished from its function, namely, rhythmical contraction. Actually, this separation between a pre-established structure and processes occurring in this structure does not apply to the living organism. . . . [In organisms] what are called structures are slow processes of long duration, [while] functions are quick processes of short duration." Ludwig von Bertalanffy, *Problems of Life: An Evaluation of Modern Biological Thought* (London: Watts & Co., 1952), p. 134. In trying to understand how neuroplasticity facilitates healing, we can regard mental acts, such as thinking, as processes that are of short duration but can have an effect on processes of long duration, the so-called structure of the brain. While thought itself cannot resurrect dead tissue, it can stimulate any remaining healthy tissue to reorganize itself to take on the lost functions of the damaged tissue.

general problems are best corrected before beginning the stages that follow for the patient to get the most benefit.

This general cellular repair stage is especially relevant in treating autism and learning disorders, and in lowering dementia risk, for example. It also applies to common psychiatric disorders. I have seen patients with depression, bipolar disorder, and attention deficit disorder make major progress by eliminating toxins and certain foods, such as sugar and grains, that they were sensitive to.

Many of these interventions involve the glial cells, which make up a full 85 percent of all the cells in the brain. The brain has a barrier around it, called the blood-brain barrier, that protects it from invaders, and it has no lymphatic system—the system of vessels that is very important for the immune system and healing elsewhere in the body. Instead, small "microglial" cells protect the brain from invading organisms, and they are one of the unique ways that the brain protects and heals itself. The glia also support the neurons by getting rid of waste products produced by the brain.

The following four stages all make specific use of the neuroplastic capacities of the brain to alter the connections between the neurons and to change its "wiring."

Neurostimulation. In almost all the interventions in this book, some kind of energy-based *neurostimulation* of the brain cells is required. Light, sound, electricity, vibration, movement, and thought (which turns on certain networks) all provide neurostimulation. Neurostimulation helps to revive dormant circuits in the hurt brain and leads to a second phase in the healing process, an improved ability of the noisy brain to regulate and modulate itself once again and achieve homeostasis. Some forms of neurostimulation begin from an external source, but other forms are internal. Everyday thought, especially when used systematically, is a potent way to stimulate neurons.

When we think particular thoughts, certain networks in the brain are "turned on," while others are switched off. This process was the basis of Moskowitz's visualization cures of chronic pain (see Chapter 1). Once a relevant circuit is turned on by thought, it fires, and *then* the blood flows to that circuit (a process that can be seen on brain scans that monitor blood flow in the brain) to replenish its energy supply. I believe that Taub's Constraint-Induced Therapy, though a movement-based behavioral therapy, involves great intentional effort and motor planning, so it too likely triggers some thought-based neurostimulation. (It also involves the final phase, *neurodifferentiation and learning*.) Pepper's conscious walking, to build up new circuits in his brain, is an example of internal neurostimulation using thought. Neurostimulation is effective in preparing the brain to build new circuits and in overcoming learned nonuse in existing circuits. Brain exercises, and many of the forms of mental practice described in *The Brain That Changes Itself,* are forms of internal neuroplastic neurostimulation.

Neuromodulation. Neuromodulation is another internal method by which the brain contributes to its own healing. It quickly restores the balance between excitation and inhibition in the neural networks and quiets the noisy brain. People with a variety of brain problems can't regulate sensation properly. They are often too sensitive to outside stimulation or, alternatively, are insensitive to it. Neuromodulation restores the balance. As we shall see in Chapter 7, neurostimulation can trigger neuromodulation, improving brain self-regulation, generally.

One way neuromodulation works is by resetting the brain's overall level of arousal by acting on two subcortical brain systems.

The first such system is the reticular activating system (RAS), which is involved in regulating a person's level of consciousness and the overall level of arousal. The RAS is housed in the brain stem (an area of the brain between the spinal cord and the bottom of the brain) and extends up toward the highest parts of the cortex. It can "power up" the rest of the brain and regulate the sleep-wake cycle. I shall show in the following chapters how stimulation with light, electricity, sound, and vibration often causes patients with a brain problem (who are usually exhausted and jittery from having a brain issue) to begin sleeping deeply, to wake up restored, and to develop a better sleep cycle. Resetting the RAS is essential to helping the brain restore its energy supplies, which it will call upon to heal further.

The second way neuromodulation works is by affecting the autonomic nervous system. Millions of years of evolution have equipped human beings with "preset," automatic, involuntary nervous system re-actions, to prepare them for nature's emergencies—as when predators suddenly attack and there is little time to think. These ready-made auto-matic reactions are built into the autonomic nervous system, called "au-tonomic" because it was thought to be largely automatic and not under voluntary control.

The autonomic nervous system has two well-known branches. The first is the sympathetic fight-or-flight reaction, which mobilizes a per-son for action and shunts blood to the heart and muscles so he or she can fight off a predator or a dangerous rival, or run away. Both fight and flight require a large discharge of energy and an increase in metabolism (to access the energy needed for immediate use). Designed for immedi-ate survival, this system focuses all a person's activities on that purpose and often inhibits growth and healing processes. Many patients with brain problems, or learning problems, are often in a state of sympathetic fight-or-flight, feeling desperate, endangered, and hyper-anxious be-cause they can't keep up with unfolding events. The problem is that a person in fight-or-flight can't heal or learn well in this state, which makes brain change harder.

The second branch is the parasympathetic system, which turns off the sympathetic system and puts a person into a calm state in which he or she can think and reflect. While the sympathetic system is often called the fight-or-flight system, the parasympathetic is sometimes called the rest-digest-repair system. When this system is turned on, it triggers a number of chemical reactions that promote growth, conserve energy, and increase sleep, all of which are necessary for healing. It also recharges the mitochondria, the power sources inside the cells (which I will discuss at length in Chapter 4), reenergizing them. Finally, and of special importance, recent studies by Michael Hasselmo and his col-leagues from Harvard show that turning off the sympathetic system ap-pears to improve the signal-to-noise ratio in brain circuits. Thus turning on the parasympathetic system is probably another way to quiet the noisy brain. Many of the techniques in this book turn on the parasym-pathetic system, and turn off the sympathetic system, rapidly relaxing people and preparing them for growth. In Chapter 8, we shall learn that the parasympathetic system also turns on a "social engagement system," which allows us to connect to other human beings, and use them to soothe and support us, and help us to regulate our own nervous system.

Neurorelaxation. Once fight-or-flight is turned off, the brain can accumulate and store the energy that will be needed for the efforts of recovery. Subjectively the person relaxes, and often catches up on sleep. Many people with brain problems are exhausted, and poor sleepers. A recent discovery by Maiken Nedergaard from the University of Rochester showed that in sleep the glia open up special channels that allow waste products and toxic buildups (including the proteins that build up in dementia) to be discharged from the brain through the cerebral spinal fluid, which bathes much of the brain. This unique channel system is ten times more active in the sleeping brain than in the waking state. This helps explain why loss of sleep leads to a deterioration in brain function: too much sleep deprivation leads to a toxic brain. The *neurorelaxation* phase appears to correct this, and can last several weeks, in some cases.

Neurodifferentiation and learning. In this final phase, the brain is rested, and the noisy brain has been modulated and is much "quieter," because the circuits can regulate themselves. The patient is able to pay attention again and is ready for learning, which involves the brain doing what it does best: making fine distinctions, or "differentiating." Many brain exercises for learning disorders and those that are based on listening therapy, for instance, involve training a person to make increasingly subtle distinctions in sounds.*

All these phases combined foster the optimal amount of neuroplastic change, but as we shall see, each of the following chapters will emphasize different states. Chapter 4 will focus on restoring general brain cell health, as will parts of Chapter 8 and Appendix 2, on Matrix Repatterning. Chapter 6 will emphasize neurorelaxation. Chapter 7 will emphasize neurostimulation and neuromodulation to reset the brain. Chapter 5 will emphasize the final stage, differentiation. And Chapter 8, on sound, will show all the phases working.

---

* Sometimes skeptics argue that the discovery of neuroplasticity is nothing new, and that neuroplastic healing is merely learning. Only this last phase involves normal learning, however, and the plastic effects of learning in the brain are not the same as the mental activity of learning.

While most people with a brain injury will have to go through each of these stages in their treatment, many of the problems in this book do not derive from brain injury; rather, they require that the patient build up circuitry that had never developed. Some, for instance, require only neurostimulation and neurodifferentiation to do this. And others will benefit from several different interventions.

An individual's progress is never, in this neuroplastic approach, dependent solely on the technique, or the disease or the problem alone. We don't treat diseases, we treat people. Because of genetics, and neuroplasticity itself, no two brains are alike, and no two brain problems—or injuries—are identical. A person with a generally healthy brain who has an injury can't be compared with a person with a similar injury who has had exposure to drugs, neurotoxins, a previous stroke, or serious heart problems. Location of harm matters: a bullet to the breathing center will kill instantly, before a person has time to "rewire"; damage to the attention centers might make it difficult to do brain exercises. Yet even attention can be neuroplastically trained, sometimes, as neuroscientist Ian Robertson has shown.

The next chapter describes an approach that triggered the first three stages for a patient who, because she was exceptionally resourceful, put together her own program to trigger the neurodifferentiation and learning stage.

Chapter 4

Rewiring a Brain with Light

Using Light to Reawaken Dormant Neural Circuits

It is the unqualified result of all my experience with the sick, that second only to their need of fresh air is their need of light; that, after a close room, what hurts them most is a dark room, and it is not only light but direct sun-light that they want. . . . People think that the effect is upon the spirits only. This is by no means the case. The sun is not only a painter but a sculptor.

Florence Nightingale, *Notes on Nursing*, 1860

A Small World

This story, of two chance encounters with a stranger, occurred within the space of a city block. The first took place at a small medical auditorium only steps from my office, to the east. The second happened in beautiful Koerner Hall, at the Royal Conservatory of Music, a few steps to the west.

In the late autumn of 2011, the Ontario Medical Association sent a playful notice to Ontario's doctors. We had a small society, the Doctor's Lounge, that met once a month in Toronto for dinner, followed by a lecture at association headquarters. The Doctor's Lounge functioned within the province's largest mainstream medical organization. Lounge members were of all ages, from very young to retired, companions in that we all had a taste for talks on the cutting edge of medicine and science.

Once there was a doctor's lounge in every hospital, where surgeons in scrubs and hair bonnets, or physicians after a long day on the wards, would, in a rare and lyrical mood, unwind with unguarded conversation, talk about their shared patients, and discuss the latest news in science and medicine. The lounge was a space with a nineteenth-century feel. But in a hurried age, as modern managers, administrators, and "efficiency experts" made sure there would be no "lounging around," the lounges began to disappear from hospitals. So we, in defiance, resurrected the lounge at our association headquarters, as a place to think free-style, with the open-mindedness that first drew us to study medicine and the wonders of the human body.

Even our organizer Dr. Harold Pupko's announcement was unlike the starchy prose of most large organizations, which so often take painstaking care to appear lifeless, as though a deadening formality might better convey seriousness of professional purpose. It was called "From Darkness to Light: Clinical Explorations," and it opened with a quote from a fictitious Potzker Rebbe: "And God said: Let there be paradox. And there was light." It read:

> What are the properties of light? Wave? Particle? Clinical tool? Yes, yes and yes. The therapeutic applications of light therapy range from the well-established (e.g., neonatal jaundice, psoriasis) to emerging popular trends (e.g., light therapy for seasonal affective disorder), but, chances are you are not aware of effective light therapy options available to your patients for conditions ranging from wound healing to brain injury....
>
> Date and Time: December 8, 2011, 7:30 p.m.

The notice continued, explaining that the lecture would emphasize the use of light for brain injury and for other neurological and psychiatric problems.

It gave me pause. Light, to treat brain injury? How might light get into the brain, encased as it is in the bony skull? I had followed the new science of optogenetics, an almost sci-fi field in which labs genetically engineer neurons to make them light-sensitive. In 1979 Francis Crick, codiscoverer of the structure of DNA, argued that the major challenge for neuroscience was to find a way to turn on certain neurons while leaving others unaffected. Perhaps, Crick speculated, light could be used to turn specific classes of neurons on or off.

It was known that some single-cell organisms, such as algae, are light-sensitive; when they are exposed to light, a switch inside them activates the cell. In 2005 genes coding for those light-sensitive switches were inserted into animal neurons, so they could be activated by exposure to light. Some hoped it would be possible to implant these neurons into the brain of a person with a serious brain disease, then surgically thread a fiber-optic line into the damaged brain cells and use light to turn them on or off. This technique had already succeeded in worms, mice, rats, and monkeys, and it seemed possible humans would be next. But this approach is highly invasive, and optogenetics's brilliant pioneer, Karl Deisseroth, a psychiatrist and professor of bioengineering at Stanford University, worried that if we surgically inserted foreign substances such as fiber optics into the human brain, they could cause immune reactions, among other problems. Deisseroth viewed optogenetics as a basic scientific tool to understand how brain circuits work, not as something that would be useful on patients. Perhaps one day the fruits of optogenetics would save lives, but as the day of the lecture approached, I hoped it would present something more practical, a treatment that would heal by working with nature, not against it.

Light Enters Our Bodies Without Our Knowledge

Luckily, light—even natural light—does not require fiber optics and surgery to pass deeply into the brain. We think of our skin and skull as absolute barriers to light, but that is wrong. The energy from normal sunlight passes through the skin to influence the blood, for instance. The lecture notice described using light to cure "neonatal jaundice" as one example. Neonatal jaundice, or yellowing of the skin and eyes, occurs when a newborn's liver is immature, not quite ready to perform all its metabolic functions. We are always producing new red blood cells, refreshing our supply; the new ones replace the older ones, which have to be broken down. Neonatal jaundice is caused when a chemical called bilirubin (from the bile), produced by old red blood cells when they break down, builds up in the body. About half of newborns have jaundice. It generally lasts only a few days, but if it persists, it can become a serious condition, and if untreated, it can lead to a buildup of bilirubin in the brain, causing permanent brain damage.

As physicians became better at saving the lives of premature infants, neonatal jaundice became a growing problem. In Essex, England, a former World War II hospital with a sunlit courtyard facing south was devoted to the care of these yellowed fledglings. Sister J. Ward, known for her skill in rearing puppies, was put in charge of the preemies. She often removed the most delicate of them from their incubators and wheeled them out into the fresh air of the sunlit courtyard, though this impulse made some of the staff anxious. However, Ward's infants began to improve. One day she undressed one of them and diffidently showed the baby to the physician in charge. Its tummy was no longer yellow in the places that had been exposed to the sun.

No one took her seriously until one day a vial containing a blood sample from a jaundiced baby was accidentally left on a windowsill, in natural sunlight, for several hours. When the sample came back, the blood was normal. The doctors were certain that a mistake had been made. But when Drs. R. H. Dobbs and R. J. Cremer investigated further, they found that the excess bilirubin in the sample had somehow been broken down, or metabolized, so that the blood in the vial now had normal bilirubin levels. Perhaps this explained why Sister Ward's jaundiced babies got better in the sun?

Investigations soon proved that the wavelengths of visible blue light— passing through the babies' skin and blood vessels to reach the blood and perhaps the liver too—had caused this marvelous curative effect. Using light to treat jaundice became mainstream. Sister Ward's chance discovery proved we are not as opaque as we imagine ourselves to be.

In fact, Sister Ward's and Drs. Dobbs and Cremer's discovery had already been made by the ancients, then was lost to modern medicine. Soranus of Ephesus, one of imperial Rome's best-known physicians, advocated setting jaundiced newborns out in the sun. Most pagans took phototherapy very seriously, and "heliotherapy"—as it came to be called by the ancients after Helios, the Greek god of the sun—was seen as so potent that ancient buildings were designed to capture as much pure sunlight as possible. The Romans even had right-to-light laws, to guarantee people's access to the sun in their homes (which led them to develop solariums). Ultimately, these laws ceased to be enforced, and the healing properties of light were almost forgotten.*

Not until Florence Nightingale, the founder of modern nursing, were hospitals designed to expose patients to as much sun as possible. But that brief, sunlight-friendly period in the nineteenth century ended with the invention of the artificial lightbulb, which was believed to contain the same full spectrum of light as direct sun. (Unfortunately, artificial light was neither full-spectrum nor equivalent to natural light.) Hospital designs no longer favored natural light, because science could not explain Nightingale's insight that sunlight actually heals.

THE IDEA THAT LIGHT IS a potent healer has been hidden in plain sight for millennia. Though the ancient Egyptians had little science, they did not doubt what they saw with their own eyes: that the sun was essential to growth and life everywhere. They worshipped the sun god Ra—they were literal sun worshippers—and, like most worshippers, had high hopes their god would not only protect but heal them. Ra's presence was everywhere. Even the pharaoh Ramses had Ra's name embedded in his. The Egyptians and many other ancient pagans saw the sun as the primary source of life, and they took it as self-evident that all life-forms ultimately derive their energy from the sun. (Of course, sunlight is necessary for photosynthesis, the process by which plants convert carbon

---

* But not entirely. Niels R. Finsen, a Danish physician, won the Nobel Prize in 1903 for pioneering the use of light therapy in modern times, including the red part of the spectrum to treat smallpox. He discovered he was not the first to make the connection. "In the Middle Ages," he wrote, "small-pox patients were treated by wrapping them in red coverings and by putting red balls in their beds. John of Gaddesden treated a Prince of Wales for small-pox by surrounding him with red objects . . . whilst Dr. Sassakawa reports that in Japan the patients are covered with red blankets, and children with small-pox are given red toys. This remarkable and uncertain employment of the red colour in the treatment of small-pox has naturally been looked upon as a mediaeval superstition." See N. R. Finsen, "The Red Light Treatment of Small-pox," *British Medical Journal* (December 7, 1895), pp. 1412–14.

dioxide and water into glucose, their energy source. Even organisms that do not conduct photosynthesis get their energy from eating plants, or from eating other animals that do so, so ultimately all growth on the planet depends on the sun.)

The ancients also sensed that the healing of distressed tissues requires growth. Ancient Egyptian, Greek, Indian, and Buddhist healers all used systematic exposure to the sun to foster healing. An ancient Egyptian papyrus from the Pharaonic period describes anointing painful, ill body parts with fluids and exposing them to the sun to obtain medical benefits. Thus many recent discoveries about light are actually rediscoveries, such as the finding in 2005 that placing patients recovering from surgery in a sunlit room (as opposed to an artificially lit one) significantly decreases their pain.

In 1984 Dr. Norman Rosenthal, of the National Institutes of Health, discovered that some depressions can be cured by sun exposure, and a recent study showed that a full spectrum of light could be as effective as medication for some depressed patients, with fewer side effects. These ideas were known to the ancient Greeks and Romans. The Greek physician Aretaeus of Cappadocia wrote in the second century, "Lethargics are to be laid out in the light and exposed to the rays of the sun, for the disease is gloom." And if sunlight influences mood, it influences the brain.

GRADE-SCHOOL SCIENCE TELLS US LIGHT energy enters the eye and hits the retina and the rod and cone cells within it; there it is converted into patterns of electrical energy, which then travel along the neurons in the optic nerves to the brain's visual cortex at the back of the head, producing a visual experience.

In 2002 a second pathway from the retina to the brain, with an altogether different purpose, was discovered. Alongside the retinal cells we use for seeing—our rods and cones—other light-sensitive cells were found that send electrical signals on a separate neuronal pathway, also in the optic nerve, to a clump of cells in the brain called the suprachiasmatic nucleus (SCN), which regulates our biological clock.

The biological clock is more than a mere timekeeper; it controls when the major organ systems turn on and off during the course of the day. It is both clock and conductor. The SCN is part of the hypothalamus, and together they function as a master conductor to regulate the symphony of our appetites as they rise and fall—our hunger, thirst, sexual longings, cravings for sleep—by adjusting our hormones. They also influence our levels of arousal and our nervous system.

The ancient Chinese knew that each organ system has times of day when it is most and least active. For instance, according to the Chinese organ clock, the heart and its energies are more active at midday, when we must move around, and less so when we sleep; our digestive system revs up after meals. Because our organ clock deactivates our kidneys during sleep, we rarely have to urinate at night—a convenience that wanes with age, in part because the organ clock, like an old watch, no longer keeps good time. Its neurons fire irregularly, an example of the noisy brain of old age.

Every morning when we awaken, and light enters our eyes, it passes to the SCN and rouses each of our organ systems in its turn. In humans, after the sun goes down, messages from our eyes signal that there is no more light outside; the SCN, in turn, sends that message to our pineal gland, which releases melatonin, a hormone that makes us sleepy. The pineal gland is more exposed in lizards, birds, and fish, for light striking their thin skulls directly stimulates the gland, making it especially "eyelike." (This pineal is often called the third eye.) Our evolutionary heritage thus reminds us that our bony skulls are not sealed vaults and that the brain evolved to constantly appraise and interact with light.

We tend to link light almost exclusively with vision, which we find a miraculous process almost beyond comprehension. But our relationship to light is even more basic. Light also turns on chemical reactions within living organisms—not only in plants. Single-cell organisms without eyes have light-sensitive molecules on their outer membranes that supply them with energy. For instance, *Halobacterium,* which lives in salt marshes, gets its energy from orange light, and its light-sensitive molecules transform that light into energy to do work. When these light-sensitive molecules absorb orange, the organism swims toward the light source, to harvest more light energy; ultraviolet light and green light repel it. The fact that different wavelengths of light have different effects on the organism means that light frequencies carry not only energy but also different types of information. Interestingly, these light-sensitive molecules on the organism's surface, so basic to the animal's survival, are structurally very similar to light-sensitive molecules in the human retina, called rhodopsin, which suggests our eyes evolved from them.

These same extraordinary sensitivities to color exist within the individual cells and proteins in our own bodies. In 1979 Moscow University scientists Karel Martinek and Ilya Berezin showed that our bodies are filled with numerous light-sensitive chemical switches and amplifiers. Different colors or wavelengths of light have different effects. Some colors stimulate bodily enzymes to work more effectively and can turn processes in our cells on and off and affect which chemicals they produce. As well, Albert Szent-Györgyi, who won the Nobel Prize for discovering vitamin C, also discovered that when an electron is transferred from one molecule to another within our bodies—a process called charge transfer—the molecules often change color, which is to say, they change the type of light they emit. (This process goes very far in fireflies, in which the enzyme luciferase generates large quantities of visible light.) Thus human encounters with light are more than skin-deep, and our bodies are not darkened caverns; within cells, photons flash, and energy is transferred, giving rise to colorful cascades of change. The question was, had anyone, to use Florence Nightingale's beautiful metaphor, found a way not only to "paint" the surface of the head with light and color but to use it to "sculpt" the circuitry of the brain?

The Lecture and a Chance Encounter

On a Thursday in December 2011, I finished seeing my patients at 7:15 and counted the few small steps to the Ontario Medical Association offices. I had a very specific agenda. I already knew that when there is damaged tissue in the brain, it is often possible to stimulate remaining healthy tissue with mental experience—be it mental exercise, movement, or sensing the world—to reorganize itself and form new connections, and sometimes even to grow new neurons to take over the lost cognitive functions of the damaged tissue. But the limiting factor is that there has to be *some* healthy tissue to take over from the damaged tissue. I wanted to explore whether light therapy might help to heal brain tissue that was still "sick" in some way. Could it help heal the general cellular function of the neurons? If this was possible, then light would provide a new way to heal brain problems. After the brain cells were normalized, the neurons could be trained to rewire themselves to take over lost mental functions.

As a colleague and I took our dinner from the buffet, sat down, and started to chat with fellow physicians, I saw, across the room, a slim woman with dark hair, Mediterranean features and skin color, glasses, and an intelligent face; she was making careful movements and looking frail. She approached me, deliberately, and began speaking, slowly. She told me I looked familiar, but she was not sure from where, and that she was really bothered that she couldn't figure it out. But before we could sort it out, she said, "I am Gabrielle Pollard." Then I introduced myself. She did not recognize my name, nor I hers.

I was beginning to suspect, from her careful walk—guarded and unsteady—and her slightly slowed speech that she might be struggling with a brain injury. Perhaps she had come to the lecture for very personal reasons. And then the lecture began.

The first speaker was Fred Kahn, a general and vascular surgeon. Slim and fit, Kahn had a white shock of hair that swept across his forehead. Though he appeared to be in his midseventies, he was eighty-two and still worked sixty-plus hours a week. He looked as if he got his share of sun—especially compared with the audience members, who were mostly younger, pale-faced, skin-cancer-wary heliophobes who knew the sun could be dangerous but had forgotten that human life could not have evolved without its rays. Kahn made a point of getting four hours of healthy sun during the week, and more on weekends. He swam four times a week and went for long walks in the fresh air. He wore casual attire, but he looked as though he would have been more comfortable in scrubs than dress clothes and couldn't stand the feeling of a necktie. He had the mild, flat, dry, matter-of-fact drawl of someone raised in rural Ontario, into which he packed his story, his irony, and a few deadpan asides.

Kahn, as I was to learn later, had been born in Germany in 1929 into a Jewish family. He had lived through Kristallnacht, November 9–10, 1938, when the Nazis set nearly all of Germany's synagogues on fire and put thirty thousand Jews in concentration camps. Three weeks before World War II broke out, his family made a daring nighttime escape by car and train, bribing German officials to cross into Holland, leaving all their possessions behind. The Kahns ultimately moved to Uxbridge, Ontario, becoming farmers. Fred was raised on a farm and went to a little red schoolhouse, trudging six miles in the snow each winter day to get himself there and back. As a boy, he worked for hours in the summer sun with his shirt off. He started driving a Fordson tractor, quite illegally, when he was ten, and he developed a farmer's virtues, becoming ever mindful of nature, its dictates, majesty, harshness, and power.

He won a scholarship to medical school at the University of Toronto. When he graduated, unimpressed with the drugs that internists prescribed, he became a general surgeon and ultimately chief surgeon at a huge mining operation in northern Ontario. With his extraordinary energy, he replaced four other surgeons at the mining hospital and ran two operating rooms around the clock. He went to Massachusetts General Hospital to study vascular surgery, then to Texas to study at Baylor with one of the finest surgeons in the world, Denton Cooley, who performed one of the first heart transplants. In California he practiced vascular and general surgery, operating on abdominal aneurysms, doing bypass procedures, and clearing clogged carotid arteries. He was a consulting surgeon to the U.S. military. As lead physician he went on to establish a 250-bed hospital, becoming chief of staff and then chair of the department of surgery. In those years, he performed over twenty thousand major surgical procedures.

"I GOT INTO LASERS, OVER twenty years ago," he told us, beginning his lecture, "because I was an avid skier and had damaged my shoulder, and it had become a chronic problem." He had skied the great mountains, including the Alps, and got a serious rotator cuff injury. For two years it had been difficult to do any physical activity, let alone ski. Steroid injections didn't help. "My surgeons said, 'You are going to need surgery on that shoulder.' And I thought, 'I am a surgeon. And I *know* what they are going to do to that shoulder, how they are going to cut it up, and I know the likely poor results. No thanks.'" So he suffered, until one day a chiropractor he knew said to him, "Why don't you try my Russian laser?"

The chiropractor had an old Russian machine. It was 1986, and the Cold War was still on, but a few of these simple contraptions had made their way to the West. So Kahn let the man use the equipment on him, and in five sessions the shoulder that had been aching and stiff for two years was cured. The laser was a low-intensity laser, not the "hot" high-intensity kind that can burn through flesh.

Kahn was intrigued. When he reviewed the scientific literature, he found that these low-intensity laser treatments worked by helping the body marshal its own energy and its own cellular resources to heal itself, with no side effects. Lasers, it seemed, could treat a number of conditions that nothing else could and could decrease the need for medication or surgery. He was so intrigued that even though he was at the top of his game as a surgeon, he gave it all up to study lights.

Low-intensity laser therapy—largely unknown to mainstream practitioners—is based on a scientific literature of more than three thousand publications and more than two hundred clinical trials with positive results. Most of the early studies were done in Russia or in eastern Europe—countries closer to China, Tibet, and India. Because the East was generally more interested in the role of energy in medicine, the earlier studies remained relatively unknown in the West.

Much of Kahn's lecture that night in 2011 was about the science of light and how lasers work to stimulate healing at a cellular level. He explained the difference between the two kinds of lasers. Lasers that burn are high-intensity lasers (or hot or thermal lasers). They can destroy flesh and are used in surgery to cut away diseased tissue. Low-intensity lasers (also called soft lasers, or cold lasers, or low-level lasers)—the only ones Kahn used—promote healing. They give off little or no heat and work by producing changes in cells, mostly by helping sick cells to energize and heal themselves.

Normal light energy is one part of the huge electromagnetic spectrum, which includes many kinds of waves, each with different wavelengths—including radio waves, X-rays, microwaves—most of which we cannot see with the naked eye. But we can see wavelengths of 400 to 700 nanometers. (A nanometer is one billionth of a meter.) Visible light, from one end of the spectrum to the other, consists of violet (400 nanometers), which contains the most energy, then indigo, blue, green, yellow, orange, and finally red (700 nanometers), which has the least energy. Natural light is a mixture of all these wavelengths. The frequency most often used for laser healing is red light, at a wavelength of 660 nanometers. But infrared light is also used typically at highly specific wavelengths of 840 or 830 nanometers; they can't be seen with the naked eye because they fall outside the visible range. (The idea of "invisible light" may seem counterintuitive, but it, too, is light and consists of photons and light energy. Night-vision goggles, used by special forces to "see" in the dark, collect infrared light, which humans normally cannot see, and amplify it.)

A unique characteristic of lasers is that they can produce light of unrivaled purity, meaning a wavelength accurate to a single nanometer. Lasers are thus said to be monochromatic, of a single color. A laser can produce a light beam that is, for example, 660 nanometers, or 661, or 662, and so on. With low-intensity lasers, precision is key, because sometimes a particular wavelength will help tissue heal, but a slightly different wavelength will not.

Another characteristic of lasers is that they can direct their beam in a single direction, and their light energy can be concentrated in that narrow beam. Most light sources, such as incandescent bulbs or the sun (natural light), produce light that disperses over distance.

A further characteristic is the intensity of laser light. A 100-watt lightbulb, seen from thirty centimeters away, will shed only a thousandth of a watt of energy on your eye. But a one-watt laser is thousands of times more intense than a 100-watt bulb. These characteristics give lasers their focus, compared with natural light (which is why we say someone has a "laserlike focus"). A laser pointer can produce a pencil-thin beam that remains concentrated when it falls on its distant target. Such lasers can be aimed by astronomers at the heavens to pinpoint stars.

When the theoretical portion of his presentation was over, Kahn showed his before-and-after slides, and almost everyone was astonished.

His slides showed people with wounds so serious that the skin was unable to close over them, and bones and muscle were sticking out. Many of these patients had remained with open festering wounds for over a year, and all known treatments had failed. Some had been told by their doctors that their limbs would have to be amputated. However, after a few laser treatments, the body started healing those wounds, and over the following weeks, the wounds closed. Kahn showed slides of people with incurable diabetic ulcers, open gashes from car accidents, terrible herpes infections, shingles, horrendous burns, disfiguring psoriasis, appallingly severe eczema—which would not heal with standard medical treatment but were healed with laser light. Unsightly scars called keloids could also be improved, as could the normal sagging wrinkles of aging, because lasers trigger the development of collagen tissue.

Other slides showed black, gangrenous limbs, dying from severe atherosclerosis (poor blood supply) or frostbite, that were saved from amputation with lasers—they had returned to a healthy plump pink. As a vascular surgeon, Kahn had frequently been called upon to try to rescue gangrenous or infected limbs, and wounds that wouldn't heal by transplanting blood vessels from one part of the body to the dying limb. Now he rescued them with light. All these problems had occurred because these patients' bodies were unable to supply their damaged tissues with blood. As a vascular surgeon, he knew good circulation is always necessary for the body to heal itself. But improving circulation is only one of many ways lasers help.

He showed slides of conditions that had been unexpectedly healed by light: torn hamstrings, ripped Achilles tendons, and even degenerative osteoarthritis, which occurs when cartilage wears away. Cartilage acts like a pillow between our joints, but as osteoarthritis develops, the cartilage disappears, leaving bone scraping on bone and causing tremendous inflammation and pain. For decades, medical schools have taught that once cartilage is lost, it can't be replaced, so conventional treatment for osteoarthritis is to give patients painkillers, which are often addictive, and anti-inflammatory drugs, which have significant adverse effects over the long term.* And for osteoarthritis they must be given long term, because they alleviate symptoms but don't cure the disease.

Yet here were pictures of patients whose cartilage had been regenerated by laser therapy. Kahn cited reliable studies showing that lasers trigger regrowth of normal cartilage in animals with osteoarthritis and also increase the number of cartilage-producing cells. Low-level lasers have also recently been shown, in several randomized, controlled studies, to be effective in treating osteoarthritis in humans.

Kahn also showed cases of people with rheumatoid arthritis, including the severe juvenile form, who got better with lasers. A seventeen-year-old girl who had juvenile rheumatoid arthritis since age thirteen made major improvements. In twenty-eight treatments her unusable, deformed, sausagelike fingers, which she couldn't close, re-formed themselves into normal hands that she could use. Astonishingly, people with herniated discs, when treated with lasers, were healed, the body somehow restoring those discs. Lasers helped various pain syndromes and fibromyalgia. People whose immune systems were so suppressed that their feet had been infested with warts and looked like stubs of cauliflower were healed. All sorts of sports injuries to knees, hips, and shoulders, as well as repetitive strain injuries, responded. Patients were able to avoid knee and hip joint surgery. And in passing, Kahn said that there were now positive results in the treatment of traumatic brain injury, some psychiatric disorders, and nerve injuries.

During the lecture Gabrielle, who was sitting behind me, fidgeted and got up and left several times. She had difficulty holding up her head and seemed overwhelmed by the sounds, the flashing slides of open

---

*In the United States, more than 16,500 people die each year from these drugs, which cause gastrointestinal bleeding—more than die from AIDS. M. M. Wolfe et al., "Gastrointestinal Toxicity of Nonsteroidal Anti-Inflammatory Drugs," *New England Journal of Medicine* 340, no. 24 (1999): 1889.

wounds. As I was soon to learn, she was not a physician and so was not desensitized to them.

THE SECOND SPEAKER, ANITA SALTMARCHE, focused specifically on studies of light therapy used for traumatic brain injury, stroke, and depression. Saltmarche is a registered nurse with a research background and became active in light therapy while working with an Ontario laser company. She got interested in the use of light for the brain when a chiropractor, who had attended her full-day training session, called to consult her on a laser case. The chiropractor was working on a professor, a woman with a Mensa-level IQ, who seven years before had been in a car accident. While she was stopped at a red light, she had been rear-ended by a vehicle going fifty-five miles an hour. Her knee smashed up against the dash, leaving her with arthritis. Her head had lurched forward and back, giving her whiplash and a traumatic brain injury.

Her brain injury symptoms were typical and disabling. She could no longer concentrate or sleep. If she spent more than twenty minutes on the computer, she would be exhausted and unable to focus. She couldn't complete tasks, to the point that she had to quit her job. When she tried to speak, the right words wouldn't come to her, and she lost her ability to speak two foreign languages. She developed angry outbursts and felt deep anguish at all she had lost. After her second attempt at conventional neurorehabilitation failed to improve her functioning, she attempted suicide.

She actually went to the chiropractor for laser treatment of her arthritic knee and was quickly helped. Then she asked whether the light, which had so helped her knee, might also be used on her head.

The chiropractor, before proceeding, asked Saltmarche for her opinion about the safety of shining the lights on the woman's head. "There was an almost forty-year history of low-level laser therapy being safe and having no significant side effects," said Saltmarche, so she thought it would be safe. Knowing which brain areas were involved in the woman's cognitive deficits, Saltmarche suggested eight areas on her head on which to focus the lights. The lights used were not lasers proper but LED lights, in the red and infrared range, which have some laserlike properties.

After the woman received her first treatment, she slept eighteen hours—her first sound sleep since the accident. Then she began improving significantly. She was able to work again, to spend hours on her computer, and even to start her own company. Her foreign languages began to come back. Her depression lifted—though she was still easily frustrated when she tried to multitask, the only area that was still challenging. She also found she had to continue treatment to maintain her improvements, and when she stopped (as she did when she had a terrible flu one time, and a fall another time), her symptoms returned. "Interestingly," said Saltmarche, "when she started her treatments back up again after the 'light holiday,' she improved from her previous level." Her physicians acknowledged her improvement, but couldn't believe light therapy was responsible.

Saltmarche told us she was now involved in a study conducted by Dr. Margaret Naeser and colleagues from Harvard, MIT, and Boston University, including Harvard professor Michael Hamblin, a world leader in understanding how light therapy works at the cellular level. Hamblin, at Massachusetts General Hospital's Wellman Center for Photomedicine, specializes in the use of light to activate the immune system in treating cancer and cardiac disease; he was now branching out into its use for brain injuries. Building on lab work that applied laser therapy to the top of the head (transcranial laser therapy), the Boston group had studied its use in traumatic brain injury and found laser treatment helpful. Naeser, a research professor at the Boston University School of Medicine, had done studies using lasers for stroke and paralysis and was one of several pioneers using "laser acupuncture" by placing light on acupuncture points.

For thousands of years, the Chinese have argued that the body has energy channels, called meridians, that give access to the internal organs, and that these channels have access points on the surface of the body, called acupuncture points because they are traditionally stimulated with acupuncture needles. The ancient Chinese knew these points also responded to pressure or heat. In recent years it was discovered that electricity and even laser light could achieve the desired influence on the meridians through the acupuncture points. The lasers harmlessly and painlessly pass light energy into these channels. Naeser was intrigued to learn that in China, acupuncture was routinely used to treat strokes. So she did a complete training in acupuncture and in 1985 went to China, where she saw lasers being used, instead of needles, to treat paralysis in stroke patients. On her return to the United States, she did a study that showed that patients paralyzed by stroke made significant improvements in their movement when lasers were used to stimulate acupuncture points on the face and other areas—if less than 50 percent of the brain's movement pathways were found to be destroyed on a brain scan.

One person treated by the Boston group was a high-ranking female military officer on medical disability who had suffered multiple head concussions in the military and from rugby and skydiving accidents. A magnetic resonance imaging (MRI) brain scan showed that part of her brain had actually shrunk from the brain damage. After four months of light treatment, she was able to go off disability and to function—so long as she continued to get light treatment. If she went off it, she regressed. Saltmarche was now participating in a larger U.S. study, with the Boston group, in which both brain injury and stroke patients were recovering lost cognitive functions, sleeping better, and getting control of their feelings, which had often become intense and unpredictable after brain injuries.

Gabrielle Tells Her Story

At the end of the lecture, Gabrielle went over and spoke to Anita Saltmarche, told her about her neurological and cognitive difficulties, and said she'd be pleased to offer herself as a Canadian subject for the U.S. study. Saltmarche said she would look into it.

I lined up to ask Kahn what kind of brain problems he'd used lasers for—since he hadn't given details. While I was waiting in the line, Gabrielle came over to me with an elderly gentleman, whom she introduced as her father, Dr. Pollard; he was bespectacled, with a delicate, distinguished English accent. As a young man, he had studied medicine at Cambridge on a scholarship. He was now eighty-one years old, a year younger than Kahn.

Dr. Pollard said he recognized me as the author of the book Gabrielle had been reading since 2007—for the last four years—and she realized she knew my face from the jacket flap that she used to hold her place. "Normally, I have a very good memory for faces," she said wistfully. Then she told me the story of how she had lost so many of her mental faculties.

Gabrielle, divorced and living alone, had supported herself with her own successful tutoring business, helping children who suffered from learning disabilities. Music was central to her life, and she sang in a choir. In 2000 she began to experience hearing loss and was sent for a CT scan of her brain, followed by an MRI. Both revealed an abnormal structure in her brain, toward the back, but her doctors weren't certain what it was. They decided not to operate but to observe the abnormality with repeated MRI scans. Gabrielle was thirty-five years old.

In 2009 the lesion was diagnosed as a brain tumor—most likely benign. But benign tumors can grow, and depending upon where they are, they can kill. The tumor extended from inside her skull out through the hole at the bottom of the skull that contains the spinal cord. That hole is small, and as the tumor grew, it compressed all the neural structures that passed through it. Her tumor grew in such a way that her spinal cord, to accommodate its presence, had to partially wrap around it, and her cerebellum, a part of the brain involved in fine-tuning movements and thoughts, was gradually being compressed. Her brain stem, the lowest part of the brain, which sits just above the spinal cord, was also being compressed and moved to the right. The tumor was diagnosed as a choroid plexus papilloma, meaning it was made of the same kinds of cells that produce the cerebrospinal fluid in the brain.

She would require extremely delicate, challenging brain surgery, in a very small area where most nerves are crucial to survival. "By the time I got to the neurosurgeon," Gabrielle told me, "I already knew I could die as a result of my surgery." She was told she could lose her hearing on one side, and "that after the surgery I could develop trouble swallowing, might not be able to eat or drink for the rest of my life, might have trouble talking, or walking, or have a stroke." She recalled her surgeon telling her, "There is a three to five percent chance you will be really mad I did your surgery." When she asked what would happen if she didn't go through with it, she recalls him saying that the chances of her being mad at him would rise to "one hundred percent." The expanding tumor would eventually strangle her breathing centers, and she would die. But the surgeon also told her that after surgery, she would likely feel better than she had in ten years.

She had the surgery in November 2009, and it saved her life. The tumor was cut out, and it was indeed benign. She was delighted to have sensation in all her limbs. But she soon noticed trouble swallowing and eating and was constantly nauseous. She now had balance problems and difficulty walking. Over a year and a half later "I was still in rehabilitation, couldn't hold my head up, and was throwing up." She slurred her words and had problems pacing her speech and producing a normal volume, so that people could "barely hear me speak." But "the most terrifying experience was losing my mental functioning—my cognitive abilities and memory. I would picture something, but couldn't get the word for it. If I headed for the word *fork,* it came out, in speech, as *knife,* and I knew it wasn't right. And I couldn't multitask anymore."

She had lost her short-term memory. She would put something down for a second and wouldn't be able to find it. Sometimes what she couldn't find was in her hand, and she'd forgotten she'd picked it up. If she took off her glasses and put them aside, it could take two hours to find them in her fifteen-hundred-square-foot condominium. When anyone spoke to her, she had to ask them to repeat their words several times because she'd forget them almost immediately. "I couldn't recognize objects," she said, "and I could see only what was directly in front of me. My mom would take me to the supermarket. If I was looking for orange juice to make fruit salad for a friend and I saw two liters of it in front of me, I'd know that was too big. But I couldn't look to the left to see the one-liter size. I once had a pair of black sweatpants, which I kept at the edge of my musical keyboard, with something much smaller on top of them. It took me three weeks to find the sweatpants, even though they were right beside my keyboard, which I used every day. I could only see surfaces."

She had trouble with visual tracking. "I had seen written music all my life. Normally, I could sight-read. But the first time I went back to choir, it was just a page of notes, with no meaning. When I got to the end of a line, I didn't know I had to go to the line underneath."

Sound—as is often the case for people with brain injuries—posed a special problem. She was hypersensitive to all sounds, which now seemed unbearably loud. Shopping malls with piped-in music, cacophony, and buzz drove her crazy. Music, which had been her chief joy—she sang every day—was now unbearable: "It had no tonality or pleasure. It was more like noise than notes." She couldn't participate in any group where more than one person spoke at a time. Her balance was so bad that she had to run her hand along the wall to walk.

And she was chronically exhausted.

"I AM A VERY STRONG person," Gabrielle told me. "I have had a lot of difficult life experiences that led me to this point, I was always a religious person, and I had always felt I was not alone, and whatever the difficulty, I felt there would be a gift of the same magnitude."

She began to focus on learning from her experiences, hoping they would not go to waste, so at the very least others might be helped. She studied her mental fatigue, the energy component of her condition. "After the surgery I felt that the energy had been sucked from every cell in my body," she said. "This lasted ten months." After doing the slightest activity, she would have to rest, sometimes for days. She had no reserves.

"I have always thought of my brain as where my thoughts were. I never thought of it as a physical organ, in charge of everything I do. So I didn't realize that I only had one energy for both my brain and my body, and if I used energy for an intellectual activity, I then didn't have the ability to speak, or move my legs, or to stand up.

"I knew it was time for a portable phone when I was lying down on the couch, and my phone rang, and I felt like I was on a desert island and didn't have the energy to get up, or move my limbs to go answer it. I was completely spent.

"Every time I reached a new skill level in recovery, there wouldn't be enough energy to run other things, because my energy had already gone into building and incorporating that new skill. If I had a setback, it could take two weeks to go from not moving, to doing a little bit of exercise, to adding the next level."

Now as people were leaving the lecture room, Gabrielle told me something she found quite odd. She said when she was looking at things, certain patterns had become quite unbearable. When a clinician at rehab wore a shirt with black and white stripes, "the horizontal contrast was like a visual scream for me. I asked her to put a towel over that shirt."

At this point I started to put things together in my head. Almost all of Gabrielle's current problems could be explained as the result of brain stem damage and malfunction. The brain stem processes the flow of signals from most of the cranial nerves that govern the human face and head. A cranial nerve controls the balance system and receives signals from the semicircular canals inside the ear. Damage to the brain stem areas that govern that nerve would help account for her tentative walk and her balance problems.

Her hypersensitivity to sound was also likely related to the brain stem. The ear has within it the equivalent of a zoom lens that allows us to focus on some frequencies and dampen others. People with damage to this system hear booming, buzzing confusion because they have lost control of that regulating mechanism (described in Chapter 8). Thus, Gabrielle couldn't tolerate malls, echoes, and Muzak, and preferred listening to one person at a time.

A damaged brain often cannot integrate different incoming sensations. For instance, maintaining balance involves integrating input from the semicircular canals in the ear (which signal position) with input from the eyes (which visually track horizontal lines in the environment, also, in part, a brain stem function) and with input from the soles of the feet. When those systems are out of sync because one or more of them are damaged, the person becomes confused and disoriented and has what is called a sensory integration problem.

I surmised that the "visual scream" that Gabrielle experienced while looking at the woman's striped shirt occurred both because, in her off-balance state, her brain was desperately seeking horizontal lines to orient her in space, and because her visual system, part of that damaged balance system, was also misfiring. When a sensory part of the brain is damaged, it tends to fire too easily, and we feel overloaded by the sensations.

The sensory systems consist of two kinds of neurons, those that get excited by external sensations and those inhibitory neurons that dampen sensations so that the brain is not overwhelmed and just the right amount is filtered in. (For instance, when an alarm clock goes off, the brain is very stimulated, because the excitatory neurons fire. But should the stimulation become too intense, it is good to have inhibitory neurons to "lower the volume" so that the person is not overstimulated.) When the inhibitory neurons are damaged, the patient experiences sensory overload, and sometimes sensation actually hurts. When I told Gabrielle about these sensory integration problems, she said, "Oh wow," explaining that it was a relief to learn that all her symptoms fit together and were part of a package.

As we were chatting, Gabrielle's father saw that Dr. Kahn was free and went to speak to him. Gabrielle's father knew that for the two years since her surgery, she had also suffered from a chronic postoperative infection called folliculitis—an inflammation of hair follicles on the back. Neither antibiotics nor other medical measures had worked. Since Kahn had had so much experience treating skin problems, Dr. Pollard, at her request, told Dr. Kahn about Gabrielle's folliculitis. "Might the laser light help it heal?" Dr. Pollard asked. Kahn assured him it would. "Stop by anytime," he said.

AS WE WALKED OUT, Dr. Pollard offered me a lift home, with Gabrielle—their car was parked just past my office. The brief distance that I had skipped across so lightly and quickly an hour and a half before was now traversed, in reverse, with slow labored steps, as Gabrielle struggled to walk. We slowed to her pace. We reached the car, and in the few minutes' ride to my home, we discussed how impressed we were by the lectures. I thought light therapy might succeed for Gabrielle, because her surgery might well have cut through tissue and caused scarring and inflammation in the surrounding areas. I suspected that she was suffering from a noisy brain and learned nonuse, and that not all the neurons in her brain-stem-related circuits were in fact dead; some might be damaged and firing pathological signals, while others were dormant. If the lasers could heal the inflammation and provide better circulation and more energy to those cells, she—like those who had traumatic brain injuries—might benefit. We agreed to stay in touch.

Visits to Kahn's Clinic

In the weeks that followed, I frequently visited Kahn's clinic and research laboratory, to see how lasers worked, talk with staff, try the equipment myself, and then train to use it. Kahn's clinic, called Meditech, had a staff of forty-five people, mostly clinicians, and also a laboratory that designed the lasers. The ultimate goal of my visits was to see how lasers might influence the brain, but first I wanted to understand how lasers worked and see what serious laser treatments could do for common bodily afflictions.

Kahn told me that after the lights cured his shoulder, he reviewed all the scientific literature on lasers. He had been confused by all the many different light protocols—the different wavelengths, frequencies of treatment, and doses of light that various clinicians or companies were using for different conditions. He then spent time with the Russian scientist Tiina Karu, head of the Laboratory of Laser Biology and Medicine, at the Institute on Laser and Informatic Technologies, Russian Academy of Sciences. Karu is one of the world's leading experts on how lasers heal tissue. In 1989, following his time with Karu, he worked with engineers at Ryerson Polytechnical Institute in Toronto to develop an adjustable laser called the BioFlex Laser Therapy System that could produce an infinite number of light protocols and be used for both basic and clinical research. Kahn then spent years trying to determine which types of light would benefit different patients, given their skin color, age, body fat composition, and kind of illness, and he developed numerous protocols for use with the equipment he developed.

Physics of Lasers

Laser stands for Light Amplification by Stimulated Emission of Radiation. Since the 1600s, light has often been understood to behave like a continuous wave—traveling through space the way waves travel through water. (This is why scientists speak of "wavelengths" of light.) But Albert Einstein showed that light could also be understood as behaving like a particle, which ultimately came to be called a photon. A photon is like a small package of light, smaller than even an atom.

Two key concepts explain how lasers are produced from photons. The first, familiar from high school physics, comes out of the model of the atom that the physicist Niels Bohr proposed. Simply put, every atom consists of a nucleus, with electrons that orbit around it, at different distances from the nucleus. If an electron is in a close orbit to the nucleus, it has a low amount of energy; if it is farther away from the nucleus, it has a higher amount of energy. (These high-energy electrons are said to be in an "excited" state.) Thus each electron orbit is associated with a different energy state.

In most atoms, most of the time, the population of electrons in low-energy inner orbits (close to the nucleus) is larger than the population of excited electrons in the high-energy outer orbits (farther away from the nucleus). Whenever an electron falls from the high-energy orbit to a lower-energy orbit, a photon of light is given off, called a spontaneous emission of light radiation. This spontaneous emission occurs randomly in normal light (for instance, within a typical electric lightbulb).

But by bombarding atoms with an outside energy source, such as an electrical current or a beam of light, we can create atoms where more of the electrons are in the excited high-energy state. Now the population of electrons in the excited state is higher than the population of electrons in the resting state in the low-energy orbit. This so-called population inversion is the first key concept for understanding lasers.

The second key concept is stimulation. In lasers, atoms are artificially stimulated—*bombarded* is a better word—by an outside energy source, to bring about population inversion.

Normally, when atoms are bombarded with energy, they release photons. Bombarding atoms where population inversion has occurred, as happens in lasers, leads to a large release of photons. These photons, in turn, stimulate other nearby atoms to release more photons still, so that a cascade of photons is released. A way to enhance this process is to surround the photon-emitting atoms with mirrors, so that once emitted, the photons hit the mirrors and bounce back into the atoms with population inversion, hitting still more atoms and stimulating them to emit even more photons. Hence the name Light Amplification by Stimulated Emission of Radiation.

There are many ways to make lasers. If you look inside a small laser pointer of the kind used by lecturers (or inside your computer's CD reader), you will find an energy pump, in the form of batteries or an electrical source, that supplies a pulse of electricity for stimulation. You will also find a small laser diode, which is where the population inversion occurs. A typical laser diode consists of a sandwich of two solid materials that partially conduct electricity. They are called semiconductors for that reason.

There is a small space between the two semiconductors. One semiconductor is made of a material that has a relative surplus of electrons; the other is made of a material that has a relative deficit of electrons. Population inversion is created in this sandwich. When electromagnetism of a particular frequency is passed through these semiconductors to stimulate them, it triggers the cascade of light amplification. Mirrors in the space between the two semiconductors capture those photons and augment the cascade of light, which can then be projected in the form of a laser light beam. The exact frequency of light emitted can be controlled by adjusting the frequency of the energy pumped into the system.

The first laser—developed by Theodore H. Maiman at the Hughes Research Laboratories in Malibu, California, in 1960—was a hot laser. Within a year, hot lasers capable of burning tissue were being used in surgery in place of scalpels, and by 1963 they were being used to destroy tumors in laboratory animals. Lasers became widely known when the movie *Goldfinger* (1964) had a scene in which James Bond was strapped to a table, legs splayed apart, while a hot laser, looking like an oversized, glowing syringe and emitting a thin, focused red light, threatened to cut him in two:

> GOLDFINGER (*not overly impressed by Bond's special high-tech car*): I too have a new toy. . . . You are looking at an industrial laser, which emits an extraordinary light, not to be found in nature. It can project a spot on the moon. Or at closer range, cut through solid metal. I will show you. . . .
> BOND: Do you expect me to talk?
> GOLDFINGER (*jubilant*): No, Mr. Bond, I expect you to die.

How Lasers Heal Tissue

By 1965 it was known that low-intensity lasers could heal. Shirley A. Carney, working in Birmingham, England, showed that low-intensity lasers could promote the growth of collagen fibers in skin tissues. Collagen is a protein that makes up our connective tissue, helps give it form, and is necessary for healing. In 1968 Dr. Endre Mester, in Budapest, showed that lasers could stimulate skin growth in rats, and a year later that lasers could radically improve the healing of wounds. By the mid-1970s, the USSR had opened four large-scale research and clinical facilities to use lasers to stimulate living tissues, a technique that, by the 1980s, was common in the Communist bloc, though rare in the West.

Not until the end of the Cold War did medical lasers become more common in the West, and not until 2002 did the FDA approve the first low-intensity laser therapy device in the United States.

WHEN PHOTONS ENCOUNTER MATTER, ONE of four things can happen. They can be reflected away from the matter, they can pass through it, they can enter it but scatter within, or they can be absorbed without dispersing a great deal. When photons are absorbed by living tissue, they trigger chemical reactions in the light-sensitive molecules within. Different molecules absorb different wavelengths of light. For instance, red blood cells absorb all the nonred wavelengths, leaving the red ones visible. In plants, green chlorophyll absorbs all the wavelengths except green.

Human beings tend to think that light-sensitive molecules exist only in the eyes, but they come in four major types: rhodopsin (in the retina, which absorbs light for vision), hemoglobin (in red blood cells), myoglobin (in muscle), and most important of all, cytochrome (in all the cells). Cytochrome is the marvel that explains how lasers can heal so many different conditions, because it converts light energy from the sun into energy for the cells. Most of the photons are absorbed by the energy powerhouses within the cells, the mitochondria.

Amazingly, our mitochondria capture energy originating 93 million miles away—the energy of the sun—and liberate it for our cells to use. Surrounded by a thin membrane, the mitochondria are stuffed with light-sensitive cytochrome. As the sun's photons pass through the membrane and come in contact with the cytochrome, they are absorbed and stimulate the creation of a molecule that stores energy in our cells. That molecule, called ATP (adenosine triphosphate), is like an all-purpose battery, providing energy for the cell's work. ATP can also provide energy that can be used by the immune system and for cell repair.

Laser light triggers ATP production, which is why it can initiate and accelerate the repair and growth of healthy new cells, including those that make up cartilage (chondrocytes), bone (osteocytes), and connective tissue (fibroblasts).

Lasers of slightly different wavelengths can also increase the use of oxygen, improve blood circulation, and stimulate the growth of new blood vessels, bringing more oxygen and nutrients to the tissues—especially important for healing.

Kahn uses four different methods to get light into the cytochrome molecules. The first is red light, generated by 180 light-emitting diodes (LEDs), laid out in rows, mounted on a soft plastic band the size of an envelope. Typically, the therapist will cover a body surface with red light for about twenty-five minutes. This red light penetrates one to two centimeters into the body and is always used first, to prepare the tissue for deeper healing, and to help improve circulation.

Next Kahn uses an infrared band of LEDs for about twenty-five minutes. Its light penetrates about five centimeters into the body, spreading the healing light deeper still.

LED lights have laserlike properties, but they are not lasers, and thus you can look directly at them with no ill effects.

Then Kahn uses the pure beam of lasers, beginning with a red laser probe, followed by an infrared laser probe.* A laser probe can deliver much more power than LEDs, in a focused beam that goes very deep. By the time the laser probe is applied, the superficial tissues have already been saturated with so many photons from the red and infrared LEDs that the laser creates a cascade of photons in the tissues, reaching as deep as twenty-two centimeters into the body. The laser probe is applied for a short time, in various spots. A total treatment with the probe darting over many points may last about seven minutes. As is not the case with LEDs, looking directly at the laser light from a probe can be dangerous, and patients and clinicians wear special glasses when using them. The energy of a "dose" of light depends on two things—the number of photons the light source gives off, and the wavelength or color of those photons. As Einstein showed, the color of a light is a measure of how much energy it contains.

In the immune system, laser light can trigger helpful forms of inflammation—but only where required. Where inflammatory processes have become stuck and "chronic," as happens with many diseases, laser light can unblock the stalled process and quickly move it to a normal resolution, leading to decreased inflammation, swelling, and pain.

So many modern diseases, including heart disease, depression, cancer, Alzheimer's, and all the autoimmune diseases (such as rheumatoid arthritis and lupus), occur in part because our body's immune systems produce excess chronic inflammation. In chronic inflammation, the immune system stays on too long and may even begin to attack the body's own tissues, as though they were outside invaders. The causes of chronic inflammation are many, including diet and, of course, the

---

* The LED red lights are 660 nanometers; the LED infrared lights are 840 nanometers; the red laser probe is 660 nanometers; the infrared laser probe is 840 nanometers.

countless chemical toxins that become embedded in the body. Chronically inflamed bodies produce chemicals, called pro-inflammatory cytokines, which contribute to pain and inflammation.

Fortunately, laser light fights excess inflammation by increasing the anti-inflammatory cytokines that bring chronic inflammation to an end. They lower the number of "neutrophil" cells that can contribute to chronic inflammation, and they increase the number of "macrophage" cells in the immune system, the garbage collectors that remove foreign invaders and damaged cells.

Lasers also decrease a stress on the tissues caused by oxygen. The body constantly makes use of oxygen, producing molecules called free radicals that are highly active and interact with other molecules. When they are in oversupply, they cause damage to cells and can bring on degenerative diseases. Another unique aspect of lasers is that they preferentially affect damaged cells, or cells that are struggling to function and need energy the most. Cells that are chronically inflamed, or that have only a limited blood supply and oxygen due to poor circulation, or that are multiplying (as happens when tissues are trying to heal themselves) are more sensitive to red and near-infrared low-intensity lasers than are well-functioning cells. For instance, a skin wound is more sensitive to low-intensity lasers than is normal tissue. In other words, lasers have a good effect where they are most needed.

To heal, the body often needs to make new cells. The first step in cell reproduction occurs when DNA replicates itself. Laser light can activate DNA (and RNA) synthesis in cells. Human cells in a petri dish will synthesize more DNA and grow in response to specific wavelengths of light. *E. coli,* a very simple form of bacteria, responds to some but not all of those. Yeasts respond and grow to still other wavelengths. There is thus a whole language of light energy, in which the specific wavelengths are the words, to which living cells respond.

But how might lasers influence the brain? Even normal sunlight affects the brain's chemicals. Serotonin, a brain neurotransmitter, is known to be low in some depressions; studies show that normal sunlight causes the body to release serotonin, which is one reason people living far from the equator feel rejuvenated and in a good mood on sunny holidays. Laser light also releases serotonin, as well as other important brain chemicals, such as endorphins, which lower pain, and acetylcholine, which is essential for learning—and which might help an injured brain relearn mental abilities that have been lost. Kahn, Naeser, and the Harvard group believe that laser light affects the cerebrospinal fluid as well. Kahn believes that the cerebral spinal fluid and the blood vessels carry the photons into the brain, where they influence the brain cells, as they might other cells. The scientific research on this pathway is in its infancy.

To fully appreciate Kahn's clinical work, I had to overcome a prejudice.

It is not difficult now to make a simple, inexpensive, "one size fits all" laser. Chiropractors and other health professionals will often use small lasers for a few minutes in their offices after a chiropractic correction, almost as an afterthought. I had tried such procedures myself and been unimpressed. I told Kahn this, and he was not surprised: "These short application times are not nearly long enough for lasers to heal anything."

Kahn's lasers are different from most small handhelds. Some of his devices cost tens of thousands of dollars and are attached to sophisticated computers. His staff members are constantly hovering over patients, changing their settings and varying their treatments.

In his twenty years of work, Kahn and his staff have observed the effects of almost a million laser treatments to determine which protocols work best for which conditions and for which kind of patient. Kahn himself still sees 95 percent of patients who come to his clinic and follows up on them. A patient's skin color, age, and amount of fat and muscle all affect how much light is absorbed. As a patient responds, the practitioner adjusts the frequency of the light pulse, waveform, and the dose of energy (number of photons passed to each centimeter of tissue over time). As Michael Hamblin observes, "There is an optimal dose of light for any particular application, and doses higher or lower than this optimal value may have no therapeutic effect." Sometimes, however, "lower doses are actually more beneficial than higher doses."

...

I FIRST GOT TO KNOW what Kahn's lasers could do by observing their effects on the conditions they were best known for. One woman I observed had a rotator cuff injury in her shoulder, usually caused by a tear to the muscle or ligament. For a year, she had had massage, chiropractic, and osteopathic help, with little benefit. After four laser sessions, her pain disappeared, and her strength and flexibility normalized.

Professor Cyril Levitt, a sixty-six-year-old anthropologist and sociologist, walked poorly because of osteoarthritis in his hips and knees, which he had had for six years, and a torn Achilles tendon. Osteoarthritis is often treated with hip or knee replacements. In four laser treatments, over the course of a week, he was pain-free in his hips and knees without medication, going up and down stairs again without discomfort; with more treatments, over a number of months his arthritis healed completely, as did his torn Achilles tendon. Several cases of sciatica, ankle problems, and chronic pain from shingles were cured. A physician who had completely ripped a shoulder tendon and was scheduled for surgery got so much better he canceled his operation. Another person, referred for chronic sinusitis, found that it improved, along with his hearing, while the ringing in his ears decreased. The improvements in all these people were permanent, so they didn't require ongoing treatment. A few people didn't get better, but they all stopped their sessions after only a few of them.

One of the neuroplasticians I described in *The Brain That Changes Itself,* Barbara Arrowsmith Young, who had healed her many learning disorders with brain exercises, also visited Kahn. As a younger woman, she had had severe endometriosis, a condition in which the cells lining the womb grow elsewhere in the body; it can cause pain and bleeding and rendered Barbara unable to have children. Multiple surgeries for it led to the development of tremendous scarring inside her abdomen, called postsurgical adhesions. The scar tissue was so extensive that she was left with continuing pain and monthly bowel obstructions, some life-threatening. Every time the surgeons went in to fix it, the scarring got worse. She suffered for decades. Finally, a test revealed that she had a genetic abnormality that caused her to form excessive scar tissue.

With all this scarring and surgery, she developed a chronic pain syndrome, with incapacitating abdominal pain, which Michael Moskowitz and Marla Golden helped to diminish. But she was still prone to severe bowel obstructions.

Knowing that low-intensity lasers can help scar tissue heal normally, I told Barbara about Dr. Kahn. After a series of treatments, her problem—which she had been told would be permanent—radically improved. Her bowel obstructions became very infrequent, only several a year, and were less dangerous, enabling her to travel, and her pain went down. Kahn has also achieved outstanding results treating endometriosis, and was able to control it in some patients so well that they were able to cancel surgery they had scheduled. I found it painful to realize that Barbara might have been spared multiple operations, infertility, and decades of living in fear of obstructions had lasers been better known.

Kahn showed me the barely visible remnants of a lesion on his own face, typical of the elderly, caused by too much sun exposure. "As a boy on the farm," he told me, "we always worked outside without shirts, hats, or sunscreen." Now he was paying the price; his dermatologist had told him that the skin lesion (called actinic keratosis) was precancerous. Typically these lesions are cut out or burned off with a hot laser. But instead of having it burned off, Kahn used the low-intensity laser, and the skin normalized itself in several sessions. Many less severe skin cancer lesions, he told me, such as some basal cell cancers, can also be healed by low-intensity laser light.

I was becoming convinced that lasers, in Kahn's and his colleagues' hands, were rapidly healing all sorts of things that should not be healed—cartilage, badly torn tendons, ligaments, and muscles.

Among the people I observed who completed treatment, the overwhelming majority got better. What might he do for brain problems? I wondered.

The Second Meeting

The next time I heard from Gabrielle was when I opened an e-mail from her on February 24. "Gaby," as she sometimes called herself, wrote that she had been busy. She had been in touch with Anita Saltmarche to set up some sessions and had become part of the Boston study. Saltmarche said the treatment would involve shining lasers over the top of her head for short periods. Gaby understood that she would need to treat herself with light for ten minutes a day for the rest of her life, starting in a few weeks. In the meantime, she had also decided to see Kahn for her folliculitis, because he had had so much experience with skin infections and wounds.

Gaby never discussed the idea of Kahn's working on her brain problems, because he had mostly shown slides of wound healing. But when he heard about her cognitive symptoms, he, as a surgeon, was quite certain they were secondary to the trauma of surgery, because no matter how meticulous a surgeon is, particularly in intracranial surgery, considerable bleeding usually occurs, resulting in scar tissue, especially in the protective layers surrounding the brain called the meninges. He also thought there was damage directly to the brain cells, leading to her symptoms.

"When I was sitting in the chair," Gaby told me, "doing the lights for folliculitis, [Fred] said, 'I can help you with the brain stuff too, I have been doing this for years.' He just shrugged his shoulders matter-of-factly as he said it. You know Fred."

Since 1993 Kahn had been treating the cervical spine, the higher part of the neck, in people with neck issues, and he noticed, unexpectedly, that when a patient also had a central nervous system or brain problem, those symptoms often improved too. He realized that the brain's cerebrospinal fluid, which flows around the spinal cord, was probably flowing back to the brain after being irradiated by the light.

Gaby asked Kahn what the treatment would involve, and he said that in the sessions when he was treating her folliculitis, he could shine another light high up on her neck, focused on her brain stem. His review of the literature had proved to him that lower doses of light, over longer periods, were effective for regenerating tissue and reducing pathological inflammation, as well as increasing the general circulation of blood in the brain—something that he, as a vascular surgeon, knew was essential to healing. The initial sessions would last longer than an hour, but he didn't think Gaby would need the lasers for life.

At the first treatment, he put the lights high on her neck and down her spine. Afterward she was exhausted, even though all she had done was sit in a chair. She needed to sleep—a typical response as the brain begins to recover. It's nothing like the exhaustion that occurs with radiation treatments for cancer, in which cells are destroyed. As I described in Chapter 3, I believe it happens because the injured brain, which has been in the sympathetic fight-or-flight response, enters the parasympathetic state; it turns off the fight-or-flight reaction, calms and neuromodulates itself, then enters the healing state of neurorelaxation.

AFTER THE SECOND TREATMENT, GABY knew her life was changed. She noticed she could concentrate longer. By the end of three weeks, she noticed memory improvements and greater energy—she was able to brush her teeth for a whole minute. Her nausea stopped. And she had strength to open the refrigerator door.

Eight weeks later she wrote me:

> I can now remember, concentrate, and multitask. I have mental clarity. I can fully rotate my head to the left and bend over. I can listen to the radio, sing, use the shredder, and go into restaurants and shopping malls. I returned to synagogue (the microphones don't bother me anymore), and I'm back doing exercises in the swimming pool. (Screaming kids, ghetto blasters, and hair dryers are no longer an issue for me.) I can walk faster than my dad on good days, and I'm a lot stronger. . . . I'm hoping . . . I will be able to drive again. . . . It's very exciting to go from any change requiring months to take hold, to having changes every two or three days. . . . I'm not counting any chickens yet, but I haven't thrown up in 2012.

Then she added a little P.S.:

> The concert: Beethoven and Your Brain: with Daniel Levitin is this Saturday night at Koerner Hall.
>   Thank you for your interest and help.

Daniel Levitin is one of the world's leading experts on how music influences the brain. He would be appearing with the conductor Edwin Outwater and the Kitchener-Waterloo Symphony Orchestra, which would play Beethoven. Levitin would explain how the music was affecting the audience's collective brain. Levitin was no disinterested academic. He had had a serious career as a musician, performing with Sting, Mel Tormé, and Blue Öyster Cult, consulting with Stevie Wonder and Steely Dan, and having been recording engineer for Santana and the Grateful Dead. Then he—like Kahn—made a big switch and became a research psychologist, investigating how music interacts with the brain. He was now head of McGill University's Laboratory for Musical Perception, Cognition and Expertise and author of *This Is Your Brain on Music*. I immediately got tickets, and because we had not met, I called his secretary in Montreal to invite him for dinner at my home that very evening, the night before the concert. She said she'd try to reach him, but he was traveling from L.A.

That evening Daniel Levitin knocked on our door while we were having dinner with friends. The conversation, well under way, was animated, about the modern German and the ancient Greek philosophers. During dessert, Levitin spied two guitars standing against the wall like two maidens hoping to be asked to dance. We spent the rest of the evening singing and playing together, songs by others, songs we had written. Not a word was said about the brain.

The next night at the concert, Levitin was *very* verbal, and he and Outwater were great witty fun together, both having a bit of the standup comic in them. Koerner Hall is built of beautiful woods that curve and sweep out from the walls and ceilings, giving the feeling that one is inside a beautiful musical instrument built to resonate.

Levitin, Outwater, and the orchestra marched through the Egmont Overture, the fourth movement of Symphony No. 9, the second movement of Eroica, and all of Symphony No. 5. While the orchestra would play the Beethoven passages, the audience used small digital devices to register in real time the specific emotions that the passage of music evoked; meanwhile a computer tallied all the results. It was fascinating how large a majority of the audience, hearing a particular passage of wordless music, would experience the same emotion, be it sadness, grief, or joyful anticipation. We all know that certain musical passages seem happy, sad, or frightening, but here was a truly lucid demonstration of how different oscillations of sound can have similar impacts upon many different brains. Levitin explained how the music—its timbre, pitch, variations, and expected and unexpected flourishes—influences the brain to lead to those emotional reactions. When the concert ended to uproarious applause, the evening wasn't over. Instead of rushing off, people mingled in the foyer overlooking the tree-lined Philosopher's Walk, listening to an exceptional Asian pianist play for everyone.

Then I saw her. I had never dreamed that Gaby, with all her problems with sound and listening to music, would have attended a Beethoven concert, because he wrote thunderous music—not what a woman who had been so damaged could tolerate. Though just the day before I had read her letter claiming she was feeling improved, I hadn't taken in the extent of her recovery. She moved quickly across the hall toward me, with an assured step. Her face was beaming, and her eyes were bright.

After introducing me to two of her friends, she said, "The last time I dared come to one of these concerts, I was so disoriented by the sound that I had to sit in my chair for about half an hour afterward. Then, when I got up"—she pointed from where we were standing, overlooking Philosopher's Walk, to the far exit, about twenty-five yards away—"it took me twenty minutes to go from here to there, and that was with people assisting me."

This woman's brain was being rewired with light.

KAHN WAS LEAST SURPRISED BY Gaby's progress. In early April, she and I met again at Kahn's clinic, and he showed me how he positioned the lights on her head, over the skull areas closest to her brain stem and cerebellum. As he placed them on her head, she lifted her hair, and I could see a five-inch-long scar behind her ear—the cut into her skull that had saved her life.

Over the next eight months, I kept in touch with Gaby. She had had her first light treatment in late December 2011 and began getting treatments twice a week. By early March 2012, she was down to once a week and declared that she had both her short- and long-term memory back, could multitask, and most important, could think clearly. Her terror of losing her mental functions was over.

She did various forms of exercise, including aqua-fitness and tai chi, an ideal exercise for a woman with balance problems.

Never passive, she was the ideal patient. The lights were healing her tissue, but she still had to relearn tasks she once could do, by engaging her neuroplasticity with repetitive training involving focused attention. What she found difficult to explain to healthy people about recovering from a brain injury was that each time she made a small step forward, she was often set back, exhausted for days, because "small steps" are not small at all. They felt as momentous to her as if she were learning each step for the very first time, because the neurons doing the activity often were doing it for the first time, since those that did it in the past had died. But once she started the lights, Gaby noticed that the setbacks were few. When the woman she was working with wore a top with alternating horizontal stripes of white and black, Gaby said, "I can tolerate it, and I didn't need her to put on anything to cover it. Still not perfect, but it isn't a visual scream anymore!"

She continued, "A week ago I got the music back!" Not only was music no longer tormenting and draining her, it was now invigorating her. "That is huge for me, because music has been so big for me . . . and I can dance!" she explained, now that she had her balance back.

"Last week I saw someone I knew from choir," she added. "He saw me when I used to move and speak like molasses. And he said, 'Oh my God you are walking!' And I said, 'It is so nice when someone notices improvement.' And he said, 'You don't understand, this isn't improvement, this is a whole other universe.'"

Proof Lasers Heal the Brain

In the past, Kahn had helped people who had brain and other nerve-related problems such as headaches from concussions, vascular dementia (dementia caused by blood vessel problems in the brain), migraines,

Bell's palsy (a paralysis of the facial nerve), and tinnitus (ringing of the ears). He emphasized he was influenced by research that had been done in Israel on light therapy and the brain.

Dr. Shimon Rochkind, a neurosurgeon at Tel Aviv University, originally pioneered work using lasers to treat injuries in the peripheral nervous system, that is, all the nerves in the body except those in the brain and spinal cord. Injury to peripheral nerves can lead to problems sensing or moving. For one hundred years, it has been known that peripheral nerves are neuroplastic and often can regrow after injury. Usually surgery is used to repair these nerves—provided it can be done within about six months of the injury. Rochkind has shown that applying low-intensity lasers to peripheral nerves can help them heal, and that the light improves nerve-cell metabolism, increases sprouting of new connections between nerves, enhances the growth of new nerve axons (which conduct electrical signals) and of myelin (the fatty covering around the nerves that allows them to send faster signals), and decreases scar tissue. Rochkind showed that in both animals and human beings, low-intensity lasers helped damaged nerves stop degenerating and start regenerating themselves. Working with an American team, he also showed that a cranial nerve could be healed.

The big question for Rochkind was: Could these wonderful changes, and new neuronal growth, also occur in the central nervous system—in the spinal cord and brain?

He next showed that some severe spinal cord injuries responded to laser therapy. The team cut the spinal cords of rats, simulating a severe spinal cord injury. They then injected spinal cord stem cells into the space between the cuts and lasered the area in the treatment group but not in the control group. The cut sections of spinal cord that were lasered regenerated, grew together, reestablished their electrical connection, and began signaling properly. In another study, he showed that lasering rat brain embryo cells led them to sprout new connections and migrate to places in the brain where they would be of use.

More breakthrough studies of this kind continue to come from Israel. Tel Aviv University zoologist Uri Oron has been studying the use of lasers to regenerate damaged brain, muscle, and heart tissue. In 2007 he and his colleagues showed that lasers can stimulate ATP production in human neural progenitor cells, which are like baby neurons, or precursors to fully developed human neurons, by aiming low-intensity lasers at human cells in a petri dish. In another experiment, Uri Oron, Amir Oron, and their colleagues from Israel and the United States tested this same laser on mice with traumatic brain injuries caused by dropping a weight on the mice's heads. The injuries were deep inside the brain. Then, four hours after the head injury, the researchers used low-intensity laser light, passing it just over the outside of the animals' heads. A control group did not get the laser treatment. Immediately after the trauma, there were no differences between the two groups, but by five days after the injury, the laser-treated mice showed far fewer neurological deficits. These advantages persisted. When, a month after the injury, the team examined the brains of the mice, the size of the injury was significantly smaller in the mice that had had light exposure.

The Orons and their Israeli and American colleagues next conducted similar experiments with rats that had had strokes. They blocked off an artery, causing a stroke, much like ones that humans suffer. Then twenty-four hours after their strokes, some of the animals had a laser laid on their heads. They had fewer neurological losses than those that weren't exposed to light. They also had more newly formed neuronal cells.

To my mind, every emergency room should have a low-intensity laser for people with stroke or head trauma. This therapy would be especially important for head injuries, because there is no effective drug therapy for traumatic brain injury. Uri Oron has also shown that low-intensity laser light can reduce scar formation in animals that have had heart attacks; perhaps lasers should be used in emergency rooms for cardiac events as well.

Eight years ago Kahn had chest pain during an incipient heart attack caused by narrowing in a coronary artery. After getting emergency room treatment, he used a low-intensity laser on his heart. His vessel narrowing disappeared on a later nuclear scan. He's now off all cardiac medication and is symptom-free. Since then, he has found that use of lasers has helped many patients with coronary artery disease, and that symptoms often disappear after six months to several years.

Using Lasers for Other Brain Problems

I visited Kahn's clinic on a regular basis to see patients who had brain problems. Often my guide was Kahn's forty-year-old clinical director, Dr. Slava Kim, a general surgeon from Kazakhstan. Kim is half Korean and half Russian-Ukrainian: he was very familiar with traditional Eastern energy medicine, which the Koreans brought with them to Russia; he is holistic in his approach to patients and a tae kwon do champion in his age class. In Kazakhstan, serious laser treatment has been commonplace in surgery since the Russian researchers Meshalkin and Sergievskii introduced low-intensity laser irradiation of the blood, a treatment unheard of in the West even today. In 1981 they began applying light to patients with cardiovascular problems.

The first time Kim saw irradiation work was with a patient who had septicemia—a life-threatening blood infection. The man had not responded to antibiotics and was at death's door. Knowing that light helps the body heal itself, the doctors inserted a fiber optic laser carrying 632 nanometers of laser light into the patient intravenously, through a tube in his vein. The approach had been copioneered by Tiina Karu, from Moscow, from whom Kahn had learned so much. When Kim checked the man's blood tests, he saw a rapid dramatic decrease in white blood cells, meaning that his infection had subsided. Suddenly the antibiotics that had failed him started working. The man achieved a full recovery. It is hard to think of a more graphic demonstration of the new fusion of conventional techniques and energy medicine: the use of an IV to administer not a drug but light.

In Kazakhstan, Kim frequently prescribed IV lasers after he performed abdominal surgeries to fight infections and speed wound healing, because lasers support the immune system; with lasers, he found he was able to shorten his patients' hospital stays. The power of lasers to heal was driven home to him when he, a fiercely devoted surgeon, under constant stress, developed an ulcer and collapsed from internal bleeding. When his gastroenterologist put an endoscope into him, she saw a large ulcer in his duodenum and that there was a serious risk that the acid from his stomach would burn through it, causing it to penetrate through his intestinal wall.

Normally the condition requires emergency surgery, but she began to treat him on the spot: she passed a low-intensity laser down the endoscope and shone it on the ulcer. After only eight such treatments, he was healed, without surgical scarring, which thus protected his digestion. This approach was far less invasive than surgery. Among other ingenious ways to administer light, I have seen an Ontario-manufactured intranasal low-intensity laser deliver light inside the nose (where the blood vessels are close to the surface, and the brain) to rapidly cure a wicked bout of insomnia.

With Kim and Kahn, I saw many remarkable recoveries, which usually didn't start out as brain treatments. One elderly man I met, Allan Hannaford, got treatment because of advanced osteoarthritis of the neck. He also had trouble seeing, because, years before, a stroke in his visual cortex had wiped out parts of his field of vision. Allan's neck improved with treatment. But the surprise was that his field of vision expanded too, because the lights for the neck had been placed close to the visual cortex at the back of the brain. Allan's improved vision has remained.

Kahn and Kim took this approach to a whole new level when they helped treat a young African-Canadian man I'll call "Gary," who had had meningitis (an infection of the tissues that surround the brain) when he was twenty-two, leaving him totally blind and deaf. Inflammation and swelling from meningitis can lead to high pressure on the brain, causing irreversible brain and optic nerve damage. Gary was thirty-two when we met. He had a sweet face and short hair and wore a blue jacket and shirt. He was a warm person and bobbed his head the way singer Stevie Wonder often does. His right eye seemed stuck, looking up at the ceiling.

Gary was accompanied by a longtime friend I'll call "Suzanne." By coincidence, Suzanne was a laser therapist, and one day it occurred to her that lasers might help Gary. Kim and Kahn supervised her and a colleague who treated him. They initially put the lights over the back of Gary's neck. Gary soon began to regain touch sensations around his ears and reported having new pulsations and sensations in the muscles of his face. Then about two months into treatment, astounding things began to happen. He regained some sight.

Since Gary was deaf and blind, the only way I could communicate verbally with him was through the "print on palm technique." I'd ask a question, and Suzanne would write each word on Gary's palm at lightning speed, and he would answer.

"Could you see anything at all before you tried the lasers?" I asked.

"I didn't notice anything before. It was dark."

"Could you see shadows?" I asked.

"No."

"And since using the lasers?" I asked.

"After I have been using the lasers, now I notice shadows, but it clicks in and out. For instance, after the lasers, I was in the kitchen and I could see the outlining of my mom and my nephew by the window." The ambient light of the window had allowed him to see his first silhouette in a decade. "I can't actually see the faces," he added, "but I can see the brown outline of them moving, then it cuts out."

Gary was overjoyed and overwhelmed with excitement, because he never expected anything of the kind to happen. Hearing this, Kahn recommended that Suzanne cover Gary's entire head and all the lobes of the brain with lights. When we met a second time, after several of these head treatments, Suzanne said that there were changes again, and that Gary had heard his niece speak into his ear. I asked Gary to elaborate.

"I was upstairs with my niece and I said something to her—she kept on coming up to me and hugging me, and her face was beside my face, and she said something, and I went 'Ah!' because I felt a loud-pitched noise entering my ear. So then I said, 'What did you say?' So she puts her face up against mine and she said something, and I felt a loud high-pitched noise. As soon as she spoke, it was like going through my ears and making me go Ahh!"

For the first time since going deaf, he had heard a human voice, however indistinctly. He also said he had begun to associate vibrations he felt on his body with sounds he was beginning to experience.

At first, most of the sounds were coming in one ear, and but a month later they were coming in both. Though he couldn't yet sort out specific words, he was now able to differentiate how many words were spoken. It hurt Gary to hear—a sign that his brain, which I saw as awakening from learned nonuse, couldn't yet modulate the incoming sensation. His pain is a sign of a hypersensitive system and might be addressed by neuroplastic exercises I describe in Chapter 8.

I saw many other marvels in the following months. I met with a half-dozen patients who had traumatic brain injuries, from falls, sports injuries, and car accidents. Many had symptoms like Gaby: brain fog, memory problems, fatigue, movement, balance, and vision problems, but also, typically, headaches. All were disabled and not recovering, in most cases for years, until they were treated with lasers. Almost all improved and resumed everyday activities, and those who were not yet 100 percent better said, "I got my life back." In other cases, mood improved. A man who came with a neck problem noticed that not only did it diminish, but his depression lifted, so that he could lower his medication for it. His scores on brain tests improved to the point that he was astonished. (Such cognitive benefits had already been shown to occur with light in a study at the University of Texas, Austin.) Another man, so depressed that he had been on disability for a year, found that with lights his depression lifted, and he was able to go back to work. With the latest data showing that in some cases of depression the brain is chronically inflamed, it makes sense that a treatment that unblocks chronic inflammation could help.

This brings us to the latest area being explored in connection with low-intensity lasers: Alzheimer's disease, the commonest kind of dementia. The Alzheimer's brain is also inflamed, and the mitochondria have difficulty functioning and show signs of aging called oxidative stress, which is a kind of "rusting" of the molecules. Lights, which improve general cellular functioning in the brain, can improve all three conditions—inflammation, mitochondrial problems, and oxidative stress.* The hallmark of Alzheimer's is that the neurons build up excess misshapen proteins, called tau proteins and amyloid proteins, to form plaques that lead to degeneration.

---

*Inflammation is also a major factor in other forms of dementia. There is general agreement that at least some vascular dementias—the second most common form—are caused by vasculitis (inflammation of the blood vessels). But evidence increasingly shows that inflammation may play a role in most blood-vessel disease. If so, it would play a role in most cases of vascular dementia. So low-level lasers may be protective for vascular dementia as well.

A team from Sydney, Australia, has lowered levels of these proteins using light. They implanted human genes associated with Alzheimer's into mouse DNA, so that the animals developed abnormal tau proteins and amyloid plaques. Then they treated them for a month with low-level light therapy, simply by holding the light one to two centimeters above the animals' heads. Using the same spectrum of near-infrared light that has helped in traumatic brain injury, Parkinson's disease, and retinal damage, they lowered both the pathological tau proteins and the amyloid plaques by 70 percent in key brain areas that Alzheimer's affects. Thereafter signs of "rusting" decreased, and the mitochondria, the powerhouses of the cells, improved their function.

A second animal study showed that light therapy improves damaged connections between neurons in Alzheimer's by increasing brain-derived neurotrophic factor (BDNF). We need human studies urgently. In the meantime, it is clear that low-intensity lasers are a powerful way to foster general cellular health in the brain, and, in combination with the exercise regimes and techniques in Chapter 2, and the other measures to preserve general brain health in Chapter 3, make sense.

THROUGHOUT THIS PERIOD OF IMMERSING myself in the healing power of laser light, I couldn't help noticing the extent to which people deprive themselves of natural light and its benefits. Hospitals often seem recklessly indifferent to the role of light in healing—they no longer have the sunlit courtyards inspired by Florence Nightingale's observation, during the Crimean War, that more patients died in the hospital buildings than in the temporary field hospitals, where they were exposed to natural outdoor sunlight and air. Hospital wards influenced by her work—called Nightingale Wards—had multiple windows strategically placed so patients were exposed to light throughout the day.

Recent studies show that light not only speeds healing but decreases pain and improves sleep; because it improves vitamin D levels, light may also decrease some cancer risks. Today a hospital patient is lucky to have a window with direct sunlight. Increasingly windows in enclosed spaces where people spend the most time, such as cars, apartments, schools, and businesses, are colored to screen out the full spectrum of natural light in order to save money on air-conditioning. Indoors, the flickering, pasty hues of "energy-conserving" cool-white fluorescents illuminate us with a ghostly glow that is so unnatural that some sensitive patients feel ill when bathed by them.

This is not the first time in history that "energy-wise" policies have hurt public health. The Industrial Revolution's use of coal polluted the great cities of Europe and America, inducing the physician Caleb Williams Saleeby to lament, in the early 1900s, that the "malurbanized millions" lived in darkened cityscapes even when the sun was out. Infectious disease became rampant, which physicians determined was, in part, related to an absence of light—not just overcrowding. In 1905 in New York, tuberculosis infections declined with the introduction of a law restricting coal smoke.

A trend began. Boston passed a "blue sky law," and children with TB were put aboard a floating hospital on a ship, where they could be exposed to sunlight to heal. The Swiss physician Auguste Rollier took patients to the Alps and exposed them to sun in his sanatorium, resulting in remarkable cures. The decisive factor was not just the fresh mountain air; its coolness meant that people could tolerate longer exposure to the sun. All but forgotten are the great strides that were made in heliotherapy, before the discovery of antibiotics in the 1930s, as a way to heal infection and strengthen the patient's own immune system. Now that our overuse of antibiotics is leading them to fail against the resistant organisms they are spawning, we may have to relearn these techniques.

Our skies may be bluer again, but our indoor spaces are ever more deprived of natural light, in ways we cannot perceive, because the counterfeit light we use is often not composed of the frequencies that preserve life. We need full-spectrum light not just for elegant atriums and lobbies for show, but for everyday living and work spaces. The damage caused by living a light-impoverished life is hidden. We can tolerate gloom for a time, but the buoyant joy we feel when we enter light-bathed spaces signals not just an aesthetic pleasure: it is an indication that we require light to flourish.

...

ON OCTOBER 7, 2012, GABY WROTE: "I drove by myself for the 1st time in approx 3 years. . . . I have no problems turning my head or with my hand-eye coordination. . . . I will add the highway later on, for now I will use alternate routes."

She wrote me again: "All the Will and No WAY: It's very strange. Before I got sick, I always thought where there's a will there's a way. I have since learned even if there's a will, sometimes there's no way. If your brain can't run it, you can't do it. It still surprises me sometimes. . . .

"I apologize for the delay in getting back to you. . . . Unfortunately, my father has not been well."

Gaby has begun tutoring again. She drives, sings, lives. Her long, painful, daily dependence on her parents has come to an end, as has their aching, abiding fear for her future, and their heartbreak on her behalf. Now she is pleased to help care for her octogenarian father, Dr. Pollard, and her mother. The customary arrangement of noble obligations between the generations that occurs in tight families such as theirs has been restored. Meanwhile, Fred Kahn hasn't taken a sick day in fifty years. Now eighty-five, he still has things to do.

Chapter 5

Moshe Feldenkrais:
Physicist, Black Belt,
and Healer

Healing Serious Brain Problems
Through Mental Awareness of Movement

Escaping with Two Suitcases

In June 1940 a young Jew escaped from Nazi-occupied Paris, just hours ahead of the approaching Gestapo. He was carrying two suitcases. They contained French scientific secrets and materials, including two liters of a newly discovered material, heavy water, which was essential for producing nuclear energy and weapons, as well as plans for an incendiary bomb. His task was to prevent them from falling into German hands and his hope was to reach England. He was stout, barrel-chested, about five foot four, extremely strong, and an athlete of some repute. A decade-old soccer knee injury made it hard for him to walk.

The man, Moshe Feldenkrais, just turned thirty-six, was a physicist who was completing his Ph.D. at the Sorbonne. He had worked on French atomic secrets in the laboratory of the young husband-and-wife team Frédéric and Irène Joliot-Curie. Several years before, in 1935, the couple had been jointly awarded the Nobel Prize for producing artificial radioactive elements. In March 1939 the lab split an atom of uranium, setting up a chain reaction that released immense amounts of energy that came to be called nuclear power. It was Feldenkrais who built the device that generated the particles that bombarded the atom. The same year Albert Einstein wrote to U.S. president Franklin D. Roosevelt that "through the work of Joliot in France," a new kind of bomb was possible; he warned that the Nazis were following this work and had begun to accumulate uranium.

A few days before his June 1940 escape, as the Nazis were marching into Paris, Feldenkrais noticed that for some strange reason his injured knee was acting up. It became swollen so badly he could barely get out of bed to go to work. True, the recent mental stress had been extreme, but he could not explain how an event occurring in the brain might cause his knee to swell. Within hours of the invasion, the Gestapo would come to search the Curie lab and force the entire staff to go down into the courtyard. Usually, in these circumstances, they would separate out the Jews and the Communists and cart them off to concentration camps. Frédéric told Feldenkrais that because he was a Jew, he would not be safe. Frédéric quickly got him papers from the French government.

With his two suitcases, Moshe and his wife, Yonah, began a desperate cross-country dash to find a ship to England. But as they drove from one port to the next, they found that either the port was closed or the last boat had left. The Nazi Luftwaffe was bombing the roads, which were crowded with desperate people fleeing for their lives in cars, because trains weren't running. Soon the roads were so damaged they were impassable. Moshe and Yonah began walking, but she had been born with a hip problem, and he had his bad knee. As she succumbed, he managed, by force of will, to push her in an abandoned wheelbarrow until they were able to join an Allied naval evacuation operation. It was commanded by a British officer, Ian Fleming, who later wrote the James Bond novels. Fleming put them aboard the HMS *Ettrick,* the last boat to escape occupied France. Because the ship was so crowded, Feldenkrais had to throw his suitcases onto a large pile of baggage, to be reclaimed on arrival.

WHEN FELDENKRAIS AND HIS WIFE arrived in England in the last week of June 1940, he searched for the suitcases but could find only one, which he turned over to the British Admiralty. But he now had a new problem: the name *Feldenkrais* sounded German. The British, fearing the Nazis were planting spies among the refugees, detained him and put him in an internment camp on the Isle of Man.

One of Britain's key scientists, J. D. Bernal, had been charged with finding scientists to help in the war effort. He had once visited Joliot-Curie's lab and now discovered that Feldenkrais was being held. Bernal got him released to help the British deal with a new vulnerability: Nazi submarines were sinking British ships. In France, Feldenkrais had done important research on sonar, a kind of underwater radar that could be used to detect submarines. After the British sonar project stalled, Feldenkrais was recruited to work with a strange assortment of scientists in Fairlie, an isolated village on the west coast of Scotland. In a matter of days, he went from being a suspect alien to being a scientific officer of the Admiralty, working in British counterespionage. By day, he worked on top secret projects. At night, he taught his colleagues judo.

In Paris he had helped set up the Judo Club of France, was among the first Western black belts, and had written books on judo, which showed, using physics equations, how it was scientifically possible for a small person to throw a much larger one. Word of his expertise spread when a commander took his judo course and asked Feldenkrais to train his home guard platoon, then a battalion. He was soon training British paratroopers in hand-to-hand combat without a weapon as they prepared for D-Day.

Origins of the Feldenkrais Method

Feldenkrais had shown a preternatural independence of mind and willfulness from a young age. He was born in the small town of Slavuta, in what is present-day Ukraine, on May 6, 1904. In 1912 his family moved to Baranovichi, in what is today Belarus. For decades, Jews in the Russian Empire had been victims of government-sponsored pogroms, murderous attacks on Jewish villages. In 1917, in response to the plight of the Jews there and elsewhere, the British, who controlled Palestine, issued the Balfour Declaration, which said, "His Majesty's Government view with favour the establishment in Palestine of a national home for the Jewish people, and will use their best endeavours to facilitate the achievement of the object." When Moshe was fourteen, he set out alone to walk from Belarus to Palestine. A pistol in his boot, a math text in his sack, and with no official documents or papers, he crossed marshes and endured temperatures of 40 degrees below as he traversed the Russian frontier in the winter of 1918–19. As he walked from village to village, other Jewish children, intrigued, joined him. At one point, to survive, they joined a traveling circus, where the acrobats taught Moshe tumbling and how to fall safely—skills he would one day perfect with his judo. By the time he reached Cracow, fifty children had joined the much-admired boy on his way to Palestine, then more, until over two hundred young people were following him. Eventually adults joined his children's march through central Europe to Italy and the Adriatic, where they boarded a boat. It arrived in Palestine in 1919, in late summer.

Like many new arrivals, Feldenkrais was penniless. He worked as a laborer and slept in a tent. In 1923 he began to attend high school and supported himself by tutoring children with whom other tutors had failed; he displayed an early aptitude for helping people overcome blocks in the learning process.

In the 1920s Arabs attacked Jewish villages and cities in British Mandate Palestine. Feldenkrais's cousin Fischel was among those killed. The Jews requested from the British either more protection or the right to arm themselves—and were refused. So young Feldenkrais began to study how to defend himself without a weapon. Arab attackers usually came at their opponents with knives, striking from above, and directing their thrusts to the neck or solar plexus. Many Jews were killed in these encounters. Feldenkrais tried to teach them to block a blow, then grab and twist the attacker's arm so that he dropped the knife. But his students were unable to resist the natural, anxious neurological reflex response of lifting their forearms up to protect their faces or turning their backs to the blow. So instead of fighting these spontaneous responses of the nervous system, Feldenkrais designed a block that used them. He now *insisted* that his students, when attacked, follow the instinctual tendency to block their faces, and he then sculpted that movement into a better block. He then photographed people being attacked from different angles and crafted blocks that molded their frightened, spontaneous reactions into effective defenses. The method worked and would become a template for his future approach to the nervous system: work with it, not against it.

In 1929 he circulated *Jiu-Jitsu and Self-Defense,* in Hebrew, the first of his many books on unarmed combat. It became the first self-defense manual used to train the armed forces of the fledgling Jewish state. That was the year he injured his knee, and while recuperating, he became fascinated with mind-body medicine and the unconscious. He wrote two chapters for a book called *Autosuggestion,* which included a translation of a book on Émile Coué's modifications of hypnosis. In 1930 he moved to Paris, where he completed a degree in engineering and began a Ph.D. in physics under Joliot-Curie.

One day in 1933 he heard that Jigoro Kano, the founder of judo, was in Paris for a lecture. Kano was a very small, frail person who had often been attacked by others when younger. Judo, a modification of jujitsu, trained its practitioners to use an opponent's own power to knock him off balance and throw him. Judo, which means "the gentle way," was also a holistic way of life, both physical and mental. Feldenkrais showed Kano his book on hand-to-hand combat.

"Where did you get this?" asked Kano, pointing to a picture of the block Feldenkrais had developed to use one's spontaneous, anxious nervous response to protect oneself.

"I developed it," Feldenkrais answered.

"I don't believe you," said Kano. So Feldenkrais asked Kano to attack him with a knife, and Kano did. The knife went flying.

Kano took the book and digested it over months. Then he told Feldenkrais he'd train him to be one of the elite students whose distinction was that when Kano threw them through the air, they could always land in a controlled way. Kano soon decided he had finally found the person to help popularize judo in Europe. Two years later Feldenkrais cofounded the Judo Club of France. To finance his Ph.D., he taught judo to Joliot-Curie and other physicists.

During his time in France, his knee problem became serious. On bad days, he was confined to bed, sometimes for weeks. He noticed that some days were better than others, and wondered why this should be and why this physical problem was worse in times of mental stress. Clearly, the cause of his knee problem wasn't chiefly psychosomatic. His knee was injured so badly that his thigh muscle had nearly wasted away. Exams showed that his meniscus, the cartilage inside the knee, was severely torn, and the knee ligaments were completely destroyed. He finally saw a senior surgeon, who told him he couldn't possibly function without surgery. Feldenkrais asked, "Is there any likelihood that the operation will fail?" The surgeon answered, "Oh yes, it's about fifty-fifty," but even if the operation succeeded, his knee would always be stiff. Feldenkrais said, "Good-bye. I won't do it."

Then one day he had a strange experience. He went out alone, hopping on his good leg, slipped on an oily patch, and hurt his good leg. He struggled home, fearing he'd be completely immobile, went to bed, and fell into a deep sleep. When he awoke, he was surprised to find that he could stand on the leg with the injured knee: "I thought I was going insane. How could a leg with a knee that had prevented me standing on it for several months suddenly become usable and nearly painless?" His neuroscience reading helped him realize that his brain and nervous system were the cause of this seeming miracle. The acute trauma to Feldenkrais's "good leg" led his brain to inhibit the motor cortex brain maps for that leg to protect it from further injury should he move. But when one side of the brain is inhibited, often the other takes over its functions. The inhibition of the motor cortex maps for the good leg caused the motor cortex map of his damaged leg to "fire up" whatever muscle he had left, so it could be more useful. This experience taught him that his brain, not solely the physical condition of his knee, was in charge of his level of functioning.

Later, on duty in the antisubmarine program in Scotland, Feldenkrais was frequently on wet, slippery decks, and his knee was often swollen. He had no choice but to deal with his problem himself. He needed to discover what triggered his brain and knee on his "bad days."

He took note that while other mammals can walk moments after birth, humans learn such basic skills as walking over time. To Feldenkrais this meant that walking was "wired in" to the nervous system through experience and involved the creation of habits of movement—habits he was now going to try to change. He began by developing a kinesthetic awareness of how he used and moved the knee. Kinesthetic awareness is a sensation that informs a person where his or her body and limbs are in space and what it feels like to move. Feldenkrais had learned, both from judo and from his neuroscience reading, that when a human stands, a group of muscles—the antigravity muscles of the back and the quadriceps—holds a person up.

Each person has habitual ways of standing that are partially learned. Every time he stands, he enacts these habits unconsciously. Since bad postural habits exacerbated Feldenkrais's problem knee on his bad days, he decided to observe himself lying down, so as to eliminate the action of gravity on his body and his need to use the antigravity muscles and the standing habits he had acquired. He spent many hours on his back, moving his knee ever so slowly, to see where the pain or restriction began, lifting his leg ever so slightly, many hundreds of times. He later told his student Mark Reese that he was observing himself "so that he could feel all the subtle subconscious connections between all parts of himself."

"No part of the body can be moved without all the others being affected," Feldenkrais wrote. This holistic insight would later distinguish his approach from other forms of bodywork. Since the bones, the muscles, and the connective tissue form a whole, it is impossible to move one part, however slightly, and not influence all the others. Extending an arm and raising a finger, by even the smallest amount, requires muscles in the forearm to contract, and other muscles in the back to stabilize those muscles, triggering reactions in the nervous system and the body that anticipate how this movement will subtly alter overall balance. All the muscles, under normal conditions, even when supposedly "relaxed," show some contraction, or "muscle tonus." (Muscle *tonus* is not the same as muscle *tone*. Muscle *tone* often colloquially refers to the defined look or visual definition of a muscle on a thin person. Muscle *tonus* is a medical term, referring exclusively to the general state of contraction of a muscle; and tonus can range from high levels of contraction to low.) Altering the tension in any single muscle affects the tension of the others. For example, contracting the biceps requires relaxing the triceps.

Using his kinesthetic awareness of tonus and breaking his walking down into minute movements, Feldenkrais could now go weeks without knee trouble. "I was far more absorbed in observing how I was doing a movement than I was interested in what that movement happened to be," he wrote, to describe his use of ongoing mental awareness of movement to give himself feedback, which would alter his functioning and his brain.

As he analyzed his gait he found that over the years he had made many adaptations to how he walked, and that these changes had made him forget some of the movements he could do before his injury, so his repertoire of movement had become restricted without his noticing. Thus many of his movement restrictions were caused not only by his physical limitations but also by his habits of movement and habits of mental perception. He had learned from Kano that judo was a form of mind-body education, because mind and body are always related. "I believe," Feldenkrais wrote, "that the unity of mind and body is an objective reality. They are not just parts somehow related to each other, but an indispensable whole while functioning."

This insight helped explain to Feldenkrais the mysterious fact that his knee had swollen up when the Nazis occupied Paris. For the third time, after the Russian pogroms and the attacks in Palestine, his life had been threatened because he was a Jew. His physical problem, he saw, could be made worse by mental stress. Terrifying experiences and memories could trigger nervous system, biochemical, and muscular reactions throughout his mind and body—even swelling in his knee.

During the war, he wrote a book that began as a meditation on the work of Freud, whom he greatly respected; unlike many clinicians of his time, Freud emphasized how the mind and the body always influence each other. But, Feldenkrais noted in *Body and Mature Behavior*, Freud's treatment, talk therapy, focused little on how anxiety or other emotions are expressed in posture and in the body, and Freud never suggested that analysts work on the body when treating mental problems. Feldenkrais believed that there were no purely psychic (i.e., mental) experiences: "The idea of two lives, somatic and psychic, has ... outlived its usefulness." The brain is always embodied, and our subjective experience always has a bodily component, just as all so-called bodily experiences have a mental component.

When the war ended, Feldenkrais learned that all but a few of his relatives had been murdered by the Nazis. Luckily, his parents and sister had survived. He finished his Ph.D. dissertation and graduated. But on returning to France he found that the Nazis, with the collusion of a French and a Japanese judo colleague, had written him out of the history of the judo club he had cofounded, again because he was a Jew. So he settled in London instead, pursued some inventions, wrote another book on judo, called *Higher Judo,* and began a book, *The Potent Self,* in which he developed his healing method, which he was now using to help fellow scientists and friends. As a physicist, he had met the greats: Albert Einstein, Niels Bohr, Enrico Fermi, and Werner Heisenberg. He was deeply torn: should he continue in nuclear physics or, given the wonderful results he was getting, pursue healing? He chose healing. His mother said half-jokingly, "He could have got a Nobel Prize in physics, and instead he became a masseur."

But his plans for staying put and pursuing his method were again interrupted. In 1948 the United Nations divided Palestine into two areas, one Jewish, to be called the State of Israel, and the other Arab, called Palestine. Within hours, six well-armed Arab nations attacked the Jewish state. A stream of Israeli scientists went to London and persuaded Feldenkrais to return, in 1951, to direct the Israeli Army's department of electronics, in top secret projects, which he did until 1953. Only then, at last, was he free to refine his life's work. In Israel he met a chemist, Avraham Baniel, who became a lifelong friend. Baniel persuaded Feldenkrais to come and give classes in his and his wife's apartment every Thursday night, saying "We can be a laboratory for you."

Core Principles

Over the course of mastering his knee problems and writing *Body and Mature Behavior,* and now seeing clients regularly, Feldenkrais refined the principles that formed the basis of his new methods. Most of them are related to facilitating what I have called the stage of neurodifferentiation (described in Chapter 3), one of the key stages of neuroplastic healing.

1. The mind programs the functioning of the brain. We are born with a limited number of "hardwired" reflexes, but the human being has the "longest apprenticeship" of all animals, during which learning takes place. "Homo sapiens," he wrote, "arrives with a tremendous part of his nervous mass left unpatterned, unconnected, so that each individual, depending on where he happens to be born, can organize his brain to fit the demands of his surroundings." As early as 1949, Feldenkrais wrote that the brain could form new neural paths to do so.* In 1981 he wrote, "The mind gradually develops and begins to program the functioning of the brain. My way of looking at the mind and body involves a subtle method of 'rewiring' the structures of the entire human being to be functionally well integrated, which means being able to do what the individual wants. Each individual has the choice to wire himself in a special way." When we have experience, he wrote, "the neural substance [the neuronal connections in the brain] organizes itself." Feldenkrais often said, as his student David Zemach-Bersin points out, that when there is a neurological injury, plenty of brain matter usually remains to take over the damaged functions. Moshe Feldenkrais was one of the first neuroplasticians.

2. A brain cannot think without motor function. Wrote Feldenkrais, "My fundamental contention is that the unity of mind and body is an objective reality, that these entities are not related to each other in one fashion or another, but are an inseparable whole. To put this more clearly: I contend that a brain could not think without motor functions."

Even thinking of making a movement triggers the movement, even if very subtly. When he got a pupil to simply imagine a movement, he noticed that the tonus in the relevant muscles increased. Imagining counting would trigger subtle movements in the throat's vocal apparatus. Some people can barely speak if their hands are confined. Every

---

* That neuroplastic point was already a theme in his *Body and Mature Behavior,* Chapter 5. In 1977 one of Feldenkrais's students, Eileen Bach-y-Rita, introduced him to her husband, the neuroplasticity pioneer Paul Bach-y-Rita (see Chapter 7). Feldenkrais read Paul Bach-y-Rita's work and actively began to integrate his concepts, which fit well with his own. In 2004 Bach-y-Rita developed a project to study Feldenkrais's results with head injuries but died before he could complete it. E. Bach-y-Rita Morgenstern, personal communication; also see her article "New Pathways in the Recovery from Brain Injury," *Somatics* (Spring/Summer 1981).

emotion affects facial muscles and posture. Anger shows in clenched fists and teeth; fear, in tightened flexors and abdominal muscles and in holding the breath; joy, in a lightening of the limbs and buoyancy. People may believe they can have a pure thought, but in a deeply relaxed state, Feldenkrais pointed out, they will observe that every thought leads to a change in their muscles.

Every time the brain is used, four components are triggered: motor movement, thought, sensation, and feeling. Under normal circumstances, we don't experience one without the other three.*

3. *Awareness of movement is the key to improving movement.* The sensory system, Feldenkrais pointed out, is intimately related to the movement system, not separate from it. Sensation's purpose is to orient, guide, help control, coordinate, and assess the success of a movement. The kinesthetic sense plays a key role in assessing the success of a movement and gives immediate sensory feedback about where the body and limbs are in space. Awareness of movement is the fundamental basis of Feldenkrais's method. He called his classes Awareness Through Movement lessons (or ATMs). It may seem "magical" to think that movement problems—especially in people with serious brain damage—can be radically changed simply by becoming more aware of the movement, but it seems magical only because science formerly thought of the body as a machine with parts, in which sensory functions are radically separated from motor functions.

This focus on self-awareness and monitoring of experience is based in part on Feldenkrais's exposure to the meditative aspect of Eastern martial arts, and it reveals him anticipating the current Western interest

---

* One of the hottest current theories in neuroscience, the motor theory of thought proposed by the neuroscientist Rodolfo Llinás, was anticipated by Feldenkrais. Llinás points out that nervous systems are not essential for life but are for complex movement. Plants don't need nervous systems because plants are not mobile. The link between movement and the nervous system, and the brain, becomes particularly clear in the simple sea squirt, called Ascidiacea. In early life, in its larval form, it moves around, like a tadpole, and has a primitive brainlike group of 300 nerve cells that receives sensory information from a primitive vestibular apparatus and a patch of skin. It eventually finds a stationary place in which to feed, and ceases to move for the rest of its life. No longer needing to move, it no longer needs a brain, and so it digests its own brain and primitive spinal cord, as well as its tail with its musculature. R. R. Llinás, *I of the Vortex: From Neurons to Self* (Cambridge, MA: MIT Press, 2001), p. 15.

in mindfulness meditation by about fifty years. Feldenkrais's insights have been reaffirmed by the neuroscientist Michael Merzenich, who showed that long-term neuroplastic change occurs most readily when a person or an animal pays close attention while learning. Merzenich did lab experiments in which he mapped animals' brains before and after different kinds of learning tasks. When the animals performed tasks for rewards automatically, without paying attention, their brain maps changed, but only temporarily.

4. *Differentiation—making the smallest possible sensory distinctions between movements—builds brain maps.* Newborns, Feldenkrais observed, often make very large, poorly differentiated movements based on primitive reflexes, using many muscles at once, such as reflexively extending their entire arms. They also cannot discriminate among their fingers. As they mature, they learn to make smaller, more precise individual movements. But the movements do not become precise until the child can use awareness to discern very small differences among them. Differentiation, Feldenkrais would show, would be key to helping many people with strokes, children with cerebral palsy, and even autism.

Feldenkrais found, repeatedly, that when a body part is injured, its representation in the mental map becomes smaller or disappears. He relied on the work of the Canadian neurosurgeon Wilder Penfield, who showed that the surface of the body is represented in the brain by a map. But the size of an individual body part in the brain map is proportional not to its actual size in the body but rather to how often and how precisely it is used. If the body part performs a simple function—the thigh, for example, mainly does one thing, moving the knee forward—the representation is small. But brain maps for the fingers, often used in precise ways, are huge. Feldenkrais understood that it is a use-it-or-lose-it brain, and that when parts are injured—and thus are not used often—their representation in the brain map decreases. By making very finely tuned—differentiated—movements of these parts and paying close attention while doing so, people experience them subjectively as becoming larger; they take up more of their mental maps, and lead to more refined brain maps.

5. *Differentiation is easiest to make when the stimulus is smallest.* In

Awareness Through Movement, Feldenkrais wrote, "If I raise an iron bar I shall not feel the difference if a fly either lights on it or leaves it. If, on the other hand I am holding a feather, I shall feel a distinct difference if the fly were to settle on it. The same applies to all the senses: hearing, sight, smell, taste, heat, and cold." If a sensory stimulus is very great (say, very loud music), we can notice a change in the level of that stimulus only if the change is quite significant. If the stimulus is small to begin with, then we can detect very small changes. (This phenomenon is called the Weber-Fechner law in physiology.) In his ATM classes, Feldenkrais instructed people to stimulate their senses with very tiny movements. These small stimuli radically increased their sensitivity, which ultimately translated into changes in their movements.

For example, Feldenkrais would ask people, as they lay on their backs, to tilt their heads very subtly up and down, about twenty times (or more), making the smallest possible movement—a hundredth of an inch—with as little effort as possible; they were to be aware only of the effect the movement had on the left side of the head, neck, shoulders, pelvis, and the rest of the left side of the body. Observing those changes will lead to decreased muscle tonus in the entire left side of the body (even though both sides of the body move when the head is tilted). This change happens because the awareness itself helps reorganize the motor cortex and the nervous system. If the person were to scan his body before and after the exercise, he would discover that, mentally, the left side's body image now feels lighter, also larger and longer and more relaxed, than the right side. (The cause is that the brain map for that side is now more differentiated and represents the body in finer detail. This technique of changing body tonus and brain maps is helpful because many movement problems often arise because areas of the body are not well represented in the brain maps.)

6. *Slowness of movement is the key to awareness, and awareness is the key to learning.* As Feldenkrais put it, "The delay between thought and action is the basis for awareness." If you leap too quickly, you can't look before you leap. He took this principle, of moving slowly in order to be more aware and learn better, directly from Eastern martial arts. People learning tai chi practice their movements at glacial speed, with

virtually no physical effort. In his early books on judo, such as *Practical Unarmed Combat*, Feldenkrais had emphasized the need to repeat actions very slowly and calmly and noted that hurried movements are bad for learning.

Slower movement leads to more subtle observation and map differentiation, so that more change is possible. Remember, when two sensory or motor events occur repeatedly and simultaneously in the brain, they become linked, because neurons that fire together wire together, and the brain maps for those actions merge. In *The Brain That Changes Itself*, I described how Merzenich discovered how subjects can lose differentiation in the brain, and he explained that "brain traps" occur when two actions are repeated simultaneously too often: their two brain maps, meant to be separate or differentiated, merge. He showed that when a monkey's fingers were sewn together and thus forced to move at the same time, the maps in the brain for those two fingers became fused.

Maps also fuse in everyday life. When a musician moves two fingers simultaneously often enough while playing an instrument, the maps for the two fingers sometimes fuse, and when the musician tries to move one finger alone, the other moves too. The maps for the two different fingers are now "dedifferentiated." The more intensely the musician tries to produce separate movements, the more he will move both fingers, strengthening the merged map. He's caught in a brain trap, and the harder he tries to get out of it, the deeper he gets into it, developing a condition called focal dystonia. We all are prone to less dramatic brain traps. Sitting at a computer, for example, we lift our shoulder unconsciously as we type. After a while we may find—as I did—that the shoulder is often up when it needn't be. Neck pain soon follows. One way to begin to deactivate the process is to learn to redifferentiate the muscles that elevate the shoulder from those involved in typing. This first requires awareness that the two actions are being done simultaneously.

7. *Reduce the effort whenever possible*. The use of force is the opposite of awareness; learning does not take place when we are straining. The principle should not be *no pain, no gain*. Rather, it should be *if strain, no gain*. Feldenkrais thought the use of willpower (of which he obviously had plenty) was not helpful in developing awareness. Nor was any kind

of compulsive driven action, which increases muscle tonus throughout the body. Compulsive effort leads to mindless, automatic movement that becomes habitual and unresponsive to changing situations. Compulsion is the problem, not the solution. We can eliminate a lot of muscle tension in the body by using awareness to spot how we often, without intending to do so, tense and use muscles that are not necessary for that movement. He called these movements superfluous or "parasitic."

8. *Errors are essential, and there is no right way to move, only better ways.* Feldenkrais didn't correct errors or "fix" people. He emphasized: "Do not be serious, eager, avoiding any wrong move. The kind of learning that goes with Awareness through Movement is a source of pleasurable sensations, which lose their clarity if anything dims the pleasure of it all. . . . Errors cannot be avoided." To teach people to leave a problematic habit behind, he encouraged them to try random movements until they found one that worked better for them. Instead of correcting errors, he encouraged them to notice lack of flow in barely detectable movements. They learn, he insisted, from their own movements, not from him. In ATM lessons he encouraged pupils to set aside the critical faculty: "Don't *you* decide how to do the movement; let your *nervous system* decide. It has millions of years of experience." In a sense, he was asking his pupils to perform a psychoanalytic free association—using movement, instead of words—so that their own spontaneous movement solutions would emerge.

9. *Random movements provide variation that leads to developmental breakthroughs.* Monumental gains, Feldenkrais discovered, are made not by mechanical movement but by the opposite—random movements. Children learn to roll over, crawl, sit, and walk through experimentation. Most babies learn to roll over, for instance, when they follow something with their eyes that interests them, then follow it so far that, to their surprise, they roll over. They learn to roll over by accident, based on a random movement. Infants sometimes learn to sit up because they are trying to put their feet into their mouths, not because they want to sit. Learning to stand and walk are momentous breakthroughs that infants make without training. They learn by trial and error, when they are ready.

Years after Feldenkrais made this discovery, Dr. Esther Thelen, arguably the world's leading scientist of motor development, demonstrated that every child learns to walk *in a different way,* by trial and error, and not, as was thought, through a standard "hardwired program" applicable to all. Thelen revolutionized the scientific understanding of motor development, but when she discovered that Feldenkrais had said as much, she was "totally awed" by his clinical discoveries and told Feldenkrais's students, "I think that the science may seem rather crude compared to the kind of intuitive, hands-on, brain . . . knowledge you people have." She then trained as a Feldenkrais practitioner.

These insights contrast with the approach of many conventional physical therapies or the use of machines for rehabilitation, which generally give patients with "biomechanical problems" repetitive exercises, based on the assumption that there are *ideal* movements for lifting, walking, getting out of a chair, and so on. Feldenkrais hated it when his ATM classes were called exercises, because mechanical repetition of action was what got people into bad habits in the first place.

10. Even the smallest movement in one part of the body involves the entire body. In a person who is capable of effective, graceful, efficient movement, the entire body organizes itself, as a whole, to do the movement, no matter how small. Consider the following paradox. We can lift a finger with ease; we can reach out to shake a friend's hand or lift a glass with equal ease. When we unconsciously shrug our shoulders, as we speak, we do so with the same ease. Yet how can these movements all be of equal ease? A finger is much lighter than a hand and forearm, and a hand and forearm are lighter than the entire arm. They are of equal ease because, in practice, when done with grace, we use the entire body for each action. When the body is well organized, muscle tension is limited throughout, and the load for all the actions is shared across the muscles, skeleton, and connective tissue. Feldenkrais had learned from Kano that the great judo masters are always relaxed and that "in the correct act there is no muscle of the body which is contracted with greater intensity than the rest. . . . The sensation is of effortless action." The practitioner need not be stronger than his opponent as long as his body as a whole is more coordinated or, as he would later say, better "organized."

11. Many movement problems, and the pain that goes with them, are caused by learned habit, not by abnormal structure. Most conventional treatments assume that function is wholly dependent on the "underlying" bodily structure and its limitations. Feldenkrais discovered that his pupils' difficulties were caused as much by how their brains *learned* to adapt to their structural abnormalities as by the abnormalities themselves—and sometimes more so, as happened to him with his knee. His original adaptations to his knee initially helped him to get around somewhat, but he learned even better ones by creating a new way to walk—which served him well for the rest of his life, and he never needed surgery. There is always a brain component to a movement difficulty.

FELDENKRAIS FIRST TAUGHT PEOPLE TO use his principles the way judo was taught, in ATM group classes. Participants typically had various problems—sore necks, headaches, sciatica, herniated discs, frozen shoulders, postsurgical limps. Feldenkrais would get them to lie down on judo mats. The huge antigravity muscles (the extensors of the back and the thigh muscles) would relax, and all the habit patterns triggered by "fighting" gravity to stand up were eliminated. He got them to scan their bodies attentively, so they became aware of how they felt, and what parts of their bodies made contact with the mat. He often told them to pay attention to how they breathed. Often subjects hold their breath the moment they get into a movement difficulty.

Then he had them explore a minute movement on one side of the body for much of the lesson, sensing subtle differences in how they made each minute movement. It was at this point that Feldenkrais's knowledge of hypnosis and Émile Coué came into play; as he spoke, he gave almost hypnotic suggestions to encourage them to do the movement with least effort, with greatest ease, so that it felt very light. Typically he chose movements that were crucial at some point in early development, such as lifting the head, rolling over, crawling, or finding easy ways to come to a sitting position. "As a teacher I can accelerate your learning," he wrote, "by presenting the experience under the conditions in which the human brain learned in the first place." He might spend fifteen minutes getting his class to roll their heads gently to one side and notice what they felt, how far they could roll them. Next, he would ask them only to imagine rolling their heads, and notice what they felt *throughout* their bodies. Often their muscles would contract, just at the thought of making the movement.

Then something odd would happen. Toward the end of the lesson, he asked them to close their eyes and scan their bodies again. The side they had worked on was generally closer to the mat and felt longer and larger. Their body images had changed, and they could roll their heads much farther. Tight muscles released. In the short time remaining, they switched to working on the other side and found that many of the gains made on the first side quickly transferred.

Feldenkrais would often ask pupils to spend most of the session focusing on the side of their body that was less distressed, discovering ways to move it with even greater ease. Then, pupils found it as though this awareness of how to move gracefully was spontaneously transferred to their distressed side. Feldenkrais sometimes said that the troubled parts of the body learned not from him, but from the side of the body that was moving comfortably.

If during a class a student found she had a restriction when she did a movement, she was only to notice it, not judge it negatively. She should not attempt to "push through" a restriction or "correct" an error. Instead, she was to explore different kinds of movements, to see which felt best, which seemed most efficient and graceful. "It is not a question of eliminating the error," Feldenkrais would say. "It is a question of learning." Thinking in terms of error and negative judgment puts the person's mind and body into a tense state that doesn't help learning. The pupil was to explore, and learn new ways to move, and in the process develop and reorganize the nervous systems and the brain, not fix them.

These classes were deeply relaxing, and people would get up from them noticing they had much less pain and a far greater range of movement. Soon people came to Feldenkrais for work with him, one on one, for help with their aching necks, knees, and backs, or for their postural and postsurgical movement problems. He began to have great success, using the same principles, one on one, gently moving their bodies on a table instead of telling them to do so.

•••

Functional Integration became Feldenkrais's term for a half hour spent, one on one, with a client on the table. The goal was for the pupil to become able to function well, regardless of any underlying structural problem, and for the mind and all the body's parts to find *a new integrated way* of *functioning* together. Hence the name "Functional Integration." Since he conceived of this method too as a form of "lessons," he called his clients "pupils." Unlike the ATMs, when he suggested various movements, these sessions were almost completely nonverbal, except at the beginning, when the pupil might tell him his or her problem.

Feldenkrais would begin by positioning the pupil on the table in the posture that created maximum comfort, relaxation, support, and sense of safety to lower bodily tension. Often people habitually "hold" parts of their body tight without being consciously aware of doing so. To reduce strain or muscle tension in the lower back, he would place a small roller under the head, or knees, or elsewhere on the body. Whenever there is the slightest strain in the body, muscle tonus increases, making it harder for a person to detect the subtle movement differentiations essential for improvement, and to learn new movements. When the pupil was comfortable, and his muscle tension was as low as it could be, Feldenkrais believed the brain was most available for learning.

Feldenkrais would sit beside the pupil and begin communicating, by touch, with the pupil's nervous system. He began with small movements, so that the observing mind and brain would begin to make differentiations. This was touching not to impose on but to communicate with the brain. If the person's body moved, he would move with it, responsively, never using more force in his movements than necessary. He did not knead the muscles or press hard, as in massage or in an authoritarian manipulation of the joints. He would rarely work directly on a painful area; that approach only increased muscle tension. Thus he might start working on a part of the body farthest from where the pupil thought the problem was, often on the opposite side. He might begin to gently move a toe, far from a painful upper body part. If he felt a restriction, he would *never* force it. What he discovered was that the brain would sense this relaxation in the toe, and the person would become immersed in that image of relaxed movement, which would soon generalize, so that that entire side of the body relaxed.

Feldenkrais's approach differs from some conventional body therapies in terms of method and goals, insofar as they focus on specific parts of the body and hence are "local" in orientation. For instance, some forms of physiotherapy will use exercise machines, to engage specific body parts to move through stretching and strengthening. These approaches, often extremely valuable, are arguably more inclined to treat the body as though it were made up of individual parts and are therefore more mechanical in orientation. They may prescribe particular protocols for particular problem areas. Feldenkrais claimed, "I have no stereotyped technique to apply ready-made to everyone; this is against the principles of my theory. I search and, if possible, find a major difficulty which can be detected at each session and which may, if worked upon, soften and be partially removed. I . . . go slowly and progressively through every function of the body."

Feldenkrais's reputation grew. A friend of Avraham Baniel's, Aharon Katzir, a scientist who made major contributions to neuroplasticity, took a great interest in Feldenkrais's work. He passed the information on to the Israeli prime minister David Ben-Gurion, and in 1957 Feldenkrais took Ben-Gurion on as his pupil. The seventy-one-year-old Ben-Gurion suffered from sciatica and low-back pain so severe he could barely rise to speak in Parliament. After some lessons, Ben-Gurion was able to leap up onto tanks to give speeches to the troops. Since Feldenkrais's house was near the sea, Ben-Gurion, before turning to matters of state, would go for a morning swim, then see Feldenkrais for his lessons. Once, Feldenkrais had him stand on his head. A photo of the elderly prime minister on his head on a Tel Aviv beach was used in an election and seen all over the world. Soon Feldenkrais was traveling and giving Functional Integration lessons worldwide, including to pupils such as the violinist Yehudi Menuhin and the British film director Peter Brook.

As Feldenkrais worked with more pupils, he discovered that his way, as he called it, of "dancing with the brain" could improve many conditions in which serious brain damage had occurred—such as stroke, cerebral palsy, severe nerve damage, multiple sclerosis, some kinds of spinal cord injuries, learning disorders, and even cases where parts of the brain were missing.

Detective Work: Figuring Out a Stroke

Feldenkrais was frequently invited to Switzerland. On one visit, he met a woman in her sixties, Nora, who had had a stroke on the left side of her brain. His book about her treatment is his most detailed account of his technique.

In a stroke, a blood clot, or a bleed, cuts off blood supply to the neurons, and they die. In Nora's case, her speech was slow and slurred, her body stiff. She wasn't paralyzed, but her muscles were spastic on one side. Spastic muscles are muscles that have too much tonus and are too quick to contract. Spasticity—related to the word *spasm*—is thought to occur when the neurons in the brain that inhibit muscle contraction are damaged. This leaves only the excitatory neurons firing, and so there is too much muscle tension. It's a classic sign of a poorly modulated nervous system.

A year after the stroke, Nora's speech had improved, but she couldn't read a word or write her own name. After two years she still required around-the-clock monitoring, because she'd often go out and be unable to find her way home. She was deeply depressed about her lost mental functions.

Feldenkrais first met her three years into her illness and had no idea of how he would approach her problem. Every stroke with cognitive problems is unique, and figuring out exactly which brain function is damaged often requires the skill of a detective. He understood that reading is not natural—the learning process requires wiring together many different brain functions. He also understood that when a stroke affects a neuronal network that processes a function, it does not mean the entire network is damaged: "When a skill cannot be performed as before, only some of the cells which were essential to the skill performance do not function." It was often possible to recruit other neurons and to teach them to differentiate "to perform the skill, though usually in a different manner."

Feldenkrais could give Nora only a few lessons before returning to Israel, so her family decided, because she was making no progress with conventional treatment, that she should go to Israel to work with him.

In his early work with Nora, Feldenkrais was trying to find out *why* she couldn't read and write. He also wondered about her body awareness and orientation: she kept bumping into things; when she tried to sit on a chair, she often sat on the edge of the seat; when she left his room, which had several doors, she often chose the wrong one. At the end of one half-hour lesson, he put her shoes, which she had taken off for the lesson, in front of her feet, with the toes facing her, without telling her why. She looked very confused, couldn't put them on, couldn't tell her right shoe from the left, and fumbled for five or six minutes. This mistake told him that her brain damage was preventing her from telling left from right, which would also interfere with her ability to read. He would have to deal with the left-right problem first because children must learn to differentiate left from right long before they can learn to read.

But before he could address Nora's orientation problem, he had to quiet her noisy, hyperexcited brain, which he knew was a problem because when he lifted her limbs, he couldn't bend them—they had excess muscle tension. He corrected the problem by having her lie on her back; he put supportive wooden rollers covered with sponge under the nape of her neck and the backs of her knees. This reduced the muscle tonus of her spastic body. Then as he gently moved her head back and forth, his touch lighter and lighter, her body relaxed, settling her brain and nervous system so that she would be in a state of heightened awareness. With so little stimulus coming into her brain, it would be easy for her to differentiate small sensory differences and learn. Next he simply touched her right ear and said, playfully, "This is the right ear."

As she lay on her back, she saw there was a couch to the right of the table she was on. He touched her shoulder and said, "This is the right shoulder." He went down her right side, touching her this way for several days running. He never used the word *left* or touched the left side. In a following session, he had her lie on her stomach, and again he touched her right side. But she was confused, because she equated "right" with the way the room looked when she was on her back, with a couch facing her "right" side. Now that she was on her stomach, the "right" side was away from the couch. (We forget that as children we must learn this distinction.) He spent a number of sessions teaching her to learn where her right side was when she was in different positions. It was his genius to realize that a concept as seemingly simple as orientation was actually complex.

Then he took her a step further and had her cross her right leg over her left. She did so, but now she thought her left leg was her right leg, because it was now on the same side as the right. It took them two months of such lessons to experiment with the different right and left positions, until she could understand left and right in all their complexity. All the while her brain was forming a new map of body awareness of left and right. Sometimes she would relapse between lessons, and he'd have to start at the beginning, but slowly the relapses became less frequent.

Only now was he ready to introduce text. Nora said she couldn't "see" the words. He sent her to an ophthalmologist, who said her eyes were fine, confirming that the reading problem was in her brain, not in her eyes. Feldenkrais gave her a book with very large print. She trembled. He handed her a pair of glasses, but she fumbled. She did not know how to orient them to put them on her face. "I was annoyed with myself," he wrote, "for not having realized that even the transfer from body awareness to external objects needs training"; a baby, grabbing its parent's glasses and trying to put them on, has the same trouble. So he trained her to orient the glasses properly to her head so the left lens was over her left eye and the right lens was over the right eye.

Because she said she could not see, Feldenkrais, instead of asking her to read (which might stress her), simply told her to look at the pages, close her eyes, and say whatever words came to mind—in Freudian free association. After she finished looking, he searched the pages he had shown her and found that all the words she had said were on the left-hand side of the page, near the bottom, usually the last three words in the line. He said, "I was exhilarated. She did read words but did not know where she read them."

Nora had told Feldenkrais, "I cannot see," not "I cannot read." He was beginning to understand what she meant. He took a straw and put one end between her lips and the other end between her fingertips, positioned over a word in a book. He wanted to make a direct link between the mouth, which speaks, and the eyes, which see. She could see the word at the end of the straw but couldn't yet read it. But after about twenty practice trials, she spontaneously started to say the word at the end of the straw—much the way children, when they learn to read, often point out each word with their fingers. Nora was reading. Feldenkrais often sat beside Nora to her left. He put his right hand under her left arm, on her wrist, to help her hold the book. With his other hand, he helped her hold the straw between her lips. In this way, he could feel the slightest change in her body, the slightest halt in her breathing, the second it occurred. When it did, he knew that it was time for him to stop moving the straw, until her nervous system could reorganize. "It was a kind of symbiosis of the two bodies—I felt any change in her mood, and she felt my determined, peaceful, noncoercive power. I did not rush her, but would read the words out loud the instant I felt her stiffen with anxiety and lose grip. Gradually I had to read less often."

One of Feldenkrais's most important ways of helping a damaged brain learn was to use his own body to sense, match, and identify with the nervous system of his pupil. Touch was always important to him because he believed that when his nervous system connected with the other person's, they formed one system, "a new ensemble . . . a new entity. . . . Both the touched and the toucher feel what they sense through the connecting hands, even if they do not understand and do not know what is being done. The touched person becomes aware of what the touching person feels and, without understanding, alters his configuration to conform to what he senses is wanted from him. When touching I seek nothing from the person I touch; I only feel what the touched person needs . . . whether he knows it or not, and what I can do at that moment to make the person feel better."

The idea of two nervous systems in symbiosis he describes as resembling a dance, where one partner learns by following the other, without any formal instruction. Such "dancing," like any kind of dancing, is about communication between two people. When Feldenkrais touched a pupil, he was often communicating nonverbal hints of what her body might be able to do when he moved it, allowing her to sense new variations of movement that her restricted limbs might be capable of. This is especially important with older pupils, who, as they age, have repeated the same movement habits over and over, which neuroplastically reinforces these patterns; by neglecting other patterns, they lose the circuitry for them, in the use-it-or-lose-it brain. Feldenkrais was able to remind pupils of movements they once had but had lost.

After three months, he taught Nora to hold a pen and write using other ingenious techniques. She continued to improve, and the lessons ended, and she returned to Switzerland.

One year later, on a visit to Switzerland, Feldenkrais spotted Nora walking near the railway station in Zurich. She looked confident. When they spoke, he was delighted to find that the teacher-pupil relationship was over, replaced by the ordinary ease of two friends bumping into each other.

When Feldenkrais agreed to work with Nora, he was not overwhelmed by the fact that she had lost brain structure, because he knew her brain was plastic; he couldn't know what her limits might be before trying patiently to teach her to re-create her orientation, then to read and write, as one might teach a child. The key to her progress was his recognizing which brain function was missing, then teaching her to make sensory differentiations. As her mind—her awareness—noticed these differences, they were wired into her brain maps, and she became ready to make even finer differentiations.

There is great beauty in the image of these two elderly people, Feldenkrais, about seventy, sitting by Nora's side, the one teaching the other how to read, their nervous systems so intertwined and attuned, he learning, as he would write, as much as she. But Feldenkrais was very careful about the words he used to describe what he did with Nora. It was not, he said, a "recovery." "Recovery is not the right word," he wrote, "since the part of the motor cortex where writing is organized and directed was not in a state to perform as before. The better word is 'recreating' a writing ability." Because the brain map circuits originally involved in reading and writing were damaged by her stroke, those functions had to be taken over by other neurons. He didn't call what he did with Nora a "cure," even though many would have. He preferred the term *improvement*. "'Improvement,'" he wrote, "is a gradual bettering which has no limit. 'Cure' is a return to the previously enjoyed state of activity which need not have been excellent or even good." Such improvements would be dramatic in children born with brain damage who had never had "good functioning" in the first place.

Helping Children

As Feldenkrais had more experience with stroke patients, he started to see children with cerebral palsy, many of whom had had a stroke in utero or suffered a lack of oxygen to the brain during birth. Often they were unable to control their tongues and lips in order to speak. Like adults who have had strokes, children with cerebral palsy often develop rigid or "spastic" limbs, with so much muscle tension that they become too rigid to move normally or at all.

In children, rigidity creates a serious problem. At birth, we do not have finely developed, differentiated brain maps that allow us to sense and make fine individual movements. A healthy newborn will put his fist in his mouth to suck, and the entire, undifferentiated brain map for the hand fires to process the sensation and the move. As time passes, he will differentiate out a few fingers from that hand and suck them, and then perhaps the thumb alone. As he plays with his hands, his brain map for the hand is differentiating, forming separate areas for each finger to sense and move. But a child with cerebral palsy, with a spastic limb or body, can't make fine, separate movements; his limbs are too rigid. Often his hand forms a tight fist, so he can't even begin brain map development and differentiation into separate areas for each movement.

Another symptom often seen in a child with cerebral palsy is that he can't get his heels onto the ground when standing, or is held in a standing position by an adult, because muscle contractions in his calves pull his heels up. Consequently, his Achilles tendons are always tense. Other such children are knock-kneed: the muscles inside the thighs, the adductors, are so tight that they pull their knees together. Both conditions can be very painful.

Mainstream medical treatment prescribes surgery for such cases. The surgeon cuts and lengthens the Achilles tendon. Or sometimes Botox injections are used to paralyze the muscle and release the tension. But the muscle contractions continue, so operations or injections have to be repeated. For knock-kneed children, the adductor is cut to relieve the pressure. But neither of these well-meaning but drastic approaches addresses the underlying problem, because it is the brain that is firing the signal to contract the muscles. And the procedures leave the child with abnormal body mechanics—for life. Other medical approaches involve various stretching exercises, reasoning that the muscles and connective tissue get shortened and lock into place—which is true. Yet these stretches are often painful and also don't address the fact that *it is the brain* "telling" the muscles to tighten.

Feldenkrais saw spasticity as caused not only by the initial damage to the brain but also by the brain's problem in regulating sensation and motor activity, because it wasn't getting differentiated input. Thus the brain didn't "know" when to turn off the firing of the motor cortex.

Once when Feldenkrais was teaching a workshop in Toronto, he saw a little boy with cerebral palsy. Ephram couldn't walk normally, needed a wheeled walker, and was very spastic and stiff. Because his heels didn't touch the floor, he walked on his toes. But his most urgent problem was that his knees were locked together, inseparable. A surgeon had scheduled an operation to cut his adductors to pry his knees apart.

Feldenkrais started to work on the toe walking. With Ephram lying down, Feldenkrais made tiny movements on the boy's feet, then his legs, to help him differentiate the brain maps for these limbs. In a very short time, the boy began to relax and breathe more easily. Feldenkrais was sending messages to Ephram's brain, using the sensory neurons of his feet and legs. This input allowed his brain to distinguish his toes and their muscles, the calf and thigh muscles, and all the movements they could make. Only when the brain could make these distinctions could it begin to properly regulate the firing of his motor system neurons and his muscle tonus.

In a Functional Integration lesson, if Feldenkrais felt the person had a muscle that was "holding" and too tight, he would often do for the person what the disturbed nervous system was overdoing. One of his astute practitioners, Carl Ginsburg, described how often Feldenkrais, rather than trying to get a pupil to stop "holding" himself tight, would do the holding for him. "Feldenkrais's understanding of habit led him not to oppose this activity but to support it by taking over the activity directly. Feldenkrais found that once they got that support most pupils just let go of the habitual action."*

Feldenkrais was able to get Ephram to cross one knee over the other, putting them even closer together than they had been. By putting the close knees even closer, Feldenkrais was doing what the boy's disturbed nervous system was "overdoing"—teaching his nervous system that it didn't need to work so hard. In a few minutes, Ephram's spastic thigh muscles released without Feldenkrais's using force. Now that the knees were a bit separated, he put his fist between them and asked the boy to squeeze the fist with the muscles on the insides of his thighs. Then Ephram completely relaxed his muscles, and his knees completely opened. "See how much easier it is to have your knees open?" Feldenkrais said. "To close them requires work." Feldenkrais had used Ephram's body to program the brain. A 2006 study of thirty-three subjects showed that Awareness Through Movement classes can also lengthen muscles,

---

*I experienced this "support" when one of Feldenkrais's earliest American followers, David Zemach-Bersin, gave me a Functional Integration lesson. I had got into the habit of automatically raising my right shoulder while typing, putting strain on my neck, leading to pain and restriction. In the lesson, Zemach-Bersin gently lifted my shoulder toward my neck, "supporting" it in the higher position, using his nervous system to take over the task my nervous system had assigned itself. In a minute or so, I felt massive relief of the restriction and pain. This idea, of dealing with the force of a contracting muscle not by opposing it but by going with it, derives from judo principles. In judo, one doesn't overpower the opponent's force but rather uses it to steer, topple, or throw the opponent.

as much as stretching can, an approach athletes might want to think about.*

A Girl Missing Part of Her Brain

Feldenkrais's approach can radically change the life even of people who were born missing huge parts of the brain, by facilitating differentiation in the remaining brain areas. Elizabeth Natenshon, whom I interviewed, was born missing a third of her cerebellum, a part of the brain that helps to coordinate and control the timing of movement, thought, balance, and attention. Without the cerebellum, a person has difficulty controlling all these mental functions. The cerebellum, which means "little brain" in Latin, is about the size of a peach and is tucked under the cerebral hemispheres, toward the back of the brain. Although it occupies only about 10 percent of the brain's volume, it contains almost 80 percent of the brain's neurons. The technical name for Elizabeth's condition is *cerebellar hypoplasia,* and there was no treatment known to change the course of the illness.

When she was in the womb, her mother felt there might be a problem, because Elizabeth hardly moved. When Elizabeth was born, she didn't move her eyes. They flickered and were not properly aligned, gazing in different directions. At one month, they rarely tracked objects. Her parents were terrified she might not see normally. As she developed,

---

* Feldenkrais said he wanted not flexible bodies but flexible brains (which would create flexible bodies). His colleague Ida Rolf often helped people with body tensions, spasticities, and postural problems. Rolf stretched the connective tissue (fascia) to free up a person's range of motion, based on the assumption that fascial layers often get stuck together, causing "adhesions." Feldenkrais practitioners, on the other hand, claimed that it was the brain that caused the restriction. Robert Schleip, head of the Fascia Research Group at Ulm University, in Germany, and an enthusiastic "Rolfer," set up a small study. He and his colleagues examined patients with restrictions of the muscles and fascia while they were undergoing general anesthesia. The hypothesis was that if the restrictions are caused by the brain, then when the brain is partially turned off in anesthesia, the restrictions should cease. Indeed, the researchers found that "most of the previously detected restrictions appear to be significantly improved (if not absent) during the conditions of anesthesia. It seemed that what had been perceived as mechanical tissue fixation may at least be partially due to neuromuscular regulation." R. Schleip, "Fascia as an Organ of Communication," in R. Schleip et al., eds., *Fascia: The Tensional Network of the Human Body* (Edinburgh: Churchill Livingstone, 2012), p. 78.

it was clear she had a problem with her muscle tonus. At times she was very floppy, meaning she had too little or no muscle tension, but at other times she had too much tension and was "spastic," making no exploratory, voluntary movements. She received conventional physiotherapy and occupational therapy, but the treatments were painful for her.

When Elizabeth was four months old, the chief pediatric neurologist at a major urban medical center tested the electrical activity of her brain. He told her parents that "her brain had not developed since birth, and there was no reason to believe that her brain would develop." Most such children show persistent deficits, and it was believed the cerebellum shows limited plasticity. The doctor also told her parents that her condition was much like cerebral palsy, and he predicted that she would never be able to sit up, would be incontinent, and would have to be institutionalized. Her mother later recalled, "I remember he said, 'The best we could hope for would be profound retardation.'" Elizabeth's physicians were accurately describing their experience with such children who had conventional treatment—the only kind they knew about.

Still, her parents, Abigail and Lou, sought help. One day, a friend, an orthopedic surgeon, who knew of Feldenkrais's work, said, "This guy can do things that no one else can." When they heard that Feldenkrais was coming from Israel to a town near them to train practitioners—one of his major activities in the 1970s—they got an appointment.

When Feldenkrais met Elizabeth for the first time, she was thirteen months old and unable to creep or crawl. (Creeping, which usually precedes crawling, means scooting along on the stomach.) She could make only a single, voluntary movement: rolling over on one side. At her first Functional Integration lesson, she couldn't stop crying. She had had many sessions with therapists, who had tried to get her to do things she was not ready to do developmentally. For instance, many therapists had tried to sit her up, over and over, and had failed. If the children's bodies are spastic, these movements hurt them—hence the crying.

According to Feldenkrais, these attempts to leapfrog through development are a huge error because no one ever learned to walk by walking. Other skills have to be in place for a child to walk—skills adults don't think about or remember learning, such as the ability to arch the back and lift the head. Only when all these pieces are in place will a child learn to walk, spontaneously. Feldenkrais saw that Elizabeth couldn't lie comfortably on her belly, and when she was on her belly, she couldn't lift her head at all.

He noticed her entire left side was in complete spasm, making her limbs rigid. Her neck was very tight, causing her pain. The fact that Elizabeth's entire left side was spastic indicated that her brain map for that side was undifferentiated, instead of having hundreds of areas for processing different types of movements.

Feldenkrais touched her, ever so gently, on her Achilles tendon, and she was so tormented he knew he first had to do something to resolve that pain: he would have to settle her brain because otherwise it would not be available for learning.

"After Moshe examined her," her father remembers, "he said to me, 'She has a problem and I can help her.' He was not bashful. My wife asked him to explain, and he proceeded to take our daughter's foot at the ankle and bend it back, and he took my finger, and he said, 'Touch this,' so that I could feel the knot of muscle, and he said, 'She can't creep, because it hurts her to bend her leg. If we soften that up, you will see she can bend her leg. And as we do this—soften her muscles—her whole demeanor will change.' And it happened as he explained—a day or two after that, she was creeping." Soon she was crawling.

THE NEXT TIME FELDENKRAIS SAW Elizabeth, one of his young pupils, Anat Baniel, a clinical psychologist and the daughter of his close friend Avraham, happened to be there. Feldenkrais asked Baniel if she'd mind holding Elizabeth throughout the lesson. He gently touched her, to begin teaching her to differentiate very simple movements. Elizabeth became intrigued, attentive, happy.

Feldenkrais gently held her head and pulled it up and forward, very slowly and gently, to lengthen her spine. Usually, he had found this movement caused a natural arching of the back and led the pelvis to roll forward—a reaction that happens normally when a person is standing. Often, when working with children with cerebral palsy and others who couldn't walk, he would use this technique to engage the pelvis, so it would reflexively roll. But when he tried it on Elizabeth, Baniel felt no movement. Her pelvis was inert in Baniel's lap. So Baniel decided that when Feldenkrais pulled, she would gently roll Elizabeth's pelvis.

Suddenly there was movement throughout Elizabeth's spastic, locked, inert spine and body. They gently moved her spine again and again. Next, they tried subtle variations of the movement.

At the end of the session, Baniel gave Elizabeth back to her father. Usually in his arms Elizabeth would plop down on him, not able to control her head. But this time she arched her back, threw her head back, then brought herself forward, again and again, facing her father. The subtle movements of the neck and spine that Feldenkrais and Baniel had done had awakened the idea of this movement and wired it into her brain. Now Elizabeth was moving the large muscles of her spine and back voluntarily, delighted with movement.

Yet there was still much to worry about: Elizabeth was profoundly disabled and carried a horrendous diagnosis. Feldenkrais could see that Elizabeth's parents were clearly concerned about her future. He usually didn't say a great deal on these occasions. But he judged a brain not by where a child was in her development but by whether, given stimulation appropriate to that stage of development, the child could learn. "She's a clever girl," he said. "She will dance at her wedding."

Feldenkrais returned to Israel. Over the next few years, her parents heroically and tirelessly did, and put up with, whatever it took to get Elizabeth to see him. They brought her to see him in hotel rooms whenever he came to the United States or Canada, and went to Israel three times, for two to four weeks of daily visits to Feldenkrais's office. In between these intensive visits, Elizabeth consolidated her gains with everyday activities.

When Feldenkrais was seventy-seven years old, he fell ill while traveling in a small town in Switzerland. He lost consciousness, and physicians discovered that he was bleeding inside his skull. A slow leak of blood had built up in the dura (the layer of connective tissue that surrounds the brain) and in the brain itself, putting pressure on it, endangering it. Unfortunately the only neurosurgeon in the town was traveling that weekend, so surgery to relieve the pressure caused by his "subdural bleed" was delayed.

Feldenkrais's colleagues concluded that his many injuries from all the throws, falls, and concussions in judo had made him vulnerable to the subdural bleed. He recovered in France, but perhaps because surgery was delayed, he suffered some brain damage. But soon he was once again giving Functional Integration lessons. And sensing that his time was limited, he continued to teach as much as he could, hoping to transmit his latest findings.

Back in Israel, he had a stroke, which affected his speech. His students gave their master daily Functional Integration lessons. Now in his late seventies and ill, he directed more and more of the children who came to him to Baniel. Baniel gradually took over Elizabeth's care, flying in for three-week periods, giving her daily lessons. Elizabeth saw her on and off for years and did brain exercises and behavioral optometry with therapists Donalee Markus and Deborah Zelinsky (see Afterword).

TODAY ELIZABETH IS IN HER thirties and has two graduate degrees. She's petite, at five feet tall, and has a sweet voice. She walks, moving so easily that an observer would never know she had once been destined to end up immobile, in an institution, severely mentally retarded—at best. "Moshe," she tells me, "said to my dad, 'When she is eighteen, nobody is going to know that anything happened.' And he was dead on." She remembers "tidbits" of those visits to Israel, "and I sort of remember Moshe, the white hair, the blue shirt, and how smoky it was in there"—Feldenkrais smoked during lessons—"him whispering things into my ear, calming me down."

Her two graduate degrees are from major universities: she earned a master's in Near Eastern Judaic studies; then wanting something practical, she did a master's in social work and got her license. She still has some residual symptoms of the cerebellar hypoplasia. She has a mild learning disorder with numbers, and so math and science are difficult. But other than that, she enjoys learning and being intellectual, and she became a voracious reader—all of Shakespeare, most of Tolstoy, and many other classics. Today she runs a small business and is happily married.

And yes, she danced at her wedding.

Creating Speech

Over five years I followed a dozen of Baniel's "pupils," children with special needs, all with serious brain problems, and I witnessed much extraordinary progress at her center in San Rafael, California. Baniel has accumulated vast experience with challenging cases of brain and nervous system damage in children—children with strokes, Down syndrome, autism and speech delay, movement problems called apraxias, cerebral palsy, and nerve injuries.

I watched Baniel work with another girl born missing a portion of her cerebellum, who couldn't speak. When her mother was seventeen weeks pregnant, an ultrasound showed that an entire section of the fetus's cerebellum, called the vermis, was missing, and the remainder had an abnormal, disorganized shape. The consulting neurologist said that if she lived, she would likely be autistic and unable to walk. I'll call her "Hope." When Hope came to see Baniel, she was two years and four months old. She couldn't move, sit, or hold her head or body up; her eyes were crossed, and she couldn't track moving objects. She wasn't socially engaged and didn't vocalize. Traditional physical therapy was painful for her and didn't help.

"The first time she came to Anat," says her father, "she learned to crawl within ten days." Baniel got her speaking by doing gentle movements that might seem to have nothing to do with speech—touching her feet and lower back, wiggling her knees, moving her pelvis and spine and ribs. Speaking can occur only if the brain can control the breath (which it does by coordinating the movement of the diaphragm, ribs, spine, and abdominal muscles) as well as the mouth, lips, and tongue. Baniel babbled playfully so Hope would realize that there was no "expectation" for her to speak words. (This was the opposite of speech therapy, which had given her exercises and drills to repeat properly formulated, comprehensible words, and which had made her anxious, because she was not developmentally ready for that. Baniel calls it "practicing failure," because "children learn their experience; they don't necessarily learn what we intend them to.") Instead, using play, she turned on Hope's "learning switch" and helped her realize that any sound she made, however imperfect, could produce communication. Throughout the session, Hope was all giggles, occasionally saying "No!" After four sessions, Hope was babbling constantly and squealing with laughter. Today she is seven and a half and speaks in short sentences.

Hope had had no vision in her left visual field. Baniel also helped her to begin tracking objects and to see on the left side by working on the body as a whole. Interestingly, this work on eye tracking also affected the prescription of Hope's glasses. It went from plus eight to minus one. Eventually she became able to function without glasses.*

Another child I saw on multiple occasions I'll call "Sydney." Immediately after his birth, he had to spend time in the neonatal intensive care unit, where he was infected with bacterial meningitis. A CT scan showed he had a stroke, caused by the infection. In addition to destroying brain tissue, meningitis can lead to severe swelling and blockages in the flow of the cerebrospinal fluid that bathes the brain. As the fluid builds up, pressure mounts and the entire head enlarges, sometimes to almost twice the size—a condition called hydrocephalus. To save Sydney's life, a neurosurgeon put in a shunt to relieve the pressure, but the shunt failed, and he needed a second surgery.

When Sydney was first brought to Baniel's center at five months, he was completely spastic. He couldn't roll over. As with many people with strokes, his fists were tightly contracted, and his arm was bent up against his chest, immovable. "It was so tight and powerful that if you tried to move it quickly," says Baniel, "you'd break his arm." His parents were told he'd never walk. He couldn't turn his head to one side, a condition called torticollis. But at the end of his first session, he opened both hands. He made progress with each visit, eventually learning to roll over and back. Baniel told his parents, "The same brain that learned to roll over, and sit up, is going to talk."

---

* Hope had crossed eyes, and such children are often sent to have their eye muscles surgically cut, to align them—an approach that, according to Baniel, guarantees a cosmetic result, but their eyes will never work properly. Feldenkrais's work has helped many such children avoid surgery.

With his lessons, Sydney started walking at twenty-seven months. Realizing he could learn, even though his speech was still delayed, his parents took the unusual step of exposing him to three languages. (Along with English, his mother spoke to him in Italian, then sent him to Italian immersion; a Spanish caretaker spoke Spanish.)

In the first couple of years, at their most frequent, Sydney's sessions at Anat's center were four to five times a week, thirty minutes each. Baniel has found that concentrating lessons together often achieves more results than spacing them out.

When Sydney was five years old, he was getting only a few lessons a year. He was still a bit less active than most children his age, and his running was rigid. Today at nine he is very engaged. The boy who wasn't supposed to be able to walk or speak now runs around and is fluent in three languages—reading and writing English, Spanish, and Italian!*

Unconfined Until the End

In 1977, Feldenkrais set up an organization, now called the Feldenkrais Guild of North America, which today accredits training programs and certifies practitioners of his method. It is affiliated with the International Feldenkrais Federation, which represents certified practitioners throughout the world who have completed an in-depth, experiential hands-on training.

Throughout his adult life, Feldenkrais believed that genetics is only one factor determining the limits of intelligence. Much of the most important learning we do, he believed, is outside the classroom, from learning to walk (and defy gravity) to learning physics as he did (mostly in the Joliot-Curies' laboratory), to learning judo. Lifelong learning ran in his family. He was proud that his frail, eighty-four-year-old mother was able to learn to lift him and use judo to throw him. He joked with some other martial artists that the throw looked "completely fake because it is

---

* Baniel now calls her approach the Anat Baniel Method, and it has evolved from her original work with Feldenkrais and her own subsequent practice. Other practitioners trained in the Feldenkrais method also specialize in children as well as in strokes, athletes, musicians, dancers, anxiety (the subject of Feldenkrais's first book), spinal cord problems, back problems, chronic pain, and multiple sclerosis. Of course, many are generalists.

just unbelievable. . . . When she saw that people could do Judo throws and lifts, she said, 'I can do it,' and it took her about ten minutes and she learned to do it."

One of the most important things Feldenkrais took from Kano and judo was the understanding of reversibility: actions, to be intelligent, must be performed in such a way that, at any given moment, they can be stopped or reversed—turned in the opposite direction. The secret was never to move—or live—compulsively. (Living or performing actions compulsively is the opposite of doing them in a differentiated way. The compulsive action, unlike the differentiated one, is always done the same way, and ironically, because so much mental effort is used, it is often performed mechanically, with little awareness.)

He wrote in *Higher Judo,* "It is bad in Judo to try for anything with such determination as not to be able to change your mind if necessary." In judo as in life, we must never be locked in—to a habit, a way of thinking, or an attitude—and even when we think we are locked in, we often are not. In judo, even when one is pinned down on the ground by an opponent, he wrote, "one should always remember the words 'immobilization' and 'holding' do not describe the actual state of affairs—they convey the idea of finality and fixity that do not exist in action. An immobilization is dynamic and constantly changing all the time. The opponent generally frees himself as soon as you stop forestalling and checking his next move."

ONE DIRECTION CANNOT BE REVERSED: living beings move relentlessly toward death. That we do so, we cannot change; but how we do so, we can. We can approach with or without awareness. Feldenkrais was very ill and dying when Avraham Baniel came to visit him in 1984 for the last time in his Tel Aviv apartment. He noticed that Feldenkrais seemed to be listening to himself, his own body, as though listening to another. Knowing his friend's curiosity, and that his friend's attachment to life was very strong, Avraham asked him, "Moshe, how do you feel?"

Feldenkrais's face was swollen, and yet he seemed, to Avraham, to be smiling in his mind.

He answered slowly, "I am waiting to listen to my next breath."

Chapter 6

A Blind Man
Learns to See

Using Feldenkrais,
Buddhist, and Other Neuroplastic Methods

The eye standeth not still but moveth incessantly.

Andreas Laurentius,
A Discourse of the Preservation of the Sight, 1599

DAVID WEBBER, SLIM WITH A gentle voice, is sitting across from me in my consulting room. He was blind from the age of forty-three, until he cured himself using his own application of Feldenkrais's understanding of the brain and mind. For years he had taken medications and had many operations on his eyes, all of which failed to restore his sight. But today he is off eye medications and can see. The ravages of his past disease are apparent. His right eye is turned out a bit and has a bigger pupil, and the right iris is a darker greenish-brown than his left. Though he can now see, he moves carefully, making almost speculative movements, with the awareness of his body in space that the blind adopt.

When David and I first meet, in 2009, he is fifty-five years old. He is visiting from the island of Crete, where he lives in a fifteenth-century pension-boardinghouse overlooking the Aegean Sea. Born in Canada, he withdrew to Crete after his blindness cost him his job. He had already made progress on his cure before going to Crete, but he was still disabled. He needed a less urgent, less stressful life, and so he sought to live at a slower rhythm and pace, surrounded by olive trees and hoping to be invigorated by the Cretan sun and air. In Crete he could live simply, on limited savings, without the stress of being blind during Canadian winters, with the risk posed by blizzards and falling on ice.

As our conversation unfolds, we realize that our paths almost crossed years ago. Though we had not met, we went to the same high school. In university, the same philosophy teacher influenced us, though in different years. As a young man in the 1960s, Webber became a sailor but then turned to studying Plato, with our teacher, who taught him to appreciate ancient Greek thought; then he turned to a classical training in the Theravada, one of the oldest surviving Buddhist schools, seeing in it a further exploration of "the examined life" that had initially drawn him to Plato and Socrates. He studied for years with two teachers, who would one day play a role in his healing: Namgyal Rinpoche, who taught him meditation and ancient texts, and the Venerable U Thila Wunta, of Myanmar, with whom he studied and traveled building pagodas. His journey inward was intense; at its height, he followed the classic practice of meditating twenty hours a day, sleeping four hours a night.

Then he married and had a son. Needing to support a family, he discovered in himself a great aptitude for systematic thinking applied to computers. By the early 1990s, he was a computer network integrator, handling the AT&T Canada account, and a member of an international team that was developing some of the first infrastructure to commercialize the Internet.

One day at a major presentation in 1996, when he was forty-three, someone in his group said, "Your eye looks red." He went to an ophthalmologist and was diagnosed with uveitis, an autoimmune disease in which the body's antibodies attack the eyes, inflaming them. Uveitis is the cause of 10 percent of blindness in the United States. The inflammation quickly progressed, affecting his iris, the center of the retina, and his lenses. He was going blind. His autoimmune disease attacked his thyroid next: it had to be surgically removed.

Because of his immune response, fluid built up behind his retina, causing its central portion, the macula (which makes out details at the center of the visual field), to swell. He lost the ability to see details. He could not read his watch but could only sense, using his peripheral vision, that there was something watchlike on his wrist. He was vaguely aware of its colors, but he couldn't get enough information to construct an image.

For five years his eyes were treated with regular injections of anti-inflammatory steroids, between his eyes and their sockets. He also received oral steroids to suppress his immune system. But the treatment could not keep ahead of the disease, and dead inflammatory tissue filled his eyes with a shifting black screen of floaters, which blocked his vision; the improvement in his vision was marginal, and the surgery resulted in two other eye problems: raised pressure inside his eyes, causing him to develop glaucoma, which can lead to blindness, and severe cataracts, so that eventually both his lenses were removed, in two operations. He now had to wear thick glasses to replace his own lenses—but they blocked whatever peripheral vision he had left.

Afraid of being helpless and dependent, he often decided not to wear his new glasses and forced himself to ride subways or go to fairs, to become comfortable in the crowded spaces that most frightened him. Though he mostly saw only a blur, he said, "I learned to get about with blurred vision and feel quite comfortable in that state. I learned that vision is much more than simply seeing details and reading symbols . . . it is my whole self that sees, not the eyes."

Two additional operations (called vitrectomies) pried open his eye sockets and surgically opened his eyeballs from the sides to vacuum out the gel inside (the vitreous humor), which contained the buildup of dead tissue. The improvement was marginal. After one of his cataract surgeries, a postoperative infection destroyed much of his right eye. His ophthalmologist told him it was basically "dead," having no pressure in it. That eye began shrinking within his eye socket. A few years later, in 2002, he needed glaucoma surgery for the left eye, which still had some vision. A trabeculectomy, which involved drilling a hole in the left eye to drain fluid, was unsuccessful. In all, he had five surgeries without gaining any significant improvement to his sight. One eye was barely able to distinguish fingers held close to his face, and the pressure in the other eye was out of control. His physical pain was overwhelming, like constantly having something in his eye that irritated it every time he moved it. The pain went on for years, often keeping him in bed.

"And," he tells me, "there was the emotional pain. The whole period was one of terror. I lived in horrific states of anxiety, and it kept getting worse." His formerly calm voice becomes tremulous as he remembers it. "At home I was losing my ability to function, even the ability to squeeze toothpaste onto a toothbrush. I was writing notes with Magic Markers, in letters an inch high. At work, I was losing my career. I was at the top of the next big wave when my boss told me that the account was going out of control because I could not see the computer screen. I was pulled off the account. It was one thing to be going blind, and another to lose my business, because I knew there would not be another opportunity like this: the beginning of the Internet expanding. It was heartbreaking. I had to go on disability to concentrate on what was going on in my eyes and my immune system."

The steroids, it was hoped, would protect his eyes from further deterioration: he was supposed to remain on them for the rest of his life, but they caused him to develop a bloated face and a racing heart. He gained weight, shook uncontrollably, had mood swings, confusion, and forgetfulness. He felt poisoned by his medicines. Always on his mind was the question: Would the steroids protect his eyes, or would the pressure and inflammation building in them finally damage his optic nerves? They did. So now he had yet another eye disease—optic neuropathy. His ophthalmologist tested his eyes and declared him legally blind.

Normal 20/20 vision is defined as what a perfectly sighted person, standing 20 feet from a standard Snellen eye chart, can read. Legal blindness begins at 20/200. Webber was 20/800, meaning at 20 feet he could only see as much of the eye chart as a normally sighted person could see standing 800 feet away—nothing. He was able to detect only the blurry waving of fingers held in front of him. All his doctors told him he would be blind for the rest of his life.

HIS LIFE TOOK A GRIM turn. Everyone except his family and some very close friends abandoned him. "My business colleagues vanished. Anyone who needed something from me vanished because I couldn't give them anything anymore." His marriage had broken up some years before his eye problems began, and now without a job, in his forties, he had to move back in with his parents. At night, he dreamed he could see, and he'd wake in the morning remembering how blissful it was to have clear vision.

But by day, at the local society for the blind, he was given a white cane and studied how to distinguish coins by feel. He had been a great reader and experienced the loss of reading as "an unimaginable hell." Most frustrating was the fact that since he couldn't read, he couldn't research his problems. In the days before he was completely blind, he would, with longing, "wander the used bookstores of Toronto like a hungry ghost," carrying a large magnifying glass, trying to find books with type large enough, and enough contrast on the cover, that he could make out shapes, one letter at a time, to guess the title. "I bought books based on their titles, just to bring them home and put them in my shelves with the hope that someday I would be able to read them."

"What drove that hope?" I ask him.

"Blind faith," he answers, "and I wanted to see my son and watch him grow."

Glimmers of Hope

One day his general practitioner, who followed his case very closely and who knew how badly things were going, passed Webber a sheet of information about an alternative approach, developed by a New York physician, ophthalmologist, and eye surgeon. William Bates, who lived from 1860 to 1931, treated many common eye problems successfully and even, on occasion, cured some kinds of blindness using what were in effect neuroplastic exercises. Bates did for vision what Feldenkrais did for movement: he showed that it is not a passive sensory process but requires movement, and that the habitual ways the eyes move affect the eyesight.

Trained at Columbia and Cornell Universities, Bates began his career brilliantly: in 1894 he helped pioneer the medical use of adrenaline, the hormone released in the fight-or-flight reaction and in stressful and frightening situations. Thus he knew, far better than his peers, the extent to which stress can affect the body, the muscles and their tonus, and the eyes (where adrenaline enlarges the pupil, affects circulation, and increases internal pressure). Bates measured the vision of tens of thousands of pairs of eyes and realized that visual clarity—how blurry things appear—fluctuates, especially when people are stressed. He observed a number of patients who had spontaneous recoveries from vision problems and wondered, could he train people to have better eyesight? He eventually became best known for helping people see better and get rid of their eyeglasses.

Conventional wisdom—dating back to the scientist Hermann von Helmholtz (1821–94)—is that the eye is able to focus on different distances because the lens changes its shape. Helmholtz studied this proposition using a new machine called a retinoscope. He theorized that this shape change *probably* occurred because the small muscle at the margin of the lens, the ciliary muscle, contracted. What Helmholtz proposed as a probability soon became accepted in textbooks as a universal truth and the sole cause of lens change—and is still taught today.

Bates, however, questioned the idea that focusing depends solely on the lens changing shape. A minority of patients whose lenses were removed because of cataracts, and who received replacement glasses with inflexible lenses (as Webber did), could still adjust their focus, a curious fact often reported in the literature but an embarrassment to a theory that the lens must change shape to see clearly at different distances. Bates attempted to replicate Helmholtz's original experiments, using a retinoscope on fish, rabbits, cats, and dogs, and found that focusing problems occurred not only because the lens shape changed but also because the shape of the entire eyeball changed, caused by the six external muscles that surround the eyes, which were previously thought to move the eyes only to track objects. Bates demonstrated that the external muscles change focus by lengthening or shortening the eyeball. When he cut these muscles, the animals could no longer change focus.*

---

* More recent studies confirm Bates's argument that the ciliary muscle of the lens is only one component in determining the eye's ability to "accommodate," or focus and maintain a clear image, while looking at different distances. Japanese surgeons have succeeded in elongating the sclera (the white tissue of the eyeball), causing the eye to have better accommodation. Studies of

The finding that the external muscles can lengthen or shorten the eye was crucial. In 1864 the Dutch ophthalmologist Franciscus Cornelis Donders had observed that people with nearsightedness (myopia), who could see clearly only when looking at objects up close, had longer eyeballs. When eyeballs are too long, the image passing through the lens falls short of the retina and becomes blurry. Bates argued that blurry vision occurred because the nearsighted person's external muscles were often in a state of high tonus, which affected the eyeball's shape. Nearsighted people often have tense sore eyes, sensations that they tend to suppress but that they can notice if they close their eyes and pay close attention to how they feel.

Bates emphasized that eye movement was essential for clear sight. The center of the retina, the macula, which sees fine detail, moves constantly to scan a single word or even a letter. The eyes perform two kinds of movements called saccades. Some saccades are observable by others: people scanning a room, looking for a friend, move their eyes in ways that we can see. But other eye movements are too small to be observable. Charles Darwin's father, Robert, discovered that even when the eye appears to be still, it moves involuntarily. It is now known that invisible microsaccade movements occur at speeds too fast to observe without special equipment. When microsaccades are inhibited, as when a drug paralyzes the eye muscles, a person cannot see. Thus, movement of the eye is essential to vision.

How do microsaccades facilitate sight? According to the current leading theory in visual neuroscience, the retina and its affiliated neurons register information crisply for only a brief period, after which the signals start to fade. When we look at a single still object, our eyes take "multiple snapshots of it." They move into a position, then pause, so the

the cornea (corneal topographic studies) in children who have had surgery on the external muscles of the eye have shown that the tension in these muscles influences the person's refractive power and thus how light lands on the retina. "Consequently, tension and, vice versa, relaxation of the external muscles do have an influence on refraction, and we can't forget the person's state of mind and the intention in the visual process. We can easily observe that we can read a text we are interested in without getting tired." The ophthalmologist Christine Dolezal, M.D., personal communication. Despite the evidence in favor of his assertions, Bates is still repeatedly called a fraud by skeptics, who cherry-pick only evidence against his work.

image casts its light on the light-sensitive receptors in the retinas, which fire off a fresh version of the image. Then as the image is about to fade, a microsaccade moves the eye a minute distance, so that nearby receptors are stimulated to fire off a second "snapshot" of the image. Even when we think we are staring fixedly at an object, our eyes are making micro-saccades, sending multiple versions of the images to refresh the brain. (We experience such fading with touch, too. When we put on clothes or glasses we feel them against our skin, but as time passes, the sensation fades, unless we move and feel a new impression of contact. To feel the texture of a fabric, we move our fingers over it, pause, then move them again, "scanning" it.)

The eyes are not merely passive sensory organs. Movement is neces-sary for normal sight: *The eye standeth not still but moveth incessantly,* Andreas Laurentius wrote in 1599. Seeing requires an intact, *active* motor-sensory circuit, meaning the brain must be able to move the eyes, sense how that movement affects vision, and then use that feedback to move the eyes to a new position. Blindness is often not only a *passive* sensory deficit, because seeing is not just a sensory activity. Seeing is a sensory *and* motor activity, and so blindness is often, in part, a move-ment problem.

BECAUSE BATES BELIEVED EYESTRAIN AND high tonus inhibit vision, he developed exercises to relax the eyes and found that, using them, his clients could lower their prescriptions, and that many could rid them-selves of their glasses altogether. And though he often spoke in terms of the eyes, he knew that any approach that modifies muscle tonus and vi-sion *always involves the brain.*

Bates developed alternative theories about how eye problems, such as nearsightedness, farsightedness, and crossed eyes, develop: he be-lieved they are often caused by the habitual ways people use their eyes. Culture, he realized, has a huge impact on our vision. In 1867 the Ger-man ophthalmologist Herman Cohn observed, from a study of 10,000 children, that prescribing eyeglasses increased as children progressed through school, read more, and did close work. (Nearsightedness, or myopia, is the commonest vision abnormality.) In Israel, ultraorthodox Jewish boys begin studying the Torah and Talmud very young, and eventually almost all wear glasses; in Asian countries, where glasses hardly existed one hundred years ago, academic pressure has children beginning to read intensively at very young ages, and the use of glasses is on the rise. About 70 percent of Asians are now myopic. Though most medical schools still explain myopia as primarily caused by genes, the changes are happening too fast to be explained by genetics. These changes are largely due to neuroplastic changes to the brain, based on the new ways people are using their eyes.

Eyeglasses correct vision by bending the light coming into the eye so that it focuses back on the retina. Eyeglasses are a quick fix: they correct blurriness and headaches, and they are reliable. But glasses don't really "cure" the underlying problem: eyestrain and nearsightedness are still there and are getting worse (which is why most people's prescriptions get stronger over time). Not reversing nearsightedness, Bates argued, leads to worse problems, because severe nearsightedness is associated with a greater risk of retinal detachment, glaucoma, macular degeneration, and cataracts, each of which can lead to blindness. For Bates, eliminating the need for glasses by alleviating nearsightedness was preventive medicine, not merely cosmetic.*

Bates developed an international following; his students called themselves natural eyesight improvement educators. His work made a powerful impact on Feldenkrais. But local New York ophthalmologists

---

* My wife and I took a two-day seminar with the natural vision specialist Leo Angart, who uses Bates's and related techniques to improve sight. In two days, between our four eyes, we were able to drop our prescriptions ¾ diopter per eye on average. (A diopter is a measure of how much a lens bends light.) Up to this point, our prescriptions had tended to increase every few years, but we stopped that process cold and began to reverse it. After that workshop, my wife and I both wear the prescriptions we wore fifteen years ago. Angart had read, in a book titled *Trance-formations,* about the hypnosis of a man who underwent age regression and reexperienced early childhood memories. People in age-regressed states often feel childlike and even assume the posture of a child. Surprisingly, the client began to see as he had as a child, before he needed glasses. Apparently, under hypnosis, the high tonus of his eye muscles radically relaxed. In a moment of inspiration, John Grinder, the hypnotist, brought him back to normal consciousness with a suggestion he awaken with the clear eyesight of childhood. After that Angart realized that the claims of Bates might have merit and was able to train himself to dispense with glasses, after having required them for over twenty-five years.

and optometrists (who sell spectacles) felt threatened. They labeled him a quack, ostracized him, and forced him to leave his teaching position at the New York Post-Graduate Medical School. It was his misfortune to have discovered the use of mental experience to train aspects of vision in an era before mainstream medicine accepted neuroplasticity.

First Attempts

On first hearing of Bates's work in 1997, David Webber began exploring it, but his eyes were so badly inflamed, he got the impression that they presented too great a complication for the Bates method. But he continued to search and heard of an Israeli named Meir Schneider, born blind to deaf parents, who had recovered using the Bates method. Schneider had a genetic disorder that gave him huge cataracts and glaucoma. Like Webber, he had had five failed surgeries, which filled his eyes with scar tissue, and he was declared permanently blind. When he was seventeen, his vision was 20/2,000. A boy younger than himself, who had improved his eyesight using the Bates method, taught him the exercises. Though they are normally done for an hour a day, Schneider, against medical advice, did them for thirteen hours. After some time, he noted a growing contrast between light and dark: light was getting brighter, darkness darker. Next, some vague shapes emerged. By six months he could see objects and read letters with a very strong 20 diopter lens; within eighteen months he was reading without glasses. Today Schneider teaches self-healing in California and has an unrestricted driver's license, which he showed me. His vision is now 20/60; it went from 1 percent of normal vision to 70 percent.

Here, thought Webber, was someone who had problems as severe as his own and yet benefited from the Bates method. Schneider's story gave him inspiration, but he felt too ill, too depressed as he lurched from crisis to crisis, too preoccupied with his multiple doctors' visits, and too poisoned by his steroid medication, prednisone, to travel to California.

Despite his interest in Eastern thought, Webber had put all his hopes in his Western physicians, upon whom he felt dependent. Only when his ophthalmologist made clear he had little more to offer did

Webber recall, from his years of doing yoga and Buddhist meditation, U Thila Wunta's stories about yogic practices to heal the eyes, and about an eye-healing tradition that came out of ancient Buddhist monasteries. Webber visited his meditation teacher, Namgyal Rinpoche, at his home in Kinmount, Ontario, who seeing his swollen, inflamed eyes, said, "I'm going to give you the four exercises used in the ancient monasteries by monks to heal their eyes. These will help you."

It was the spring of 1999. After all the high-tech interventions he had done, the instructions were so simple and so seemingly primitive as to appear childlike, if not ridiculous. The four techniques, which had been part of the oral tradition, were the following:

First, Namgyal Rinpoche told him to "meditate on the color blue-black for a few hours a day. It is the color of the midnight sky, the only color that will totally and completely relax the muscles of the eyes, that is the most important thing. In the past, this method had healed even shattered eyes. Try lying on your back with your feet flat on the floor, knees pointed to the ceiling, with your hands resting quietly on your belly." This posture would reduce tension in the lower back and in the neck and would also allow for less restricted breathing. While doing this meditation, Webber could put his palms on his eyes to further relax them. But the emphasis of this visualization meditation was to achieve "a quiet, spacious-feeling state of mind," said Webber.

Second, Namgyal Rinpoche told him to "move the eyes up, down, left, and right, and around in circles, as well as on diagonals."

Third, he said he must "blink frequently."

And fourth, he said, "Sun your eyes. Sit at a forty-five-degree angle to the sun, in morning or later afternoon when the sun is lower in the sky, eyes closed, to let the warmth and light penetrate through all the eye tissues, like taking a warm bath for the eyes, ten to twenty minutes a day."

That was it. He was given no explanation about how this treatment would help his blindness, except that deep relaxation of the eyes was essential.

These techniques sound remarkably similar to some that Bates used for less severe conditions. For instance, Bates also emphasized covering the eyes with one's palms to relax them, blinking, and spending long periods looking into the sun with eyes closed. (Webber told me he later heard a Bates practitioner comment that Bates had learned palming from ancient Eastern traditions.)

Webber didn't really know what to do with these low-tech suggestions. He was desperately tense from the constant pain, and his fiery left eyeball felt as if it were exploding with pressure.

Simple though the exercises were, he couldn't do them. When he began to perform the key exercise, the blue-black meditation, he found, to his great disappointment, that it made him much more anxious because "I was unable to do it even for a few moments. My damaged optic nerves threw off a continuous stream of visual 'noise' in the form of white and gray flashing lights in the center of my visual field." (As I listened to his story, I thought of how these disturbing firework sensations were probably the signs of a noisy, dysregulated nervous system, which can occur when there is sensory damage. The optic nerves are the most forward extension of brain tissue in the body, and damage to them would likely have interfered with his entire visual circuit.) Simple "palming" made him restless. None of the Buddhist exercises, all of which had a meditative component, were able to calm him or relax his eyes even for a few moments, let alone hours a day.

Putting It All Together

A Feldenkrais practitioner, Marion Harris, invited Webber to an ATM class, hoping it might help him relax, though she didn't encourage him to believe it would help his eyesight. By coincidence, he had grown up a few streets over from Harris. In 1999 he started with Harris's weekly ATM lessons. "I figured one thing I could do was roll around on the floor, and I really enjoyed it." As time passed, he found that the ATMs were reducing his anxiety and overall tension. A year later he decided to train to become a Feldenkrais practitioner, a profession he could practice without using his eyes, because the lessons were conducted by speaking to clients and gently moving their limbs. As he grew blind, he had developed a subtle sense of touch—a common neuroplastic adaptation.

During his training, Webber learned that Feldenkrais had left a legacy of more than one thousand ATMs, from his weekly lessons in Tel Aviv, including a one-hour lesson on the eyes, called "Covering the Eyes." He got a tape recording of it to listen to. The lesson was billed not as a cure for blindness but as a series of exercises that could improve vision in the sighted. As is typical of an ATM, it instructed the pupil to lie down on the floor, to eliminate the strain of gravity—just as Namgyal Rinpoche had said.

He lay down on the floor and listened. Webber immediately realized that the exercise was Feldenkrais's exploration and modification of Bates and was also uncannily close to the Buddhist exercises. "I could feel the changes in my eyes the moment I started doing that lesson," he said. "I knew I had the tools to achieve a total relaxation of the nervous system and relax my eyes completely and heal my nervous and immune systems. As the lesson progressed, I experienced the eyeballs in their orbits, their weight and shape"—*orbit* being the medical term for the bony eye socket in which the eyes sit. "I could feel the backs of the orbits and the efforts of the extraocular muscles as the eyes moved about: left and right, up, down and all around. The process spontaneously released the unconscious tonus held in my eyes. When resting, my eyes felt as if they were floating, like flowers in warm pools. In the course of just one hour, my eye movements had become smooth and felt lubricated, as did the movements of my neck and back. My mind was quiet, spacious, and alert. I was happy: I had found the key. I knew that healing was certain."

In the lesson Webber was to scan his entire body, part by part, and notice any tension or holding, and aim to make his breathing gentle and quiet. Scanning his entire body was necessary, even though the lesson would concentrate on the eyes, because any movement affects the entire body. The taped voice encouraged him to perform all the instructions without exerting effort or straining.

Next, he was to begin palming, covering his eyes with his palms, so that his fingers were on his forehead and his palms were over his eyes but not quite touching them. Palming is crucial because (as Bates emphasized) most people with vision problems suffer from eyestrain as their visual system struggles to take in information. Palming blocks far more light than occurs by simply closing the eyelids, and it gives the optic nerve, and the visual circuits of the brain, a true rest. Palming slowly decreases both movement in the eyes and overall tonus.

The next instruction seemed to have been conceived with Webber in mind:

> Notice that even though your hands are covering your eyes you still see all types of shapes and different colors as in a kaleidoscope. This happens because when your optic nerve is excited it cannot record anything except colors and shapes. This shows that your whole system is not quiet.... Slowly see if, in the background of your eyes, you can find a point that is darker or blacker than its surrounding points. If you look you will slowly see black dots. Look at those black dots and think that they are big and cover the whole background.

In my terms, the excited optic nerve and the unquiet system Feldenkrais described were a sign of a noisy, poorly modulated brain that had to be quieted, in order to restore the balance of neuronal excitation and inhibition.

Next, Webber was to rest. After a long pause, the voice said:

> Uncover your eyes by removing your hands and remain with your eyes closed. Pay attention and slowly move only your eyes [i.e., not the head] only to your right. Do not move your head. Look completely to the right, as if you wanted to see your right ear. Do this movement gradually and slowly, as if your eyes were heavy. You will look forward first and then turn both eyes to the right until, in your mind's eye, you can see your right ear. Then slowly return your eyes to the front.

Moving the eyes to the right, without moving the head, was a typical Feldenkrais maneuver. Usually when a person looks to the right, he turns his head and spine, as though they are locked together. Feldenkrais was asking the pupil to differentiate eye movement from head and neck movement—to make him aware that he could move his eyes independently, with little effort.

Webber was to rest again. Then the voice asked, "Where is 'in front'? Most people find that unclear. A person can move his eyes a little right or left and still feel that his eyes are 'in front.' That is one of the things that disturbs clear vision. In your feeling, or sensations, clarify the location of 'the front.'"

Here Feldenkrais had been working on a problem Bates had found in all people with vision problems, which Bates called inadequate "central fixation." People can see fine detail only with the central portion of the six-millimeter macula, which is near the center of the retina. But the retina is not like a film in a camera. All the film used in a camera is equally sensitive to detail; not so in the eye. Only the macula, which is densely filled with cells called cones, can detect fine details. So it must be aimed precisely. But Bates discovered that because of habits of modern life, people's aim is imprecise, so the image falls on cells outside the macula, called rods, that don't detect details, contributing to the blurred vision.

Human beings evolved to use their eyes at many different distances: as hunters to spy animals far off, as gatherers to collect small seeds. Today people increasingly spend most of the day at computers and smartphones, reading hurriedly, looking only short distances ahead. Fast readers take in most of a line of text in one "eye gulp," so they cannot see all the words clearly. Repeat that thousands of times, and we wire this way of using the eyes into the brain: a sloppy use of central fixation and a neglect of distance and peripheral vision.

Bates found that when he asked a person with a central fixation problem—who didn't know how to aim her macula—to read an eye chart, he got odd results. The person might find that the letter she was looking at was blurry, but the one beside it less so. Thus her eye-aim was off. In Feldenkrais's terms, she "didn't know where the front was." By learning to aim the most detail-sensitive part of the eye directly at the object of her attention, she would be able to get a quick improvement in clear sight.

The voice on the tape continued:

> Pay attention that your movement has an equal pace and quietude. Be sure you can notice that your eyes are not jumping large distances. This is not simple. Each eye is accustomed to seeing at specific angles. It sees sharply and clearly where it stops and less clearly in other places. Those are the places where your eyes skip or jump. If you habituate your eyes to move gradually there won't be angles where your eyes don't look. Then your vision can improve. In general your eye is never completely quiet and always makes small movements in order to see.

Feldenkrais was describing saccades and microsaccades. The eye must move to see, but if the macula is not to jump over details, which leads to blurry vision, it must always move smoothly, which can't be done when tonus is high.

His next instructions emphasized more unusual, nonhabitual movements of the eyes, practiced first slowly, then quickly. As the tonus went down, Webber was instructed to scan himself for changes, to see if his nervous system had relaxed. If it had, it would show up in his ability to see black:

> Cover your eyes with your hands again and discover if you see larger patches of black. You might see one spot that is blacker than its surroundings. Think that the whole background is slowly turning blacker. Think that the inside of your eyelids are like black wet velvet. That is the type of black your whole optic nerve sees when it is calm and not doing any movement or receiving any impulses. This is the darkest black a human can see.

Webber remembers that the tape went on to describe other movement variations and visualizations, but the basic structure of the lesson promoted some of the major stages of neuroplastic healing that I have observed as necessary to quiet the noisy brain.

First, palming, by turning on the parasympathetic nervous system, allows the nervous system to settle, relax, and rest. This neurorelaxation stage allows the nervous system to rest and gather energy that will be necessary for learning and differentiation.

Second, neuromodulation occurs as the imbalance between excitation and inhibition is being adjusted. Webber first became aware of signs of excess excitation when he noticed the flashing bright colors. Then, with that awareness, he also noticed darker areas, which were associated with the inhibited parts of the visual system. By using his mind to imagine the black areas expanding, he was proactively modulating his nervous system, restoring the balance between excitation and inhibition in his visual system.

Third, once a modulated state has been reached, a series of increasingly fine differentiations can be made. The differentiations cannot be so difficult that the person leaves the settled state. They must be done with ease. But they must be demanding enough to be beyond what the brain has been previously capable of. One way to bring these differentiations about was to perform very slow, smooth eye movements, teaching the eyes not to skip over more of the visual field than necessary.

Finally, once the differentiation has been learned, the effect of these new changes on the whole nervous system is observed, appreciated, and enjoyed. This is essential, because it brings the awareness that change is possible and pleasurable, which encourages the brain to consolidate the neural networks and activities that led to the change.

When Webber finished performing the nonhabitual eye movements with sensory awareness, he noticed something pleasant and unexpected: he was now able to feel his eyeballs in their orbits. The lesson "served to bring the eyes back into my self-image, through direct sensing of my body parts. This was especially true for the 'dead' right eye." During the course of his blindness, it had disappeared from his body image. The body image has both a mental component (our subjective sensory awareness of our body) and a brain component (in the sensory neurons of our brain maps). Webber no longer had a sense of where the eye was in his head. Because it is a use-it-or-lose-it brain, when a sensory function is disturbed, the body part affiliated with it stops sending normal sensations from it to the brain. As we've seen, Feldenkrais believed the mind either ceases to represent an unused body part or alters the representation, shrinking it in the brain map. In this brilliant observation, he anticipated the work of the neuroplastician Michael Merzenich, who showed, using microelectrode brain mapping, that when an animal doesn't use a body part, the brain map for that part shrinks or is reallocated to represent other parts.

THE QUESTION ARISES: WHY DIDN'T the Bates and Buddhist exercises, which contained the fundamental insights, work for Webber without Feldenkrais's modifications? Webber answered, "I did not feel I had the skill or energy to meditate without distraction. I needed something more efficient at that time of great weakness to reorganize the neuromuscular system." Because he had so much pain, so much inflammatory and surgical wounding of his eyes, he had developed, as he put it, "all sorts of reflex ways of holding them that locked in the high tonus." The Feldenkrais method's use of nonhabitual, differentiated movements, its slow pacing, and its rest periods prevented Webber from responding with his habitual, compulsive reflexes. "The Feldenkrais lesson seemed to disarm my defenses. The constant and surprising shifts of attention throughout the lesson, and the explicit search to notice differences, kept me interested, alert, and engaged in the process. I was ripe for change." Feldenkrais's addition of movement prepared the way for Webber to make use of his meditative skills.

How Visualization of Blue-Black Relaxes the System

How visualizing blue-black may relax the eyes and tonus in the visual system, and why visualization can be so effective generally, is revealed in many recent studies. Brain scans show us that generally *many of the same neurons that fire when we perceive something in the external world also fire when we first remember that object or experience*. In the brain, imagining an act and doing it are not as different as they may seem. As discussed in detail in *The Brain That Changes Itself*, in the chapter called "Imagination," when people close their eyes and visualize a simple object, such as the letter *a*, the primary visual cortex lights up in brain scans, just as it would if the people were actually looking at the letter *a*, and this happens with complex imagery as well.*

Because visualization—which is a use of imagination and memory—activates the same neurons that are activated when we have the real experiences, visualizing negative experiences or memories triggers all the negative emotional reactions that we had with the original experience—wiring them more deeply into our brains. But on the upside, visualizing, remembering, or imagining pleasant experiences activates many of the same sensory, motor, emotional, and cognitive circuits that fired during the "real" pleasant experience. This is why hypnotists can get a very anxious person to visualize a pleasant scene and rapidly put him into a totally relaxed state; it is also why visualizing one's athletic or musical performance can improve that performance. As I showed in Chapter 8 of *The Brain That Changes Itself*, when people do mental practice, just imagining doing scales on an instrument, they improve almost as much as when they play the instrument physically. Brain scans also show that those who do "mental practice" develop changes in the same brain areas, to roughly the same extent, as those who do "physical practice."

What Feldenkrais and Bates were doing, with visualization of blue-black with eyes closed, was putting the visual system into the identical state it is in when no light is impacting it, allowing it to rest and recover its energy. But doesn't simply closing the eyes, or sleeping, achieve this state? No, because closed eyes still let some light in; and more important, imagining scenes, or dreaming with eyes closed, lights up the visual system. Thus, palming closed eyes appears to relax them more than

---

* A team of researchers from UCLA and the Weizmann Institute, in Israel, showed TV programs, such as *Seinfeld* and *The Simpsons*, to epileptic patients who were undergoing neurosurgery and who had microelectrodes implanted in their brains. The researchers showed patients a series of 5- to 10-second clips and made recordings from one hundred neurons that fired as they watched. They then distracted the patients. After some time, they asked the patients, "What comes to mind when you remember the *Simpsons* clip?" The same neurons that fired when they watched that clip now fired when they remembered it. The same thing happened with the *Seinfeld* clips—the neurons *specific* for the *Seinfeld* clips fired. In other words, the same neurons fire when one perceives an event or visualizes it immediately after the fact. See H. Gelbard-Sagiv et al., "Internally Generated Reactivation of Single Neurons in Human Hippocampus During Free Recall," *Science* 322, no. 5898 (2008): 96–101.

sleeping. That is why the palming and meditative techniques of visualizing pure blue-black were essential to healing Webber's visual system and eyes.

Vision Returns: The Hand-Eye Connection

His vision began to return. As he made slow, steady progress, doing all the exercises daily, he tapered off the steroids. He added his own innovations, teaching himself to stimulate his eyes by gently squeezing them using only his external eye muscles, in order to stimulate the draining of dead cells and lower the pressure within his eyes. On a visit to his ophthalmologist in July 2009, he had 20/40 vision in his left eye with glasses (which he needed only because his own lenses had been surgically removed). Even his right eye, which had been 20/800, had improved to 20/200.

He began tinkering with other Feldenkrais exercises and drew on another Feldenkrais concept to bring his vision to a new level.

Shortly before he died, Feldenkrais became fascinated with the hand-eye connection. Recall from the previous chapter that Feldenkrais developed an exercise where a pupil was to bend the head, with as little effort or movement as possible, while being aware of its effect on the left side of the body, and that this soon lowered tonus in the neck, which then generalized to lower tonus throughout the entire left side of the body. Performing such a small pattern with awareness, in one part of the nervous system, can soon relax the entire body and lower anxiety, by inhibiting the excess firing of the motor cortex.

Feldenkrais began exploring what happened when a person simply opened and closed a hand—the slightest bit. He asked a pupil to imagine softening her palm, then open and close the fingers, drawing them in and out, very gradually, about a quarter of an inch, or less if the fingers were tight, while observing the effects on the rest of the body. This movement could be almost effortless, because when we inhale, the fingers and the hand tend to open a minute amount, then contract on exhalation. He called the lesson "The Bell Hand," to emphasize that the hand is shaped like a bell; the opening and closing of the hand

and fingers were so small they were like the vibratory movements of a bell.

Just becoming aware of the movement, and any hand tonus, allows the tonus to diminish not only in the hand but soon in much of the rest of that side of the body and eventually in the whole body. The hand, because it is used so much, has massive representation in the motor cortex. The brain map for the hand is very close to the map for the face and eyes, perhaps because when children see something with their eyes, they reach for it *simultaneously* with their hands, and neurons that fire together wire together. "The neurological pathways," Webber said, "that link hands and eyes are like a superhighway in the brain. I speculated that by using this connection, I could spread learning, and inhibition of tonus, from the neurons representing my hands, directly to the neurons in the motor cortex that controlled the tonus and gross movements of the eyes."

So Webber began opening and closing his hands regularly, and once his hands reduced their tonus, he brought them to his eyes and palmed them. The muscular tensions and quick jerky movements in his eyes were in stark contrast to the relaxed state of his hands. Then just by observing that difference—making that sensory differentiation—his brain began to gradually release the tonus in his eyes. It was, he said, as though his eyes, in the presence of such relaxed hands, "felt safe. It was almost like the tension in the eyes just dissolved into the emptiness of the hands."

These releases occur spontaneously, without effort; indeed, trying to release tonus with effort frequently backfires. An overly tense nervous system, when supplied with correct information—a reminder of how different relaxation and tension feel—often allows tense parts to match relaxed parts. Simple awareness is an agent of change, as when a person becomes aware he is holding his breath when tense: he releases it automatically.

Webber found that by using the Bell Hand he could turn off his sympathetic fight-or-flight system quickly, which "put me into a very receptive, parasympathetic learning state that inhibited a significant amount of noise in my sensory and motor cortex, which then spread to the eyes and the rest of my system." He realized that he could use the Bell Hand exercise to enable the part of himself of which he was most consciously aware (his hand) to teach his more unconscious part (his eyes) how to move, to release tonus, and to improve.

As he normalized the tonus in his eyes, the blood circulation to them increased, as did the range and smoothness of his eye movements, allowing him to get more information to his visual cortex. He did the Bell Hand exercises one or two hours a day. After six weeks of this regimen, he returned to his ophthalmologist, and his vision was 20/20 in the left eye, with glasses. He asked the doctor, who was as delighted as he was, what he thought was causing the change. The doctor paused and said, "It must be cognitive," meaning a change in the brain. He now wears his glasses only for some activities.

CRETE SEEMED THE IDEAL PLACE for Webber to consolidate his gains. He had lived there as a young man, planted olive trees that had now matured, and knew its fresh food and its recuperative pace. He moved back in 2006 and was energized by the elements: the sea, the air, and the mountain walks through ancient villages of stone during all four seasons. He thought, in Feldenkraisian terms, that removing himself from his Toronto routine, with its hidden triggers for his habits, might free his nervous system to reorganize itself; in this respect, his retreat to Crete recalled the routine advice of physicians of an earlier time, who knew that sometimes the best chance for recovery lay in radically changing the surroundings to provide months of deep, sustained rest to strengthen one's constitution.

At first, Webber suffered great loneliness, but then he found a community. He noticed, as only one who was formerly blind could, that he was less reliant on seeing. His brain had reorganized during the period of blindness. "As I relied less and less on my eyes for organizing my world, my mind became increasingly clear and peaceful." He hoped that this Mediterranean life would further settle his nervous system, which in turn might stop his autoimmune disease from attacking more organs. Though the nervous and immune systems are sharply distinguished in textbooks, they are not in our bodies, as the new science of neuroimmunology makes clear. Stress can trigger immune reactions. Settling the neuroimmune system, he hoped, would further improve his vision and prevent relapses.

He returned occasionally to Toronto, to visit his physician. On one of his visits to his ophthalmologist, as he sat in the waiting room among so many who were going blind or had serious vision problems, he thought of all such waiting rooms everywhere, "filled with people who couldn't do anything about it. I felt if I ever get out of this jam, I want to help other people."

He now thought he might have some tools to honor his pledge. At a Feldenkrais conference, he met one of Feldenkrais's original students, Carl Ginsburg, a practitioner who lived in Germany. Ginsburg, on hearing Webber's story, wanted to learn from him and invited Webber to join him in presenting at his workshops in Mainz, Bavaria, and Vienna. Ginsburg had injured his cornea years before, which left him in much pain. A lesson from one of Feldenkrais's close assistants, Gaby Yaron, had healed him.

Thus far Webber had helped himself by doing ATMs. Now Ginsburg gave him Functional Integration lessons. Because Webber had walked and moved for years without vision, he now had to reorganize his body to integrate his new sight.

Most people in a Functional Integration lesson are almost in a trance and lack the vocabulary to describe all the subtle movements. But Webber was able to recall them, minutely. He experienced a total reorganization of how he held his body as well as an emotional reorganization, the like of which is seldom seen except in a profoundly effective psychotherapy or psychoanalysis.

In the first several of seven sessions with Ginsburg, Webber explored the difference between each side of his body and discovered that he was somewhat unstable when he stood on his right leg, and that he had a concentrated knot of muscle in his right calf. As the layers of more obvious tonus in the calf were eliminated, he became better able to feel deeper layers of tonus that he had not yet recognized in the backs of his eyes, and in his neck, back, and pelvis, all the way down to his legs. The tonus felt "compact. . . . From inside, my breathing pushed against what felt like a wall running along the plane of my back." As the work went forward, "I saw in a flash that this wall was anxiety and fear compacted. At the same time, I also felt it to be a structural phenomenon—the muscles at the back of my eyes, diaphragm, and pelvis were gripping and shaped by this density like tree roots growing in rocky ground. While the fear I felt was very real, the wonder at experiencing it in this new way dissolved my need to be afraid. I felt entirely safe to breathe."

When he stood up from the table, he felt more balanced. "When I walked about, it was obvious to me that this wall—built of fear—had been an unknown part of myself, related to my eyes, and had been defining my posture for years." Now as he walked, the fear became more transparent and began to fade in and out and then "dissolved on its own accord like smoke." Mentally recognizing the tonus he carried—the wall of tension—was enough to allow his nervous system to release it and the emotion connected to it.

In one dramatic session, with Webber lying on his back, Ginsburg gently lifted his head. Webber said: "As he made small, very delicate movements with the bones of my head, and my ears, I seemed to be unwinding deep inside my skull. My breath deepened. He brought his thumbs to the upper ridge of both temples. I suddenly felt myself going blind once again: alone, curled up in a world of sadness. In my mind I saw my right eyeball fall out of my head and disappear somewhere between my ear and the floor. I felt this as the death of sight. Grief and sorrow poured through me in waves from head to toe. Held in the space of Carl's attention, I felt safe. I was able to breathe and let the full force of these very strong and difficult feelings, thoughts, and memories pass through me in waves. As I watched, I felt muscles letting go in my lower back and warmth spread into my pelvis. My right eye came back in my awareness. I felt its weight and round shape. It found a new resting place deep in the center of the socket."

Webber felt that seeing was now reintegrated into his way of being, so that when he moved his body—to look at the horizon, for instance—his spine, ribs, neck, and pelvis made all the adjustments necessary for that to be an easy movement. He had worked through a significant part of the psychological trauma of going blind by reexperiencing, in a dreamlike fantasy, what it felt like to lose his sight. (His right eyeball falling out of his head was a beautiful symbol of his loss.) Then, having made all his unconscious fantasies, fears, and postures conscious, he emerged with a new mental and physical organization that felt free. At the end of the session, Ginsburg noticed that even Webber's face had changed: the whole right side had lengthened.

A Move to Vienna

In 2010 a Viennese ophthalmologist, Dr. Christine Dolezal, attended a workshop Webber gave in Vienna, where he shared some of his techniques. She realized that a combination of her work and Webber's would help many of her patients, and soon they teamed up. The eyes "organize" and control how we hold our heads, and our heads control how we hold our bodies; Dolezal realized that most of her patients who had lost central (macular) vision strain their eyes to see details, causing them to tighten their necks and upper bodies, and they start to feel unsafe and unbalanced.

While Dolezal gave them conventional ophthalmological treatment, Webber helped them work on their body organization and improved their ability to coordinate the use of their eyes, necks, and other body parts, which further helped their vision. Patients who worked at computers all day long had developed problems focusing and were getting headaches and neckaches; they could, with Webber's help, feel less distress, and increasingly work without glasses. He helped children with misaligned eyes (strabismus), which can lead to double vision. Often people with misaligned eyes develop a secondary problem. Their brain, in an attempt to eliminate the double vision, stops processing input from one of the eyes, leading to a condition called "lazy eye" (amblyopia). He helped those children as well. And he helped a legally blind man, who was housebound after having lost his central vision from a complication of uveitis, to improve his vision and resume a social life.

• • •

THESE ANCIENT BUDDHIST IDEAS—MODIFIED BY Bates, Feldenkrais, and Webber—have been dismissed in the West due to a lack of understanding of plasticity, brain circuitry, the role of movement in vision, and the fact that the brain is so connected to the body. In this chapter I have focused on their role in a single case of blindness. Because vision is so complex, there are many paths to blindness. I make no claim that what Webber did for himself will work in all cases. I argue only that the natural vision principles behind what he did can be applied far more widely than is done now, from the milder problems of those who have blurry vision to more serious ones, and to prevent future vision problems.

There are now new neuroplastic exercises for rewiring many aspects of the visual system. Michael Merzenich and his colleagues at Posit Science have developed computer-based brain exercises to expand peripheral vision that are used with the elderly to keep them driving automobiles into their most advanced years and to help limit car accidents. Another company, Novavision, has developed brain exercises that can help people who had strokes, brain injuries, or tumor surgeries in their visual cortex, causing their visual fields (the amount of a scene they can see) to be radically reduced. Studies show that computer-based exercises can reexpand the visual fields—sometimes modestly, but every bit helps. And we saw in Chapter 4 that low-level lasers can improve visual fields.

Related to natural vision therapy is the relatively unknown field of behavioral optometry, which for almost one hundred years has understood that vision is a group of skills that can be trained. The field relies on neuroplasticity. The neurobiologist Susan Barry, Ph.D., spent fifty years with two-dimensional vision because she had strabismus—her eyes were misaligned. As we've seen, in response to the double vision caused by the misalignment, the brain turns off input from one eye, so the visual cortex for that eye gets no stimulation. To see in 3-D, the brain needs input from two eyes, which scan the visual field from slightly different angles. With neuroplasticity-based training from her behavioral optometrist, Barry reawakened and rebalanced her visual cortex and finally experienced 3-D at the age of fifty, as she compellingly described in her book *Fixing My Gaze*. Plasticity exists, from cradle to grave.

THE VERY PLASTICITY OF THE visual system, which allowed Webber, Barry, and others to rewire their brains, has been a blessing to them; but with our frequent use of computers, we are all rewiring our visual systems, biasing them toward central fixation. North American children are thought to spend up to eleven hours a day looking at screens. Their peripheral vision is being underused.

The situation will not be improved when Google Glass recruits the small amount of peripheral vision left free, so that even when people are walking down the street, they will be able to access the Internet and be less present. Google Glass will be used not for scanning the periphery but for more "central vision" purposes, making the user less attentive to what is going on at the margins. It is at the margins where the dangers and opportunities we are not paying attention to lurk. Novelty lives *there*.

The unintended consequence of such devices, which don't take our biology into account, is to take us further from the principles of natural vision necessary to preserve good eyesight. Each new technology that adults embrace not only influences themselves but also becomes formative for the young, their "normal" experience. But what we do with our eyes molds our brains and guides its development—literally. The eyes have the power to turn brain plasticity on or off. In fact, a recent and remarkable study shows that in the visual system, neuroplastic change begins *not* in the brain but in the eyes. A team led by Takao Hensch, of Harvard Medical School, and Dr. Alain Prochiantz, of École Normale Supérieure, demonstrated that in newborn mice, the retina sends a protein called Otx2 to the brain, instructing it to enter a very plastic phase that allows accelerated learning and plastic change to take place. They were able to use labeling techniques to track the protein as it travels from the retina. Basically, as Hensch put it, "The eye is telling the brain when to become plastic." This finding—that brain plasticity is triggered by changes in the eye in response to visual stimulation—is a powerful demonstration of our core thesis that the brain and mental activity cannot be understood in isolation from the body.

WEBBER HAS FEW REGRETS THAT he restored his sight, but he has some. His greatest agony while blind was that he could no longer see or read emotion on human faces; he had much concern about his own safety and countless inconveniences. Yet as blind people will sometimes say, certain aspects of existence become richer without sight, especially some internal experiences. "It is true that you lose something by being able to see," he said. "I found there was more of a quiet feel to the mind, where I was aware of my thoughts, feelings, and sensations because my mind didn't go into as many associations, because the visual information was not there to trigger it. Without sight, sensing of my internal states was more direct." He feels that the reliance of most sighted people on central vision—especially those of us who sit most of the day at a computer, focusing on a screen a few feet in front of us—at the expense of peripheral vision has a cost. Peripheral vision, which he relied on exclusively, gives the seer context. Central vision, with its focus on detail, can cause us to lose context. "Central vision," he said, "is edges, lines, and details, but they are not in relationship with anything. The addiction to central vision leads us to a sense of nonconnectedness, and that is a fundamental problem."

I asked him, "Are you saying you felt more connected to the world when you didn't have central vision?"

Surprisingly he answered, "Yes, I did. When you feel safe, without having to see the details, you are more in the parasympathetic system. There is a shift that happens, and you are aware of your whole self, embodied in the whole body." He added that as he lost his central vision, and had to rely increasingly on peripheral vision, "my intuitive sense became more available and trustworthy."

The biggest change since getting his vision back, apart from being able to see emotions on faces, "is the sense of agency: that I am able to manipulate the world in a more efficient way. And I see things that are beautiful, and would rather be able to look in Christine's eyes than not"—referring to the fact that he and Dolezal have become romantically involved.

HE WROTE TO ME FROM Crete: his thoughts that the loss of central vision had opened up new kinds of perception for him had called to mind the archetypal figure of the blind seer, Tiresias, who spoke to Odysseus in the underworld in Homer's poem, and of course the legend that Homer himself was blind. In Homer's world, once blinded, one never returns to the land of sight, but one does "see" and even "foresee" what others cannot.

His letter displayed an awareness that sometimes the wisdom of the past can be more instructive than modern science when it goes down a dead end. The ancients (including the ancient Buddhists and perhaps earlier Yogis who first developed the exercises that helped Webber) were not shackled to a machine metaphor for the brain, like the one that has dominated modern science for the past four hundred years. They were free to see sight as a living, growing mental activity and thus to think it possible to develop and nurture vision.

One day Webber wrote me, displaying an appreciation of the visual world that only a man who had gone on his journey to blindness and back could. He described seeing a nearby olive tree, so old it is listed as a national monument: "Its age is estimated at 3,000 years. That goes back to Minoan times. It is vast in scale—the trunk is veins and networks and spaces and chasms. . . . The canopy is about 47 meters across. It is still giving fruit . . . 80 to 100 kilos of oil. Which is down, it seems, from the 220 kilos it used to give in times past. That is many generations of consistent care and attention. Imagine the stories around that tree! The area is populated with many old giants. They seem like humans who simply put down roots and quietly go about their business of living. Often they look like they are dancing—while others are standing in judgment. There is a quality of intelligence in the air in these groves of ancient trees—Athena is still speaking and teaching."

I wondered if he was writing not only of the tree but of how much he had gained from finding a natural way to heal himself, based on knowledge so ancient that for most it is dead, but that for him is totally alive.

Chapter 7

A Device
That Resets the Brain

Stimulating Neuromodulation
to Reverse Symptoms

I. A Cane Against the Wall

First he noticed it was becoming hard to sing, a nightmare because that was how he made his living and singing was who he was. Then he could barely sing at all but could still speak his lines. And then over a couple of years he began to lose his speaking voice, until it became wispy thin and trailed off, so that he could generate only short, barely audible bursts of whispered air.

"It was agonizing to watch him lose his beautiful singing voice, heartbreaking. I fell in love with that voice," said Patsy Husmann, his wife of fifty years. Ron Husmann was a singer of first rank on Broadway, on television, and in film, and throughout the 1960s and 1970s his deep baritone was everywhere. He sang in *Camelot* opposite Robert Goulet. He costarred in *The Gershwin Years* with Frank Sinatra, Ethel Merman, and Maurice Chevalier. He starred on Broadway in *Tenderloin*, and worked with the leading ladies Debbie Reynolds, Julie London, Bernadette Peters, and Juliet Prowse in more than half a dozen other Broadway shows. And he toured as the lead in *Irma La Douce, Show Boat, South Pacific,* and *Oklahoma!* At one point he was in thirteen commercials running simultaneously and appeared on *The Ed Sullivan Show* and in series like *Dr. Kildare, Get Smart, The F.B.I., 12 O'Clock High, Cheers,* and even the soap operas *Search for Tomorrow* and *As the World Turns.* Singing live, in a theater that held three thousand people, Ron could be heard by everyone in the audience without using a microphone, while the rest of the cast required one.

The bass register begins to mature in richness only in a singer's thirties, and it completely fills out in his forties. Ron was at his peak at forty-four when, as he whispered, "it stopped dead."

As with many people who are eventually diagnosed with multiple sclerosis (MS), it took doctors a number of years—nine, in his case—to realize that his lost voice and a complicated package of other symptoms were caused by MS. In MS, one's immune system, instead of attacking invading organisms as it should, turns against the brain and spinal cord and attacks the fatty sheath around the long projections of the nerves. This sheath, called myelin, functions as insulation and can increase the speed of the conduction of a nerve signal fifteen to three hundred times. After being attacked, the myelin sheath, and often the nerve it surrounds, becomes damaged and scarred. (The word *sclerosis* in *multiple sclerosis* means "hardened and scarlike.") Because antibodies can attack myelin almost anywhere in the brain or spinal cord, each patient gets a different version of MS, and each person's symptoms unfold in a different way. Ron's deep voice was stripped of its beauty in a series of onslaughts. First the middle tones began to disappear; then suddenly he didn't have the low notes, for which he was most famous. He went to all the "voice people" who serve performing artists. Onstage, directors had to mike him up so he could be heard, until there was nothing much left to amplify. By the time his singing career was ruined, he was able to hit only about eight notes around middle C.

Next, because the nerves controlling his bladder were damaged, he lost the ability to initiate or stop his urinary stream because he had no feeling in his bladder. "It's like it's disappeared, so I have to remind myself to go. It's dead, there's no signal there." Muscles throughout his body atrophied, and he developed burning and numbness in his arms and legs. Then he began having trouble walking and felt tingling in his legs. At a performance of *Irma La Douce,* Juliet Prowse, on cue, ran across the stage and jumped into his arms, and he collapsed, severely hurting his back.

As the muscles of his legs and arms wasted away, he needed to walk with a cane; then he needed two canes, the kind that go all the way up the arm; then he sometimes had to use an electric cart and gained fifty pounds from lack of exercise. Next he began to have trouble with balance. Standing with his eyes closed, he couldn't keep himself erect. He had trouble swallowing—always a terrifying symptom. He was increasingly choking on his food because the brain stem, which coordinates the rhythmical contractions of the throat muscles, was no longer working properly. His worst symptom was his unrelenting exhaustion. He got to the point where he could only whisper into the phone for perhaps a minute, until his voice broke up so badly that he imagined he would have to stop trying to whisper altogether.

The multiple areas where the nerves are inflamed and scarred and where the myelin is damaged are called plaques, and they can be seen on brain scans. MRIs of Ron's brain showed that many of his plaques were in his brain stem, which sits immediately above the spinal cord and is one of the most densely packed parts of the human brain. The brain stem, as we've seen in Chapter 4, is a subcortical area that regulates many of our most basic functions—breathing, blood pressure, alertness, temperature, and others. It is also the major neural highway—almost all signals from the brain to the body, and from the body to the brain, pass through it. The cranial nerves help regulate most of the motor and sensory functions we associate with the head: eye movements and focus, facial expression, facial movement and sensation, the muscles of the voice, swallowing, as well as taste, sound, and balance. One of the cranial nerves, the vagus nerve, descends directly from the head into the body proper. It regulates digestion and helps regulate the autonomic nervous system—and our fight-or-flight reactions. As we shall see, it even regulates aspects of the immune system, which protects the body from infection and injury.

An Unusual Device

By coincidence, perhaps, a friend of Ron's from high school also developed MS and voice problems. Now a retired professor living in Madison, the friend told Ron that a laboratory there, at the University of Wisconsin, had invented a strange device that you put in your mouth to help MS symptoms. He had tried it as part of a study the lab was doing, and it had actually helped with his voice. The inventors were using the device to treat a range of MS symptoms, not only voice problems. The lab had a strange name, the Tactile Communication and Neurorehabilitation Laboratory, and it was run by three men: Yuri Danilov, a Russian neuroscientist (and former soldier of the Soviet army); Mitch Tyler, an American biomedical engineer (formerly of the U.S. Navy); and Kurt Kaczmarek, an electrical engineer.

The founder of the lab, Dr. Paul Bach-y-Rita, had recruited them. Bach-y-Rita, who had recently died, was a legendary figure, one of the first advocates of using brain plasticity in healing. A physician who worked as a neuroscientist, he was the first of his generation to argue that the brain is plastic from cradle to grave, and he used that understanding to develop devices that facilitated positive plastic change. Devices that he developed helped blind people see and helped restore balance lost after brain damage; they also included computer games for stroke patients to train their brains to restore lost functions.

When Ron arrived at the lab, he saw a small, modestly equipped room in an old building. It had a loading dock at its entrance, the hallway was under construction, and as one patient said, it "did not look like the home for scientific miracles." Ron's attitude was "This may work, this may not. What have I got to lose?" The team reviewed his medical records and did tests and recordings to determine his ability to walk and balance. They took him to the university's voice assessment department and recorded his speech, which was incomprehensible, broken up, and appeared as little dots on the monitor. When the baseline testing was complete, they took out the device he had heard about.

It was small, fitting into a shirt pocket. It had a cloth strap attached, and some of the scientists in the lab wore it hanging around their necks, like a pendant. The part that went into the mouth and rested on the tongue looked like a wide stick of chewing gum. This flat part had 144 electrodes on its underside, which fired off electric pulses, in triplets, at frequencies designed to turn on as many of the tongue's sensory neurons as possible, by generating a pattern of stimulation that roved across the underside of the device. This flat part was attached to a tiny electronics box, about the size of a matchbox, which sat outside the mouth and had some switches and lights on it. Yuri, Mitch, and Kurt called it the PoNS, named, tongue-in-cheek, for a part of the brain stem called the pons, one of the device's main targets. The acronym PoNS stands for Portable Neuromodulation Stimulator, because when it stimulates the neuroplastic brain, it modifies and corrects how the neurons are firing.

The team asked Ron to put the device in his mouth, while he stood as straight as he could. It painlessly stimulated his tongue and its sensory receptors with waves of gentle signals. Sometimes the stimulation tingled, and sometimes it became barely noticeable, and when it did, the team would adjust the dial, turning it up. After a while, they asked him to close his eyes.

After two twenty-minute sessions, Ron was able to hum a tune. After four, he was able to sing again. At the end of the week, he was belting out "Old Man River."

What was most remarkable was that Ron's improvement, after almost thirty years of steadily worsening symptoms, was so rapid. He still had MS, but now his brain circuits were functioning so much better. He stayed at the lab for two weeks, working Mondays through Fridays, practicing with the device in his mouth, resting, and practicing again. He did six sessions a day during the first week—four in the lab, two at home. Electronic voice testing showed huge improvement, a steady stream of sound. His other MS symptoms started to improve. The day he left, the man who had come in wobbling on a cane tap-danced for the team.

I spoke with Ron two months after he returned home to Los Angeles. He had brought the device home to practice with and reinforce his gains. Now that he had his voice back, he was gushing words—at times I had to ask him to talk more slowly, so I could get it all down.

"You can imagine if you haven't sung for twenty-eight years, what it's like suddenly to sing again. The fact that I could carry a tune, and hook one note to another, after four twenty-minute sessions, was astounding and emotional—more than emotional—I broke down. They told me to hum and vocalize while the thing was in my mouth. I gradually realized my voice was getting stronger. The next day Yuri said, 'You don't need that cane.' That day I got rid of it. By the third day, I was able to stand without any support, and with my eyes closed. By the time I left, I could sing two octaves. I was a bass baritone, and I had a low E that I could sing in public, and when I did *Annie Get Your Gun*, I got up to an F sharp. And . . . I can be loud now! I was so loud in their lab, they had to put their fingers in their ears. And now when we walk our dog every night, I walk so fast my wife can hardly keep up with me."

Then he said to me, "Do you realize that we have been talking for a full hour?"

"I wasn't expecting you to sound younger than I do," I said finally. "Your voice sounds like that of a man decades younger."

He took a moment to think. "Well, maybe it should," he laughed. "I haven't used it for thirty years."

Why the Tongue Is the Royal Road to the Brain

The PoNS is in my mouth as I write these words, because the stimulation, in addition to promoting healing, seems to sharpen focus, and I want to get to know its potential. Its signals reach only 300 microns beneath my tongue's surface, turning on the sensory neurons that lie there. (A micron is a thousandth of a millimeter.) The device is providing the neurons just enough stimulation to fire their own electrical signals to the brain, as they would if I put some food on my tongue and felt it there. The team labored for years to use this mild electrical stimulation to create a firing pattern in the sensory neurons that would most closely approximate the way they fire in response to being touched, at 200 Hz, in a rhythm of three signals, pause, three signals.

But why stimulate the tongue? Because the tongue, the team has discovered, is a royal road to activating the entire human brain. The tongue is one of the most sensitive organs in the body. "When the carnivores started to move on the surface of the earth," Yuri points out, "the first points of contact with the earth were the tongue and the tip of the nose. Both are designed for exploring the environment—for close contact. A lot of animals, from insects to giraffes, use the tongue extensively, and it is capable of a highly precise movement, so the brain developed a strong connection to it." And human babies, in the oral phase, try to get to know the world by putting it in their mouths, sensing it with their tongues. There are forty-eight different kinds of sensory receptors on the tongue, fourteen on the tip alone, to sense touch, pain, taste, and so on. These sense receptors pass electrical signals to nerve fibers, then on to the brain. By Yuri's analysis, there are 15,000 to 50,000 nerve fibers on the tip of the tongue, which create a huge information highway. The device sits on the front two-thirds of the tongue, which is supplied by two nerves that receive sensory information from the tongue's receptors. The first, the lingual nerve, is for receiving touch sensation; the second, a branch of the facial nerve, is for receiving taste sensation.

These nerves are part of the cranial nerve system, which connects directly to the brain stem, which sits two inches behind the back of the tongue. The brain stem is where major nerves that enter and exit the brain converge. It is closely connected to the brain's processing areas for movement, sensation, mood, cognition, and balance. Thus, electrical signals that enter the brain stem can turn on much of the rest of the brain simultaneously. Brain scans and EEG recording studies that the Madison team has done on people using the device show that after 400 to 600 milliseconds, brain waves are stabilized, and all parts of the brain start to react, firing together. Many brain problems arise because the brain's networks are not firing together, or because some are underfiring. But often we don't know exactly which circuits are underperforming, even with brain scans. Owing to plasticity, each brain is wired somewhat differently at the microscopic level. So when brain scans show damage to an area in a given patient, we can't be 100 percent certain what goes on in that area. "But our tongue stimulation," says Yuri, "activates the whole brain, so even if I can't see where the damage is, I know the device is turning on the whole brain."

Once the team stimulates a patient's brain, they invent exercises to help a person regain whatever function was lost. The patient is always asked to use the device to stimulate the brain while doing an appropriate exercise. Ron was asked to hum; a person with balance problems would stand on a balance ball with eyes closed; someone with problems walking would try to walk, then run, on a treadmill.

There is something else intriguing about the tongue, of little interest to Western clinicians but of great interest to Yuri Danilov, the team's Russian member. For millennia, the tongue has been of central importance in Chinese and Eastern medicine for making diagnoses because it is an internal organ that can be seen from outside the body.

The Chinese believe that our bodies have energy pathways, called meridians, that convey an energy called *chi* or *qi* through them. Two of these key meridians, "the governing vessel" and "the central vessel," meet at the tongue. Martial artists, tai chi practitioners, and qigong meditators, to improve their performance, often place the tongue on the roof of the mouth, to link those two energy channels. Meridians emerge on the skin surface at acupuncture points. The acupuncture points used by Chinese medicine haven't changed in several thousand years, but as Yuri points out, it has recently been claimed that several points are on the tongue. These tongue points are now being used in Hong Kong to treat traumatic brain injuries, Parkinson's, cerebral palsy, stroke, visual problems, and other neurological problems. Acupuncturists frequently use electrical stimulation (electroacupuncture) instead of needles; possibly the device also functions as a form of electroacupuncture.

Meeting Yuri, Mitch, and Kurt

Yuri Danilov stands six feet six, has a shaved head and the high cheekbones of a Mongolian, and is huge and powerful. He was born in Irkutsk, one of the oldest cities in Siberia. He spent ten years of his childhood north of the Arctic Circle, when his parents, polar geologists, moved the family to Norilsk, a gulag city built by Stalin. Half the people there had been in the gulag, and 100,000 prisoners are buried nearby. Norilsk is the northernmost industrial city in the world, and so cold that when you spit, your saliva turns to ice by the time it hits the ground. Yuri's personal record for standing outside was in weather that was less than minus 65 Celsius, the lowest point on the thermometer. The day after he graduated from university, at twenty-two, the Soviet army stationed him for two years in Murmansk, also north of the Arctic Circle. At times his unit was sent out on exercises opposite NATO Arctic forces, just over the border.

Yuri's scientific interest in Eastern medicine began early. As he was growing up in Siberia, "there were Chinese people everywhere, and teas and Chinese herbs, and we used Chinese medicines and acupuncture in everyday life." As a young man, he created an electrical machine to locate acupuncture points on the skin by detecting the changes in electrical activity over them. He used acupuncture to treat his toothaches and headaches.

Yuri became an accomplished neuroscientist, working in the country's leading lab for visual neuroscience, the famous Pavlov Institute of Physiology, which was part of the Soviet Academy of Sciences. He earned one degree in biophysics (which enables him today to work with engineers), and a Ph.D. at the Pavlov Institute, in neuroscience. His area of greatest expertise is visual neuroscience. He did his research on the neuroplastic properties of the brain's visual system long before it was widely recognized that the brain is plastic. By coincidence, the first article he translated, in 1975, into Russian was by Dr. Paul Bach-y-Rita, the man who set up the lab in Madison where he now works. He also became quite familiar with the use of electrical stimulation to treat sleep and other problems. Electrical sleep machines, unknown in the West, were used in hundreds of clinics throughout the USSR.

When he started at the Pavlov Institute, two thousand people were there, including five hundred scientists, and it was a place of great intellectual rigor, but the economic chaos following the transition from Communism led to thirty rounds of cuts and caused the august institute almost to collapse: there was no longer money for experiments, equipment, electricity, lab animals, drugs, or salaries. In the early 1990s he left the lab to do a sixteen-university tour lecturing about neuroplasticity in the United States and briefly working there. Afterward he returned to Russia to find his lab empty. The equipment that had taken him twelve years to set up, the animals he worked with, the money for experiments, were all gone.

When Yuri arrived in America in 1992, there was no one like him. He was an accomplished, hard-boiled neuroscientist with a long pony-tail, well versed in Eastern movement practices such as yoga, medita-tion, tai chi, and the Russian martial arts, including the system perfected by Russian special forces and Stalin's bodyguards. Fifteen years later he found that aspects of these practices, in combination with the PoNS, could be extremely useful for helping neurologically ill and brain-injured patients to "reset" their brains.

At the Madison lab, Yuri works with patients, and as he discovers strengths and weaknesses in the device, he feeds that information to his codevelopers, Mitch and Kurt.

Mitch is the team's biomedical engineer and study coordinator. He is the interface between Yuri and other collaborating clinicians, and he handles the scientific and technical facets of the research. His task has been to understand how to get information across the skin.

Mitch also practices Eastern martial arts and is a second-degree black belt and an instructor in tae kwon do and a daily mindfulness meditator. He participated in the Cold War, for the United States: when the Soviets launched Sputnik, he was chosen as one of the brightest American kids, to be fast-tracked into a special stream studying math and science. Ultimately he served in the U.S. Navy, tracking Russian convoys, submarines, destroyers, and communications. Mitch and Yuri understand each other, though the understated, gracious, mellow-voiced, California-raised Mitch and the no-nonsense Arctic Yuri are like polar opposites attracting. Mitch has been learning bits of Russian since grad school, when he started reading abstracts of articles not avail-able in English.

Mitch originally trained as a high-tech engineer of electrical machines—he never took a biology course. "I was a bit arrogant," he recalls. "Who needs that soft science, cells and squishy stuff? I am an engineer! We are going to conquer the world!" After a 1981 car accident fractured his spine and left him paralyzed from the navel down, that attitude changed. "Lying in the hospital room, not able to feel my legs, I was terrified. I didn't know how nerves worked." He got a copy of *Gray's Anatomy* from his nurse, and "it became my bible and launched my interest in how I could apply my technical knowledge of circuits to biological systems."

By 1987 he had fully recovered and was working in Paul Bach-y-Rita's lab. Paul was a big-picture thinker who came up with far-out ideas, and Mitch's job was to implement them. His first task with Paul was working on one of his sensory plasticity projects, a condom for paraplegics with spinal cord injuries who had lost all penile sensation. The condom had "tactile pressure sensors" that detected friction in intercourse and transferred the stimulation it detected to electrodes that tickled a part of the body that could feel. This stimulation in turn sent signals to the man's brain. They hoped it might help the demoralized subjects, robbed of the pleasures of intercourse, become sexually excited. It worked.

Kurt Kaczmarek, Ph.D., the third member of the team, is an electrical engineer. Of the three, he worked longest with Dr. Bach-y-Rita, whom he met in 1983 as a student. He is now a senior scientist in the University of Wisconsin's department of biomedical engineering. Slim, Kurt is in his early fifties and has dark blond hair and an earnest, conscientious air. As a boy, growing up north of Chicago, he loved to design, build, repair, and improve electrical devices. He worked for years in a TV repair shop. Even today his hobby is repairing old electronic devices.

Kurt spent twenty-five years learning how to produce synthetic electrical signals that can carry complex information that can be inputted into the skin's touch receptors, then relayed to the brain. Working with Bach-y-Rita, Mitch, and the team, he constructed a device that supplied visual information from a camera to the tongue, then to the brain, allowing blind people to see (described in *The Brain That Changes Itself*). They learned to present the information on the tongue using an array of 144 electrodes and found ways to coordinate the firing sequences of electrodes in wavelike patterns. The team has learned that some wave patterns will put people to sleep, as do the Russian sleep machines; others stimulate them to be more alert, as occurs when people take amphetamines or Ritalin-like drugs.*

Kurt is the team's calculation grinder and deep analytic thinker. He is a genius at taking a concept and translating it into a working physical device. He is probably the world's leading expert on how to use electrical stimulation to speak to the brain through the human skin, a process he calls "electro-tactile stimulation." His long-term project is to use all he's learned to develop guidelines for making electro-tactile devices. But that larger task is always being interrupted now that they have invented the PoNS, because he is constantly redesigning and improving it. "I mean," he says, "people are coming in here with a cane and then walking out without one."

The Early History of the Device

Against the wall of Yuri's small office sits the one cane they have kept, the first that was left behind in this tiny lab. It belonged to Cheryl Schiltz, who came to the lab after being disabled for five years and went home actually dancing. Yuri's office once belonged to the group's founder, Dr. Paul Bach-y-Rita. The story of how Cheryl recovered, and of Bach-y-Rita's own realization that the brain is plastic, was driven by a very personal experience, which I told in detail in *The Brain That Changes Itself.*

In 1959 Paul's sixty-five-year-old father, Pedro, had a stroke that paralyzed his face and half his body and left him unable to speak. The doctors told Paul's brother George that Pedro had no hope of recovery. George, a medical student, was still too early in his medical studies to have learned the doctrine of the unchanging brain. So he began treating his father without preconceived ideas. After two years of daily, intensive, incremental brain and movement exercises, Pedro underwent a complete recovery. After he died (mountain climbing at the age of

---

* Cranial electrotherapy stimulation (CES) devices, such as the Fisher Wallace device or the Alpha-Stim device, apply the stimulation to the head. They are modifications of the Russian sleep machines, and the FDA is proposing they be approved as safe for insomnia, anxiety, and depression. They have been on the market since 1991.

seventy-two!), Paul had an autopsy performed on Pedro and discovered that 97 percent of the nerves in a key pathway in his brain stem were destroyed. Paul had an epiphany: the exercises that Pedro had done had reorganized and rewired his brain and built new processing areas and connections that worked around the stroke damage. It meant that even the brain of an old man was plastic.

Paul's research was in vision. One of his first applications of neuroplasticity was to develop a device to help the blind see. "We see with our brain, not with our eyes," he said, arguing that the eyes are merely a "data port"; its receptor, the retina, converts information from the electromagnetic spectrum that surrounds us—in this case, light—into electrical discharge patterns, which are sent down the nerves. There are no images or pictures in the brain (just as there are no sounds, smells, or tastes), just patterns of electrical-chemical signals. Based on a comparative analysis of the retina and the skin, Paul determined that the skin, too, could detect images, as it does, for instance, when we teach a child the letter A by tracing it on his skin. The skin's touch receptors convert that information into electrical discharge patterns, which are then sent to the brain.

So Paul developed a device consisting of a camera, which sent pictures to a computer, which converted them to pixels (little dots like those that make up the picture on a computer screen), and sent that information to a small plate of electrodes that fits on the tongue—the prototype of the device Ron Husmann used. He called it the "tactile-vision device." Each electrode functioned like a pixel. When the subject aimed the camera at an image, some of the electrodes would fire tiny pulses of controlled electrical stimulation to represent light and slightly fewer to represent gray, while some remained off, to represent darkness. The same image that appeared before the camera appeared on the subject's tongue. Paul and the team decided to use the tongue as the "data port" because it has no layer of dead skin and is moist, so it is a great conductor. And it has so many nerves that Paul thought it would deliver a high-resolution image to the brain.

Subjects who had been blind since birth and used the device were able, with some training, to detect moving and looming objects; they could differentiate the faces of "Betty" and "Twiggy," and they could "see" complex images, such as a vase in front of a telephone. A blind man was able to use the tactile-vision device to detect perspective and even sink a basketball. Paul called this process "sensory substitution." It was a brilliant example of brain plasticity, because circuits in the brain that processed touch reconfigured themselves to connect to the brain's visual cortex.

But the tactile-vision device was doing more than providing a new way to help a blind person see. It showed that, in principle, the brain could be rewired by a sensory experience. The senses provided direct avenues to rewire the brain.

In January 2000, team member Mitch came down with a serious infection that affected his balance apparatus, making him dizzy and unable to stand. He wondered whether the vision device might be adapted for balance problems. Paul agreed it might. Instead of using a camera, they used an accelerometer, a device like a gyroscope that can detect movement and position in space. They put it into a hat that fed information about position to a computer, then fed it to the tongue device, giving Mitch, the subject, information about where he was in space. If he leaned forward, the electrodes would give him gentle stimulation, and he would get a sensation of champagne bubbles rolling forward on his tongue; if he leaned sideways, the bubbles went to the side.

Their first patient was Cheryl Schiltz. Five years earlier, an antibiotic had damaged 97.5 percent of her vestibular apparatus (the balance organ in the ear), seriously disabling her. She was constantly disoriented and needed support to stay upright. Though she was only in her early thirties, she came to the lab with a cane.

When Cheryl inserted the device into her mouth, she was immediately oriented and calmed. The information on her tongue, which went directly to the areas of the brain stem that process *touch*, then found its way to another part of the brain stem, the vestibular nuclei, which process *balance*. The first time she wore the device, it was just for a minute, and after she took it out she was still able to stand for a few seconds and felt great. The next time she tried the device for two minutes, and the residual effect lasted forty seconds. The residual effect grew with training and practice, stretching into days, then months, until, after two and a half years of use, she no longer needed to wear the device at all. With training, Cheryl's brain was developing new circuits. She was completely cured. At this point, the account in *The Brain That Changes Itself* ended.

BUT CHERYL'S STORY DID NOT end there. She was so moved by her recovery that she decided to go back to school to become a rehabilitation professional. She did her internship at the Bach-y-Rita lab. Her job was to train people to use the device that had helped her. She never dreamed who her first patient would be. Shortly after Cheryl was cured, I received an awful e-mail from Paul. He had received devastating personal news. He had been coughing, and, though he had never smoked, he was diagnosed with lung cancer that had metastasized to his brain. He underwent chemotherapy, with cisplatin, the cancer retreated, and he was able to go back to work. But just as an antibiotic had destroyed Cheryl's balance, Paul's chemotherapy destroyed his. It fell on Cheryl to train Paul to use the device he had helped invent. His balance problem was cured, and he returned to work. But in December 2005 he wrote to me that "the cancer returned . . . I have even less energy!" He was able to work until shortly before he died in November 2006—about a year before neuroplasticity finally achieved wide recognition.

Dead Tissue, Noisy Tissue, and New Thoughts About the Device

One of Paul's last published works was a paper called "Is It Possible to Restore Function with Two-Percent Surviving Neural Tissue?" Here he reviewed his own work, as well as literature on humans and animals, and found an interesting coincidence. His father, Pedro, had lost 97 percent of the nerves that ran from his cerebral cortex through the brain stem to the spine. Doctors had shown that 97.5 percent of Cheryl's vestibular apparatus had been damaged. Evidence from other sources also indicated that it was possible to restore lost functions with only

2 percent of surviving neural tissue. Paul's theory was that in his father's case the rehabilitation had "apparently unmasked previously existing pathways that, prior to injury, had not had the same relationship to the recovered functions." Unmasking accounted for the neuroplastic rewiring.

But Paul, Yuri, and the team thought Cheryl's difficulties with balance had stemmed not only from loss of functioning tissue but also from the fact that her vestibular system had become very noisy: its damaged neurons were giving off disorganized, random signals that blocked detection of any useful signals from any remaining bits of healthy tissue. The balance device, which gave Cheryl more accurate information on where she was in space, reinforced the signals from the healthy neurons. Over time the brain neuroplastically reinforced these circuits, leading to her residual effect.

As I discussed in Chapter 3, the "noisy" brain, with a poor signal-to-noise ratio, applies to many forms of brain damage because surviving but damaged neurons don't necessarily "fall silent," but may still fire electrical spikes, just at different rates and rhythms than normal. In the brain, these aberrant signals can "mess up" the functioning of the healthy neurons they are connected to, and which are receiving chaotic input—unless the brain can shut down the damaged neurons. In engineering terms, Cheryl had a poor signal-to-noise ratio, meaning that not enough strong clear signals in her networks could be detected against the backdrop of other signals in the brain—the noise. A noisy brain can't perform its normal functions and soon stops doing so. Then learned nonuse sets in.

When asked to describe what it felt like to experience her brain before and after putting the device on, she said, "I always had this constant noise in my head, and not a noise I could hear, but this feeling of noise. If you could hear confusion, that is what it would sound like. And my brain was really, really confused because it didn't know what to do. I was so consumed with trying to stand up, and stay straight, and get from point A to point B. It is like you are in a room with a bazillion people talking all at once. That was what it felt like in my head. When I put that device in, it was just like, aaah, I had stepped out of that room, and I'm standing on the side of the ocean, and oh my gosh, it's quiet. It's still. But it feels so good. It's like I came back."

MEANWHILE YURI, THE GROUP'S SURVIVING neuroscientist, was struck by a number of things. When Cheryl was wearing the device, she appeared to enter a deep meditative state (the kind of relaxed state that I argue follows neuromodulation and is so helpful for neuroplastic healing). This was a surprise. Also, she and others who came to the lab for balance problems began to notice multiple unexpected yet welcome responses to the device. Though balance was the target, they saw improvements in sleep, multitasking, concentration, focus, movement, and mood. The treatment was showing benefits for patients who had different problems, such as stroke and traumatic brain injury. A few with Parkinson's, who had come for balance problems, found that their Parkinson's movement problems seemed to diminish.

The team's initial working hypothesis was that the device Cheryl used (which came to be called the Brain Port) provided accurate *information* to her brain about where she was in space, transmitted by the moving "champagne bubble" stimulation, and that it was this information that quieted her noisy brain, by overriding the inaccurate signals given off by her damaged tissue. The accurate information sent input to the 2.5 percent of her existing healthy tissue, exercised it, helped it build up stronger connections, and possibly recruited other brain areas to take over balance processing as well. The electrical stimulation was a medium for delivering that valuable information.

Yuri had a heretical thought. Maybe the electrical stimulation was providing a significant part of the cure. If it was only the information about where she was in space that was curative, he wondered, then why didn't Cheryl's problem get better when she looked at a wall with straight lines, or when her shoulders were touched with a finger whenever she leaned to the side? And why was the device helping so many other brain problems?

Yuri began to suspect that the energy stimulation itself was helping— as it did in the Russian sleep machines, when they cured insomnia.

"Yuri," says Mitch, "became cheerleader for the idea that it was the electrical stimulation on the tongue that was inducing the changes." At about that time, another group at another lab designed a study of the device, comparing users of the original device with a control group that got a version of the device that fired random electrical signals rather than information about where the subject was in space, on the assumption that random stimulation wouldn't provide useful information. "No!" Yuri protested, "that won't be a good control . . . the electrical stimulation alone will help." And it did.

What this suggested to Yuri was that the electrical stimulation, which *started* on the tongue's sensory receptors and sent "spikes" to balance neurons in the brain stem, didn't stop there. The neurons in the brain stem's balance system were obviously sending spikes throughout much of the rest of the brain stem and other parts of the brain, activating them all, including areas that regulated sleep, mood, movement, and sensation. This hypothesis was confirmed when a subject used the device while his entire brain was scanned. Most of the brain lit up.

This result helped explain how the device was helping other disabilities or brain problems, especially when Yuri paired its use, and the information on balance that it provided, with appropriate mental and physical stimulation and exercises. Perhaps the device would alleviate other kinds of brain damage and, who knows, even assist ordinary learning? Paul's protégés, so eager to continue his work, suddenly suspected that they had in their hands an insight and a discovery that might allow them to make an all-purpose brain stimulator. So they made a new device, the PoNS, that, instead of providing information on where the user was in space, just provided ongoing stimulation.

Yuri knew of three other kinds of stimulators that worked like the PoNS, targeting the brain with very low stimulation. In vagus nerve stimulation (VNS), an electrode is coiled around the left vagus nerve (a cranial nerve near the carotid artery in the neck), which sends stimulation to the brain stem's nucleus tractus solitarius, one of the areas targeted by the device. At times VNS works for depression, but it requires surgery to implant a pacemaker into the chest to fire electrical stimulation. Another kind, deep brain stimulation (DBS), has been used on patients with Parkinson's disease or depression, to target the circuits involved directly, with some success. But with DBS, a surgeon must implant electrodes deep in the brain. The PoNS is matter-of-factly held in the mouth as a child might hold a lollipop.

It was time to start gathering patients with different conditions and see whether this new device would help them.

II. Three Resets: Parkinson's, Stroke, Multiple Sclerosis

Parkinson's Disease

Anna Roschke has had Parkinson's disease for twenty-three years. She is now eighty years old and got her first symptoms when she was in her late fifties. She was brought to Wisconsin for treatment from Germany, where her doctors had given up on helping her further. She couldn't walk, maintain balance, pour a glass of milk without spilling, or control her tremor. Her speech was slowed, and she couldn't maintain a flow of conversation. Her son, Victor Roschke, a molecular biologist who develops drugs to fight cancer, said, "She was in bad shape. Her tremor was her worst symptom. The doctors were adjusting the doses of her medicines, and the medication was keeping the disease under control to some extent . . . but they said at this point there was nothing else they could do about the illness. Basically they had run out of options." She knew she had done well, for a while, for a person with an early diagnosis of a progressive disease, but still she dreamed she might make herself useful by doing small meaningful things, such as baking cookies for her grandchildren. But she was so frozen into the immobility of advanced Parkinson's disease that all she could do most days was to sit in front of a window and look out, or stare at television.

The team had reason to think the device might help. Brain scans of patients with balance problems had shown, to their surprise, that when patients used the device, the globus pallidus, a part of the brain that becomes hyperactive in Parkinson's disease, lit up.

After two weeks on the device, Anna recovered her abilities to speak and walk, and her tremor was diminished. She no longer needed a walker, and "she could walk quite normally," Victor says. "It was the most striking observation. We also noticed there was a remarkable improvement in how she spoke. It was our impression that, other than her tremor, she appeared like a normal person."

She continued to use the device regularly. When Victor next visited, he learned that his eighty-year-old mother had been found standing on her kitchen tabletop, painting the ceiling with *Hausfrau* thoroughness. "It was a horrifying story," he laughs, knowing how much his mother loved to be active and useful. Considering how disturbed her balance and movement had been, he says, "it was amazing she was able to do it and not fall." During the day she now goes to the park, moves around easily and quickly, and bakes cookies for her grandchildren.

She still has Parkinson's disease, yet her functioning has improved so greatly that she's not living as though she has the disease. "I was skeptical about the device," Victor says, "because I am a scientist, and I only believe in scientific data. But when I saw the effect, especially for her coordination and cognition, I came to believe this technique is wonderful."

Stroke

Mary Gaines lives in Manhattan. She's an engaging fifty-four-year-old, with blond hair, red cheeks, and large eyes. In 2007 she was head of the private school where she had worked for twenty-two years. An American raised in Europe, she spoke French, Italian, a little German, and a bit of Flemish. When she was not even fifty, she had a major stroke, caused by a blood vessel that burst in her brain. It began as a series of "small strokes." First she noticed heaviness in her arms and legs; then she started to see flashing lights. Her partner, Paul, drove her to the hospital. "I was in the MRI machine at New York–Presbyterian Hospital when I had my *big* stroke," she says. A classic left-hemisphere stroke left her with weakness on her right side and affected her language: "I couldn't speak, write, read, cough, make any noise. I was mute."

She also developed problems thinking, couldn't filter out unimportant information, experienced sensory overload, and couldn't understand conversations because she was so disturbed by background noise. When the brain is healthy, it automatically helps sort out what information is worth paying attention to. "After my stroke," Mary said, "I had to consciously assess every sound, shadow, almost every smell, to know whether it was dangerous." Her visual processing slowed so much that, as a passenger in a car, she couldn't understand traffic patterns. "I was always playing catch-up," she said. Not knowing what was safe and what was dangerous left her nervous system in a constant state of fight-or-flight.

She couldn't perform the simplest movements and gestures, like turning the stove on and off. Simple tasks exhausted her, and she became socially isolated. She began speech rehab every day at Helen Hayes Hospital for her aphasia (loss of speech) and dysarthria (inability to articulate sounds properly). "I would sit and listen to other people talking, and I wouldn't understand or follow what people were saying." After six months' leave, she tried to go back to work but couldn't handle it. "I thought I had to live with this."

Disabled, she labored four and a half years to get better, but most of her deficits remained. Then she heard about the lab in Madison, where her sister happened to live. In January 2012 she went for a two-week stint. Like many who have been ill for a long time and who have tried mainstream treatment at esteemed hospitals, she was skeptical.

"Day two at the lab I started feeling a change, and I kept that to myself," she told me, "because I was feeling, 'I want it to be true, so I am imagining it.' But when I went out for lunch that second day, it was like a comb had gone through my brain, and I didn't have any tangles anymore." Her problems with thinking and sorting out stimuli disappeared. Her fight-or-flight reaction began to turn off. Suddenly her peripheral vision was back, and she could do visual processing in real time. "I could tell which traffic was coming, and which going," she said. "On the third day, I had my energy back. And oh my God, I could talk to someone across the table and hear them. I was ecstatic, elated. I had to calm down, because I didn't want anyone to think I was crazy. The device has changed my life."

After the two weeks in Madison, she took the device home, using it three to five times a day. By March 2012 she had used the device at home for two months. With only the occasional halting pause, she told me, "I know I still have some work to do, but I feel like myself. . . . I think the biggest thing is that I can do things with 'flow,' and things come second nature to me again. I can now enjoy daily activity and just being alive." Before, she could barely get through a newspaper article, and now "I can read anything I want."

Though Mary's recovery has been life-changing, it hasn't been complete; she still gets weekly migraines. She can multitask again, but not as long as she could before; and she's still not as fast at tasks as she was. At first she thought she would use the PoNS as long as the team suggested, but she stopped after six months, when she realized that the gains she had made were holding without daily practice. "Now I practice yoga, meditate, walk, clean the house, garden, and cook with enthusiasm. My greatest delight is my freedom, and I enjoy it every second."

Multiple Sclerosis

Max Kurz, in charge of research in the department of physical therapy at the University of Nebraska Medical Center, is a scientist with expertise in biomechanics and motor control. He led the first study of the device outside the Madison lab. Yuri, Mitch, and Kurt needed to see if other groups could replicate their Madison lab results in a varied population of MS patients. Kurz's study included people with both relapsing and remitting MS and progressive MS. The eight subjects came twice a day for two weeks of training at the clinic and were then each given a device to take home for the next twelve weeks. Most came in on canes, one on a walker.

"The changes that we saw in the patients were pretty remarkable," said Kurz. "And they were really fast, faster than what we'd see normally in the clinic." All seven of the patients who had come in on canes were "now able to walk faster, longer, go up and down stairs, not having to hold on to the railing. That was very convincing to us." Not only did people improve in their balance and walking, they also improved in other MS symptoms, indicating that a more general healing process was occurring. "Patients are reporting improved bladder control and an improved ability to sleep," he told me. "Those are things we're not treating, but they're changing." A patient who was confined to a wheelchair became able to transfer from the chair to the bed, roll over in bed, get up on his knees, sit on them, and balance himself independently. "These are things that you just don't see happening in that type of patient," said Kurz.

"One woman had a lot of shaking, and head and arm tremors, that went away." No medications had been able to help her tremors. "Her walk," Kurz said, "when she came in was uncoordinated. She came with a cane, and she got rid of it. She was able to walk, and then run, at the end of the study. She was able—within a couple of weeks—to jump rope. That's crazy. Here you have balance problems, and with training on the device you are able to jump rope. Some of the things are just unexplainable!"

The woman he spoke of was Kim Kozelichki. She's been able to stop her decline, then radically improve. Kim, an avid athlete and tennis player, went to college on a tennis scholarship. MS struck when she was twenty-six years old, when she was working as a manager. The onset was insidious. First, she felt tingling in her feet, which spread to her hands. Then she developed neuropathic pain in her feet, hands, neck, and back. Next the MS affected her balance, so that she regularly stumbled into walls, and started dragging her leg when she walked. She developed double and triple vision. When she swung at a ball on the tennis court, she would miss by a foot. She had played the piano but had to give it up. Her head tremors became so bad, she always looked as if she was shaking her head to say no. Her knees started turning in, and she eventually needed a cane; then her husband, Todd, a homicide detective, had to push her in a wheelchair on longer walks. Her fatigue and her inability to think or remember words, or process events in real time, were so bad that she had to quit work. An MRI scan showed MS lesions all over her brain and spinal cord.

Kim's nurse-practitioner recommended that she participate in Dr. Kurz's study. Athletes and musicians often make good patients, because they know about incremental practice. Within a couple of days of using the PoNS, Kim says, "I was better balanced, not bumping into the walls, feeling stronger. I felt normal again—as normal as can be expected with this disease." When she started with the device, she could walk 1 mile per hour on the treadmill, clinging to the handrails. After two weeks, she was going 2.5 miles per hour. At home with a PoNS, she trained for two twenty-minute sessions a day, one for balance, and one while walking and doing housework. By her fourth week, she was up to 3.5 miles per hour without using the handrails. "What freedom!" she says. After eleven weeks, Todd was throwing balls at her on a tennis court so she could swing. "She was zinging those things back at me so fast," he says, "I was ducking to get away."

A year later she now walks without a cane and can play the piano again. She's not all better—her fatigue and cognitive issues persist to the point that she still can't work. But she is much more functional, suffering much less, and has hope. She and Todd are able to go to movies, go out to eat, take walks, and enjoy life together.

III. The Cracked Potters

Jeri Lake

Since the PoNS was helping people with Parkinson's and MS—both of which are degenerative and progressive diseases—the team next wondered, might it help people who had had a brain injury? They put out the word that they were interested in working with traumatic brain injury patients who had not gotten better with conventional approaches.

Jeri Lake, a forty-eight-year-old nurse-practitioner, had been riding her bike on a cold February day. "I was commuting into work six years ago," she says. "We had a small amount of snow on the roads. But I always biked in all kinds of weather. I stopped at an intersection and hit the pedals to proceed, but then a car began coming toward me and, without putting on a turn signal, turned into my path. I had to do a rapid stop, and it flipped the bike. I have no idea what happened after that. The car didn't hit me, but I ended up on the side of the road and my helmet was broken."

The weekend before, she had been on a 35-mile ride, after which she and her son had worked out for another hour, getting ready for the 500-mile race they did together every summer. Even when she wasn't in peak training, Jeri rode 75 to 100 miles every week because "that was how I cleared my head." She is a pert, compact woman with trim brown hair; a rugged, high-energy person, she comes from a family of self-described "energy junkies . . . the type of people who don't do inactive." She specialized in nursing midwifery and was the lead partner in a practice in Champaign, Illinois, that did deliveries at all hours of the night. When she wasn't working, raising four children, or spending time with her husband, Steve Rayburn, who teaches Shakespeare, she was camping and hiking. She rode her bike twelve months of the year.

After her accident, she actually rode the rest of the way to work. There a coworker was disturbed by her condition and took her to the emergency room. Jeri was nauseated, vomiting, and not thinking clearly. The break in her helmet was behind the right ear, indicating a likely point of impact in the parietal and occipital areas. There were bruises on her right shoulder and right hip. The doctor diagnosed her with a concussion, sent her home with some pain meds, and told her to rest. That was on a Wednesday. She slept straight through the next few days. That Saturday she was on weekend call; her husband didn't want her to go to work, but Jeri said, "You don't avoid call when partners are involved." She went anyway.

"When I started getting reports from the midwives who were going off duty," she says, "none of it made any sense. I just didn't know what they were telling me, and I started crying. Over the rest of that weekend, I was in a fight-or-flight response all the time, incredibly anxious."

She had become hypersensitive to soft sounds. She couldn't bear to eat because the clattering of the cutlery and plates startled her. And once her startle response was initiated, it didn't stop: "If anyone made any sound, they had to scrape me off the ceiling, and I started twitching and sobbing uncontrollably, and the only way it stopped was if I went to sleep." She was also overstimulated by light and had to be in a darkened room. It was as though her brain could no longer filter out noise, motion, light, or any kind of distraction, and when she tried to, she got severe headaches. Multitasking was out of the question.

Then she lost muscular control. A significant part of her injury was to the right side of the brain, which governs the movement of the body on the left. Jeri started dropping things, having most trouble with the muscles on the left side of her body. "My arm and leg on that side were twitching, and I had a tremor."

By Monday, her face was numb. One of her partners, fearing she might be having a slow bleed inside her brain, took her back to the emergency room. Though they diagnosed her as having a traumatic brain injury (TBI), she felt she was not being taken seriously. "The doctor said my face was numb because I was hyperventilating, but I knew that wasn't right, because the numbness had come before I was so upset. But they wouldn't listen. The nurse said I wouldn't do higher math for six months, and the doctor said that he would pray for me that I would calm down. My husband said he had never seen me so angry."

JERI BEGAN TO HAVE MANY more problems than doing higher math. In a dizzying descent, she lost all sorts of cognitive functions. When she tried to speak, sometimes no words came out, or she'd gasp, or she'd look at the sink and call it a "shoe." She had no balance, fell backward all the time, and couldn't catch herself.

Her vision was off. She couldn't see objects to her left and began walking into things on that side. She lost all depth perception, the sense the world has three dimensions. Being a passenger in a car was suddenly horrifying for her because she couldn't judge where other cars were: "I would scream all the time, because I thought cars were going to hit us. Everything looked like it was on top of us." To drive Jeri somewhere, the family put curtains on the car windows and laid her on the backseat with her eyes closed.

When walking, she couldn't sense the position of the ground because she couldn't feel if she was on an incline, and her family had to call out "Downhill!" or "Uphill!" so she wouldn't stumble. Patterns on a rug seemed to move, as did print on a page. Because the system that aligns the eyes wasn't working, she couldn't get objects into focus and developed double vision (a problem called post-trauma vision syndrome). She was prescribed prism glasses to help with the double vision, but she still couldn't focus.

This gutsy, self-possessed athlete and leader was now inconsolable and could not regulate her senses, her movements, or her emotional responses. An obstetrician at Jeri's office, who knew how resilient she normally was, became alarmed by her deterioration. He urged her to see a neurologist, who diagnosed post-concussion syndrome—generally a condition more serious than concussion, because it means the symptoms are enduring. He told her she had to stay at home and rest for six months, which she did.

After six months, a neuropsychologist showed her a stack of photographs of people. When Jeri was repeatedly shown pictures of the same face, she couldn't recognize the ones she had already seen; she had lost the ability to distinguish and identify human faces. The neuropsychologist told her not to think about going back to work for a year, after which they would get together to see how she was doing.

At home, she felt she was falling apart; she couldn't make dinner or do laundry and felt a burden to her husband, who took care of her. Though he "never faltered," it seemed to her she no longer had a role in her family. "I had always been the mom who gathered all the kids over and loved the noise and thrived on chaos and knew my children's friends. Now Mom was this fragile thing. If any little thing happened, she would be completely overwhelmed again, crying, sleeping for another week."

After the year was up, she returned to the neuropsychologist, who saw that she had made no progress. He said, "You have permanent damage in the right hemisphere, and the frontal executive function is a mess. Not only are you not going back to your work as a health-care provider, you are not going back to any kind of work. You are unable to function.

Most recovery occurs in the first year, and you will probably get a little more in the second year." Everything was to be geared not to fixing her brain but to learning to live with her problems, or to "compensating" for them, finding ways to work around her limitations. "The message was," she says, "'Accept what you have.'" Over the next months, many clinicians reiterated: her condition was permanent.

THE TERM CONCUSSION IS OFTEN used by physicians interchangeably with *mild TBI*. Most people diagnosed with mild TBI recover to their previous level of day-to-day functioning within three months. But we really know whether an injury is mild only after the fact, if the symptoms pass. Sometimes even when patients feel better, they are not "out of the woods," especially if they have had multiple concussions, which set in motion an underlying pathogenic process that will lead to long-term problems, as we will see. If mild TBI-concussion symptoms persist past three months, the diagnosis is revised to "post-concussion syndrome" and TBI, as happened with Jeri. TBI is currently the leading cause of disability and death in young people.

Many people have come to think that concussions, because they are called mild TBIs and because they occur so routinely in sports, are nothing to be overly concerned about. They assume that they lead only to a temporary disruption or alteration in mental function, and that no serious damage has occurred, as long as the player can mouth the words "I feel okay" and rejoin the game. But recent studies of National Football League players and other athletes show that repeated concussions can lead to a nineteen-fold increase in rates of early-onset Alzheimer's disease and other memory problems, neurological problems, and depression. Multiple mild TBIs can lead to a degenerative process in the brain called chronic traumatic encephalopathy. It does not occur only in football players, who suffer many concussions. The researcher Robin Green and her colleagues at the University of Toronto have shown that TBI patients can sometimes experience a symptomatic recovery, only to deteriorate over time, probably because of a degenerative brain process.

Another reason concussion symptoms are often casually dismissed is that emergency room CT scans and MRIs are usually normal after a concussion, even when tissue is injured. When a head moving through space collides with an object, the accelerating brain within is suddenly decelerated as it smashes against the inside wall of its own skull. Then, typically, it bounces backward and up against the opposite side of the skull. These blows can cause the neurons to release chemicals and neurotransmitters, and lead to excess inflammation, disrupted transmission of electrical signals, brain-cell damage and death, and metabolic depression.

The effects of a concussion are not confined to the point of impact any more than a hammer blow to a window breaks only the part that is struck; the huge transfer of energy radiates throughout the brain. It can affect not only the cell bodies of the neurons but also the axons that connect neurons. Axonal injury can be seen only with a new kind of scan, called diffuse tensor imaging. Since axons connect different brain areas, damage to axons can cause problems in all those areas, so that many functions—sensory, motor movement, cognition, and mood—are affected, regardless of where the initial impact occurred. And perhaps this explains why people who have had blows to different parts of the head may have uncannily similar symptoms.

Jeri Meets Kathy

One day Jeri's speech therapist told her, "The weirdest thing just happened. A woman who has an injury identical to yours has just become my patient, and it was as though you walked into my office all over again." The new patient's brain injury was more recent, and she was about a year behind Jeri in dealing with it. The therapist urged the two women to get together to support each other, and they did.

Kathy Nicol-Smith, a medical technologist, middle-aged and living in Champaign, Illinois, had been driving from work when her car was hit twice. First she was rear-ended, and then, because the driver behind her couldn't stop, her car was smashed again, from the side. Kathy hit her head and had a whiplash injury. She developed amnesia. And like Jeri she was diagnosed with a TBI, because right after the accident she developed multiple symptoms, which did not lessen with time. She had severe headaches, slept a lot, found that light bothered her so she had to close her eyes in daylight, couldn't hold things or walk properly, had coordination and balance problems, had difficulty speaking, and couldn't figure out where she was in space or distinguish changing inclines. She had memory problems, such that she burned everything she cooked. She lost 3-D vision, so "everything seemed flat," and developed double vision: "I felt like someone had put Vaseline on my glasses and everything was one big blur." She couldn't read or concentrate, even to watch television: "My brain couldn't keep up with anything."

Kathy had another terrible problem. Shortly after her accident, her husband, who had been her major support, was diagnosed with pancreatic cancer. Four months later he died.

Jeri and Kathy began meeting regularly. Jeri says, "I was trying to keep her going, as she had a lot more to deal with than I had, with loss on top of loss. We both started taking pottery classes to regain eye-hand coordination and to strengthen our hands. We called ourselves the Cracked Potters because the pots aren't cracked, but the potters are." Meanwhile Jeri Googled everything she could about brain injury.

In her Web search, Jeri found out about the Madison lab. She told her neurologist, Dr. Charles Davies, who was also treating Kathy. Dr. Davies arranged to talk with Yuri. After a long wait, a call from the lab invited Jeri and Kathy to come. Jeri had already planned a visit to her ailing eighty-seven-year-old father and couldn't call it off, but she insisted Kathy go on her own. "Kathy went, and called me after two days, and I could hear it in her voice. Her speech had changed—it was fluid, there was inflection. She once sounded like I did, had a flat hesitant voice, devoid of tone and feeling. Now suddenly there was this new voice saying 'Jeri, you've got to get up here, this is amazing,' and I knew something incredible had happened to her."

Like Ron, Kathy had come in walking on a cane and left without one.

WHEN JERI ARRIVED AT THE lab in September 2010, escorted by her husband, she walked tentatively, slowly, barely swinging her arms, as she moved her feeble frame down the hall toward the lab. Wearing prism glasses, this once-spirited woman looked like a frightened, depressed mouse, stiff above the waist and wobbly beneath. Standing posture is the result of a contest between two equally ambitious, ancient forces. One is the upright, bipedal stance of humans, a gift of millions of years of evolution, which created the extensor muscle system of the spine and back, and the nervous system controls that keep us upright. The other force, a far more ancient one, is gravity. Most walking, as we have seen, is a controlled forward fall, a complex process that requires constant brain stem feedback so it doesn't go awry. When Mitch first saw Jeri, he thought her brain was "like the switchboard in the old Lily Tomlin telephone operator skit, after Lily had, out of frustration, simply pulled out all the plugs." The working diagnosis was TBI, with diffuse axonal damage.

The team made before-and-after films of Jeri, and I pored over every detail. In the film of her arrival, she constantly looks on the verge of an uncontrolled fall. Her feet are such uncertain supports that, as she walks, she keeps losing her balance. Her arms suddenly shoot out sideways, at forty-five degrees, as though she is flapping a pair of wings in a desperate attempt to stabilize herself. The trepidation triggered by each step can be seen on her tense face. As she attempts to launch a foot, it is as though the toe gets glued to the floor, and when it is finally released, the heel, instead of continuing to lift and move forward, either swings out, almost causing her to stumble, or crosses into the path of the other foot, making her stance so narrow, she is about to topple over. With each step her ankle begins to buckle. To turn, she has to reach for the wall to stabilize herself, while her feet knock into each other. If she looks up, she falls backward.

The team tested Jeri by using the Dynamic Gait Index, putting her through a standardized obstacle course. When she came to a shoebox that she had to step over, she came to a full stop—instead of taking it in her stride. She turned completely sideways (as though trying to get over a hip-high fence) and then barely made it over without falling. Going down stairs she was so uncertain that she would cling to the side railing with both hands, take a single step, rest, and then another. The team checked her balance by putting her in the "shaking phone booth," a specially designed compartment with a moving floor and sides that allows them to precisely measure a subject's balance quotient.

Jeri, like so many traumatic brain injury patients, was on four medications, as she said, "just to keep my head above water." Some were uppers and others were downers. She took Ritalin in the morning, "to have enough energy to get a couple of hours of things done"; an antidepressant kept her anxiety at bay; Ativan was one of multiple drugs she tried for sleep; and she took Relpax for migraines. She was typical of a patient with a nervous system that is spinning out of control because it has lost the ability to regulate itself.

That first day Jeri wept as she told Yuri how her clinicians had told her she would make no further progress. It had, after all, been over five and a half years since her accident, with no improvements. Now her brain was so overwhelmed by his and Mitch's baseline testing that she had a lot of trouble following him and answering his questions. Her husband believed she couldn't endure any more and thought that perhaps he should get her home for the day. She recalled Yuri turning to Mitch and saying "This is not what I expected," and she became frightened they would send her home.

Jeri put the device in her mouth, and Yuri gave her precise instructions. She was to stand perfectly straight, so that her neck wasn't cramped, and so the blood supply to her brain stem would not be blocked. He checked her hip position, fussed about her knees, and measured the distance between her shoulders and her head. Then he asked her to stand, with the device on her tongue, for twenty minutes, eyes closed. That frightened her because she always fell when she couldn't see, and she couldn't imagine she'd be able to stand the whole time.

He turned it on, and she closed her eyes. When she wobbled, someone on the team touched her on her arm or shoulder, to give her a sense of where she was in space—because the PoNS, unlike the device Cheryl had used, did not indicate her position in space. Her mind began to calm, which often happens after about thirteen minutes on the device, and she realized the team was no longer touching her when she swayed. Then, to her surprise, they told her, at the twenty-minute mark, "Time's up."

She pulled out the device and walked with an almost normal gait and no balance problems. Turning to her left as she departed the room, she realized, with a shock, that she was able to look effortlessly over her shoulder without falling. On the film, Jeri yells, "I just turned my head" and her husband starts crying. Her voice is normal, colorful, songlike, spirited. She can form words clearly—her dysarthria has disappeared. Her antigravity muscles are working, and she stands straight as an exclamation mark, her chest puffed out and moving with grace.

Then she begins to look terribly confused. Can this change have happened so fast? Can five and a half years of disability be reversed so quickly? As moment piles upon moment, she realizes that, yes, it has reversed. "I just want to go out and run!" she says. Two days later she was indeed running on a treadmill.

"It was amazing," says Jeri. "They gave me my life back—within twenty-four hours I had gone places I never believed I would go again. It was beyond my wildest dreams. I felt so much like the person I had known for the forty-eight years before the accident that it was hard to remember that I was supposed to take it easy and rest, because I had to form new neuronal pathways. When I left for Wisconsin I was sleeping eleven to twelve hours a night, and napping one to two hours during the day, and never had any energy. That first night I slept eight hours, woke alert at six-thirty a.m., and I was rested. I felt for the first time in years my brain woke at the same time my body did."

When she got up that morning, she looked out the window. "I didn't think I was screaming, but I was, and my husband came running out of the shower, and I said, 'Look at that lake! The shoreline is not a line! There are trees, and behind those trees, there are other trees, and that means there must be a bay between them!' I hadn't realized how flat my world had become, until suddenly I could see depth again. Before, it was like looking at *a picture* of a lake. Now I felt the 3-D movie has nothing on me, I felt my own 3-D! And I found I could recognize people by their faces again." Most of these changes happened for Jeri in the first forty-eight hours, and within two days she realized she didn't need to wear her prism glasses anymore.

Five days later Jeri walked down the hallway where she had taken her first gait test, for a reassessment. Now she was nimble, walked fast, flawlessly, with a swagger and a smile, her upper spine and torso fluid, swinging her arms with joy, like the graceful athlete she had been. Coming up to the shoebox, she neither slowed nor paid close attention to it but passed straight over it. She bobbed and weaved around the obstacle course, hustling up stairs and down without holding the railing. She stood on one foot. Then she went outside into the nearby hills and ran up and down them like a kid.

She returned home after a week in Madison and practiced with the portable device the team gave her for six twenty-minute sessions every day. "My cognitive speed," she said, referring to her ability to think, perceive, and make decisions, "got faster every day, the brain fog lifted, and I was amazed at the ease of getting through the day. I had so much energy that I didn't know what to do with it!" Soon she got into a car, and Steve drove her to see her granddaughter, Eva. Because her accident had occurred before Eva was born and had robbed her of the ability to recognize faces, she said, "I felt I was seeing her for the first time."

What followed were "three glorious months." Jeri was now sure that she would go back to work again. Yuri, based on his experience with Cheryl, wanted her to spend a full year and a half using the device.

Kathy, who had been to Madison a few weeks before Jeri and also had a breakthrough, was back home in Champaign. She too was using the device six times a day to stimulate neuroplastic growth. For two twenty-minute sessions a day, she used it while standing on tiptoes on a mat, or on one foot, to improve her brain's balance circuitry. She did two more sessions while walking on a treadmill to improve her movement and two more while meditating, to quiet down the noise in her brain. Her results were astonishing. She lost almost all her symptoms. She could read once again for pleasure and had no problems finding words. Her double vision and two-dimensional vision were gone, and her balance problems improved. She could multitask—she prepared a meal for twelve people at Thanksgiving.

At the end of three months, Jeri's husband, Steve, drove both Cracked Potters to Madison so that they could be retested and monitored to make sure they were using the device properly. Yuri explained to them that their brains had quieted their noisy firing and had started forming new neuroplastic connections but had not completely healed yet. Like Cheryl before them, they would need to build up the residual effect over time.

Setback

On December 27, 2010, on their way to the lab for their assessment, Jeri, Kathy, and Steve were sitting at a stoplight on University Avenue, right in front of the lab, when a car behind theirs smashed into them at full speed. Their car was totaled. When the police came, the man driving the car that hit them said he honestly hadn't known whether the light was red or green because he had been looking for his cell phone.

"I felt a stabbing pain right at the base of my skull," said Jeri, "and Steve said I told him, 'I think I am hurt.' Kathy had the PoNS in her mouth at the time! This was exactly the kind of accident that had caused Kathy's original brain injury, and I began trying to help her slow her breathing. They took us to the emergency room."

Kathy's balance problems, word-finding problems, dizziness, and need for very long periods of sleep all returned. Jeri's symptoms escalated over the next few days: her speech regressed, and she had trouble finding words again, her balance was off, she could no longer run, the double vision returned, and she lost depth perception. Her sleep deteriorated so that she woke up tired and had no energy. Her thinking problems returned. Worst of all, her headaches were back after three months without a single one, and she had the worst migraine of her life. In January 2011 her symptoms were so bad that she was sent to the ER, because the doctors again feared that she might be having a brain bleed. She wasn't. But this setback was typical of what happens when people with a partially healed TBI are reinjured.

Yuri told Jeri and Kathy they had to begin all over again. They should use the device six to seven times a day for twenty minutes, while meditating. Exercise of any kind, mental or physical, would be too taxing for their vulnerable brains.

Every neuroplasticity lab should have its own psychiatrist for times like this. Clearly most brain-injured or neurologically diseased patients have cognitive, emotional, and motivational difficulties. And how can they not, when their brains are not working? Luckily, at the Madison lab, Kathy and Jeri had wry but tender Alla Subbotin, another Soviet immigrant. They were now going to find out how this Russian-American team would push and motivate them and their twice-injured brains to emerge from this new disaster. "Alla is wonderful, a godsend, my coach, and I need her," said Kathy. "Laid back, kind, but she wants you to do what you must. Oh, they are all strict! And Yuri is the meanest and the most loving person in the world. He was so worried about me and Jeri."

Kathy went on: "You know, they don't give up on you. They live to see you live. Magic happens there for people like me. Yuri wants you to succeed. And he makes you feel bad when you don't do it right. And he is the one who gives you the biggest hug when you are crying and who gets so excited, saying 'Oh Kathy!' because it is so emotionally exciting when your life is given back to you. It's hard work and they let you know it will be. They are cheerleaders and coaches. But you have to want it really badly."

Jeri's progress was steady. By late February, after hours of meditating while using the device, she was allowed to begin gently exercising other functions, like walking around with the PoNS in her mouth or using it while reading e-mail. "By March, my progress was going straight uphill at an unbelievable pace. I was feeling great," she told me. She was running again, and doing forty-mile bike rides again. She was now functioning as well as she had been before the second accident.

In early May, Jeri and I spoke again. She was ecstatic. "My son got married this weekend. I spent from seven p.m. till midnight Saturday night, greeting guests and dancing with everyone. Eight months ago I would not have been able to be at my son's reception, I would have had to be taken home to sleep." She fell silent. "I'm going to cry. There just aren't words to tell you how this feels."

Jeri still has some issues. Multiple concussions are often much harder to treat. She still tires more easily than she did before her brain injuries. But she did complete 380 miles of her 500-mile bike ride, and she has her driver's license back, and is doing part-time volunteer work and training to administer neuropsychological testing to TBI patients.

Kathy is doing better too, walking three miles a day, and has shed the fifty pounds she gained from being unable to move. She sleeps well, is cognitively clear, and is no longer overwhelmed by noise or sensations, though she finds that when she does more than one activity, she often needs a nap, and can get overloaded by information, which is limiting: "But it's not like before when my brain literally shut down. Now I have my life back." She still needs to use the device every day, but only half as often as she did at first. A residual effect is building. It is too early to tell if steady use, over a couple of years, will lead to a residual effect comparable to what Cheryl experienced—she no longer needed it at all. But that took Cheryl two and a half years, and Kathy and Jeri each had *two* brain injuries, not one.

Kathy remains in frequent contact with Jeri. "And yes," she says, "I am still throwing pots."

IV. How the Brain Balances Itself—with a Little Help

A Woman Missing Brain Stem Tissue

Today the Madison team is working with Sue Voiles. Sue is missing part of her brain stem, and the challenge is to see if her remaining tissue can be trained to do what her lost tissue once did. Though only forty-four years old, she came to the lab on a walker.

When Sue was thirty-five, her handwriting and balance mysteriously began getting worse. A brain scan showed she had a rare cavernous malformation of the brain—a cluster of abnormal blood vessels—and one of them had started leaking. Nine years later a neurosurgeon told her that if she didn't have surgery very soon, she could die; but he also told her that with surgery there was a real risk she could end up disabled, and at best, the result might not be perfect. Sue was a schoolteacher with two sons to care for, and she opted for the surgery. I am looking at her functional magnetic resonance imaging (fMRI) brain scan now and can see that a spoonful of brain tissue has been removed from an area that is normally not much thicker than a big toe. Her life was saved, but she could no longer walk normally or control her face, balance, speech, or vision.

At the lab I watch Yuri and Mitch spend the morning putting Sue through tests to get her baseline functioning. They test her balance by putting her in the "shaking phone booth" to see how long she can stay upright. They then test her gait, using the standardized obstacle course. They put her in an fMRI machine to watch her brain activity while she's watching a virtual-reality video that makes her feel she's losing her balance. They film how she holds her head, smiles, and follows objects with her eyes—actions controlled by the cranial nerves.

Yuri now assigns Sue her first task: to stand still with the device in her mouth for twenty minutes and balance herself. The lights in the room are softened to create a meditative calm. He turns the device on. The first goal is to reset her brain and turn off noisy circuitry, through neuromodulation. She calms quickly, her face relaxes, and her balance improves.

Yuri won't let up on her stance because he wants the energy to flow properly, so she enters a meditative state while standing. She must stand as though a string were lifting her head up ever so slightly; her shoulders are down, to make sure her neck isn't crooked, cutting off the blood supply to her brain stem. She must breathe with her diaphragm, scan her body for tension, and try to relax it. Her knees must not be locked, and her hips should be aligned. Four thousand years of Eastern practice have determined the best posture for meditative relaxation, which Yuri has found helps put the nervous system into the correct state to benefit from the device.

The next day Sue is on the treadmill. She starts at half a mile per hour. Yuri ups her gradually to 1.5, then faster—this for a woman who a day ago was on a walker. She is now looking up at Yuri plaintively for a reprieve.

"You have to be dead tired—that's my job," he says.

"I have a sore back, Yuri," she says, pulling the device out of her mouth to talk.

"If you are not sore and not tired, we are doing a bad job." When he sees her posture deteriorate, he comments, "That isn't right."

She's huffing and puffing, and her face says, *I'm really really trying.*

"You want dishonesty?" he asks her, both verbally and nonverbally with his upturned hands and raised eyebrows. He gives her no nonsense, no North American sugarcoating.

He's impatient to be helpful. This neuroplastic approach, he explains, requires that she take a very active role by concentrating on each movement. He takes her off the treadmill to show her how to walk with more hip movement. As with most people with a walker, her posture has been neuroplastically altered by it, and she is stooped forward.

"Right now your body is one big block—you have to learn to move your body in parts," he says. "Pretend the most precious thing is your head, and learn how to move your lower body without moving your upper body." He shows her how to do a tai chi–like stance, to make her stiffened body come alive.

"She has all normal movements, but it is not assembled!" he tells me. "When you see a few moments of stability, that means it is possible. One of the three steps she does is normal, which means that she is capable of doing the normal steps. I am continually challenging her. Making it more difficult."

"GOOD!" he yells over to her on the treadmill.

"Well, I have to be rough," he says to me. "When I do something nice, everybody start to be worse. So I have to be nasty. Dragging. She is dragging. Means she is not lifting the heels enough. So I change the angle." He raises the elevation on the machine and yells over its roar, "I don't want to hear dragging! Lift your knees, Sue! No dragging! Longer steps! Soft landing!"

Making up for Sue's lost spoonful of tissue will be a slow process, much slower than the rapid process by which Ron Husmann brought back his singing voice. Ron had some healthy tissue to work with; it just wasn't functioning correctly. But Sue is missing tissue and so will have to rewire other brain areas to take over, and that will take much longer. Time will tell if she can permanently leave her walker behind.

Then finally her treadmill session is over.

"You are good lab rat today," he says.

"Why, thank you," she drawls with a beaming smile.

Yuri's Theory: How It Works

In Western medicine we tend to believe that each illness takes a different course, and so the treatment must be different for each. So how, I ask Yuri, is it that the device is helpful for symptoms of conditions as varied as MS, Parkinson's, TBI, and chronic pain?

"Nothing more practical than a good theory," Yuri answers, repeating the motto from the Soviet Academy of Sciences. Yuri believes that the device works by triggering the brain's self-correcting, self-regulating system that allows it to achieve "homeostasis." As I mentioned before, the term *homeostasis* was first introduced into Western medicine by the nineteenth-century French physiologist Claude Bernard, to describe the ability of living systems to regulate themselves and their inner environment, and to maintain a stable state in the body, despite the many influences, both external and internal, that tend to disrupt that state. Thus, homeostasis counteracts influences that would push the system into deviating from the optimal state at which it evolved to function best. For instance, human beings tend to have a temperature of 98.6°F, and our bodies function best in that state. If we get too hot, our bodies will attempt to return to that temperature; if our bodies cannot, we may die. Many organs contribute to our homeostasis: the liver, the kidneys, the skin, and the nervous system.

Neural networks have their own homeostatic mechanisms, which are best understood by realizing that different neuronal networks perform different functions. In the central nervous system, the *motor system neurons* are those neurons in networks that typically transfer information from the brain to the muscles so we can move them. *Sensory neurons* typically process incoming sensory information from a body part. Motor and sensory neurons are called *primary neurons,* and both involve the transfer of information via electrical signals.

Interneurons are another set. Their primary job is to modulate or regulate the firing activity of their neighboring neurons. Interneurons can perform a homeostatic-like regulation function, to make sure that the signals reaching other neurons are at the optimal level and come at the optimal time so they can be useful, neither overwhelming nor understimulating the other neurons.

"A good example of how interneurons work is the photoreceptors in the retina," says Yuri. The range of amounts of light that our photoreceptors have to process is huge, from the small amount of light in a darkened room to that on a sunny beach. Light is measured in a unit called lux. The light in a living room in front of the TV is about 15 lux. On a sunny beach, on a summer day, the light can be up to 150,000 lux. The individual photoreceptors in the human eye didn't evolve to process that wide a range, but with the help of interneurons, they can adapt to it.

If the signal coming into a sensory neuron is too low to be detected, its interneuron will excite the neuron, so it is able to fire more easily, amplifying the incoming signal. If the signal coming into the sensory neuron is too high, its interneuron can inhibit the sensory neuron from firing, making it less sensitive to the signal. Interneurons also help make signals sharper and clearer. Ultimately, the interneurons and their networks send signals to the small muscles around the pupils, adjusting their size to take in more or less light as required. (So when the pupils change size, it is a visual demonstration of interneuron feedback in action.) But it is not only the pupils that readjust to maintain homeostasis. Much of the interneuron network does as well.

BRAIN DISEASE OFTEN AFFECTS INTERNEURONS. In some brain diseases, the cells remain alive but can't produce the right amount of a particular neurotransmitter. In others, as in a stroke or brain injury, the cells die. Either situation can disrupt the ability of the interneuron system to help the rest of the brain return to homeostasis. Signals may be too low, causing the brain to miss important information. Or signals may be too high and may spread too far through the brain network, stimulating neurons they shouldn't be affecting. (We saw this when Jeri became hypersensitive to sound, light, and movement.) Or signals may last too long and become indistinguishable from ones that follow, blurring together, again making the system noisy. Sometimes the circuitry becomes so hypersensitive that it doesn't turn off (as happens with many chronic pain syndromes: a small movement can trigger a pain sensation lasting hours to days).* Ultimately, when signals remain too high for too long, they saturate the networks. Once a network is "saturated," it misses information and can't make distinctions because the network can't keep up with all the signals coming its way. (Perhaps this relates to the incredible fatigue that almost all such patients feel, and helps explain the great effort that is required for minimal accomplishment, and their sense that their brains are on overload.)

When homeostasis is disturbed, the balance of inhibition and excitation is disturbed, and the system cannot regulate a wide range of input, so such patients are at the mercy of the signals coming at them. They may experience distress from a low amount of light, such as a flashlight shone in darkness, and have to cover their eyes. They often describe feeling confusion and hypersensitivity to some stimuli but none to others. When this happens in motor circuits, they have limited control over their muscles.

Yuri's hypothesis is that the PoNS device works in so many different kinds of illness because it activates the neuronal network's general mechanisms of homeostatic regulation. His emphasis on using brain homeostasis as a new method of self-healing is unique.

---

* Another example of signals becoming too high occurs in a chronic pain syndrome called trigeminal neuralgia. It often starts when a cranial nerve that supplies the face, called the trigeminal nerve, is impinged upon by a blood vessel or pinched, causing acute pain in a small area. Over time, as the nerve is repeatedly pressed, it becomes hypersensitive; the signals become too high and spread throughout the brain network, so that the smallest movement of the face can cause excruciating pain throughout the entire face. The device doesn't correct the acute pain, but it can at times dramatically dial back the spread of acute pain into chronic pain throughout the face, giving quick relief, presumably by activating the interneuron system to stop the spread of pain.

The device, he believes, sends extra electrical spikes—signals—into the interneuron system, creating spikes in interneurons that are unable to produce spikes by themselves due to disease. This allows a network that has lost the ability to regulate the balance between excitation and inhibition to be restored.

ANOTHER MARVEL OF THE MADISON lab is that after treating two hundred people, the team has found no side effects. (Yuri originally tested the PoNS for hours on himself, to see if he would develop side effects, and he continues to use the device for thirty minutes to an hour each day, to make sure that if they do occur, he will be the canary in the coal mine.) "During the twelve years of research," Yuri says, "we see only positive results *or nothing*." That finding—positive results that return a brain to normal functioning, or nothing—is consistent with the idea that the device gets the network to correct itself through homeostasis.

"When we inject an extra million impulses into the network, we initiate a process of self-regulation and self-healing," says Yuri. "The brain stem is the crossroads between brain and spinal cord, the cerebellum pathways and multiple cranial nerves. We are delivering millions of spikes to an area of the brain that is connected to *everything*. It is the part of the brain with the highest density of different structures, and half of these are responsible for the self-regulating autonomic nervous system and other sources of homeostatic regulation."

Targeting the brain stem and its interneurons, then, is a way of targeting homeostatic regulation for much of the body, including the homeostatic mechanisms that regulate the senses supplied by the cranial nerves (such as balance and aspects of vision), which went awry in Cheryl, and the cranial nerve that, when pinched, gives rise to the chronic pain syndrome called trigeminal neuralgia. The brain stem houses the controls for the massive autonomic nervous system (the sympathetic fight-or-flight system and the calming parasympathetic system). Thus heart rate, blood pressure, and breathing are self-regulated here. The vagus nerve, which supplies and regulates the gastrointestinal tract and digestion, is in the brain stem; its stimulation turns on the parasympathetic system and calms a person down. The brain stem also houses the reticular activating system (RAS), which regulates our level of arousal, influences our sleep-wake cycle, and can power up the rest of the brain (see Chapter 3 for details). Stimulation of the vagus and the RAS, Yuri believes, is the reason most patients who use the device have found they sleep better at night and are more awake during the day.*

The controls for the voice and for swallowing (which Ron struggled to control) are in the lower part of the brain stem, in a part called the medulla. Thus, to target the brain stem is to target the body's hub for self-regulation.

The brain stem (and the nearby cerebellum) has links to other important areas of the brain that govern movement (which is why the device can be helpful for patients with Parkinson's, MS, or stroke), higher cognitive functions (which is why the subjects improve their concentration, focus, and multitasking), and mood centers as well.

According to Yuri, in a patient with an injury in the motor cortex, the motor network will give off fewer spikes in some areas. For the person to move properly, the brain requires constant feedback from the muscles and limbs, so it can "know" where they are in space and can adjust the movements as needed. These "sensory-motor loops" make up integrated circuits. In an injured brain, Yuri believes, the spike flow in the sensory-motor loops that go from the body to the brain and back is unbalanced, desynchronized, disrupted, or too low. Instead of getting, say, a burst of a hundred spikes in 100 milliseconds in order to move, a muscle will get only ten spikes in that time, so it can't contract properly, because its contraction becomes slow and weak. Before Jeri's treatment,

* Vagal stimulation by the device may also account for improvements in Parkinson's disease. Recent breakthroughs in understanding Parkinson's, from the work of the neuroscientist Heiko Braak, show it as possibly originating in the stomach from a pathogen, entering the nerves in the gastrointestinal tract that reach the vagus nerve, then passing up into the brain stem and into the same nuclei that are stimulated by the PoNS. This theory also explains why PD patients have so many autonomic symptoms and gastrointestinal symptoms that cannot be explained by the standard theory, which localizes the disease in the basal ganglia. See C. H. Hawkes et al., "Review: Parkinson's Disease: A Dual-Hit Hypothesis," *Neuropathology and Neurobiology* 33 (2007): 599–614; H. Braak et al., "Staging of Brain Pathology Related to Sporadic Parkinson's Disease," *Neurobiology of Aging* 24 (2003): 197–211.

the team recorded the number of spikes arriving at her muscles from her brain; they found that instead of arriving in a short quick burst, the spikes took much longer to arrive. In addition, Yuri reasons, because there are too few spikes per second in the system, sensory input from the muscle back to the network will be low, and slow to arrive, so both the motor and sensory parts of the circuit will carry too few spikes per second. In such a situation, the patient will have difficulty benefiting from physical therapy.

But if, during physical therapy, the device can deliver an additional hundred spikes into the affected circuitry—sensory, motor, or both—controlled movement can begin. Thus, after Jeri used the device, tests of her muscles showed that spikes from her brain arrived in the correct number and in the correct amount of time.

As the spikes go to the motor part of the circuit, the limb moves more and in return fires up the sensory part of the system, which more clearly registers limb movement and sends more spikes back to the motor system neurons for feedback. Thus, a virtuous cycle is set up.

The results improve many different symptoms for another reason, which may seem surprising to clinicians accustomed to thinking of the brain in terms of a rigid localizationism, the idea that mental functions are always performed in hardwired modules in very localized areas. According to that model, if several mental functions are damaged, a different intervention will be required for each one.

However, most mental functions take place not in isolated locations but in widely distributed networks. Even a basic function, like bending a finger to hit a key on a computer, activates areas of the frontal lobes (involved in thoughtful planning of the move), areas in the motor cortex a bit farther back (responsible for individual movements), areas deep in the center of the brain (involved in combining movements automatically, because the typing finger moves forward, then down on the key, then up), and the peripheral nerves—and that's just for one simple movement. These huge networks are called functional systems. Even a simple gesture requires a huge functional system to support it.

According to Yuri, if some harm comes to one part of a functional system required for a movement—say, a person has a stroke in the motor cortex—the effects will not be confined to the motor cortex. Because the motor cortex is connected, or networked, with many other brain areas, the *whole functional network* that underlies the movement will be affected, and signals throughout will be weakened to some degree. In other words, the dead tissue in the motor cortex will have an impact on the living tissue it is connected to, and all the components of the system will become weaker. This point has not been sufficiently emphasized in our current nonholistic, localizationist approach to brain problems, which focuses only on the dead tissue but leaves out the effects on connected living tissue, a point emphasized in the theory of brain arrhythmias.

But clinicians see damage radiating through entire networks every day. Patients with Parkinson's disease, stroke, MS, and TBI frequently have problems with balance, movement, and sleep as well as thinking and mood problems, even though all have different diseases that initially strike different parts of the brain. Parkinson's patients who lose their balance often look very much like MS patients with balance problems, even though the initial location of the primary disease differs; the illness soon affects widely distributed networks secondarily, interfering with a range of functions.

The genius of the Madison team's approach is to couple electrical stimulation of the network with rehabilitation exercises to awaken *the whole functional system*. Almost all their patients are assigned exercises that quiet sensory noise and stimulate balance, motor movement, and the sensation of movement, as well as mental exercises, regardless of whether they have Parkinson's, MS, stroke, TBI, or some other brain problem.

There are other methods of successfully stimulating the brain, such as transcranial magnetic stimulation (described in detail in *The Brain That Changes Itself*) and deep brain stimulation (DBS), but the PoNS may have advantages in many situations. Transcranial magnetic stimulation uses a noninvasive device that contains a coil of changing magnetic fields; held outside the head, it turns on a three-centimeter area of the brain but not necessarily the relevant functional networks. DBS, sometimes used for Parkinson's disease, does activate relevant networks but requires invasive brain surgery to implant the electrodes. Yuri, Mitch, and Kurt showed, using a brain scan, that they could stimulate one area that DBS targets for Parkinson's, the globus pallidus, using the noninvasive PoNS, which is probably one reason why they were able to help Anna, who had Parkinson's.

For Yuri, the best way to activate the relevant functional network is to do so naturally by getting the person to do an activity (such as balance exercises for people with balance problems) that would normally activate that network, while supplementing it with a boost of additional natural spikes.

With the PoNS, the only artificial electrical stimulation that occurs is on the surface of the tongue; it turns on sensory neurons 300 microns deep, which then send their normal, natural signals via the cranial nerves into the brain stem and on throughout the whole functional network. Thus, after that first artificial low-dose electrical stimulation of the tongue, *all the neurons in the network are stimulated by neurons in the chain,* not by electricity from the device, so that the neurons pass on their signals as they normally would, to the next neurons in their network. This extra infusion of spikes is helpful, Yuri argues, because as we've seen, some networks, affected by disease, appear to generate insufficient natural neuronal spikes to function properly. Neuronal networks that are not used waste away or are taken over for other mental activities. With more spikes circulating in the functional network, it becomes active again, neuroplastic growth processes are initiated, and synapses are maintained and increase in number. All this activity is facilitated by the introduction of spikes, which modulate, rebalance, and optimize the system and make it easier for the patients to exercise and thus reawaken their atrophied circuits.

Four Types of Plastic Change

Based on two hundred subjects and on what we know about the time frames of plastic change, Yuri believes that he has observed four types of plastic change with the PoNS.

The first type of plastic change is the response that occurs within minutes, such as when Ron's voice improved or Jeri's balance returned. Subjects start to breathe differently around the thirteen-minute mark, although they rarely notice the change themselves. Then they have a two-hour window, after using the device, when they get special benefits from any kind of cognitive or physical exercise they do. These quick changes are products of what Yuri calls "functional neuroplasticity." They are so swift because they rectify a physiological imbalance in the excitation-inhibition systems that produces symptoms. Ron's "spasmodic dysphonia" was caused by the damaged nerves for his vocal muscles constantly firing. By activating homeostasis and inhibiting those over-active neurons, the PoNS easily reversed the dysphonia. Sue's eye track-ing, which had been jumpy for many years, stabilized within minutes, and her facial symmetry improved. This type of plastic change addresses *symptoms*.

The second type of plastic change is *synaptic neuroplasticity*. Exer-cising while using the PoNS, for several days up to several weeks, makes new and more lasting synaptic connections between neurons. Yuri be-lieves that it may also increase synapse size and the number of recep-tors, strengthen the electrical signal, and increase efficiency of conduction along the nerve axon. It took Ron several days to give up his cane, and five for Jeri to begin running again. Common changes seen in the first few days include improvements in sleep, speech articulation, balance, and gait. This type of plastic change begins to modify under-lying network pathology.

The third kind of plasticity is *neuronal neuroplasticity*, so called by Yuri because it involves change not just in the synapse but throughout the neuron. It occurs after about a month or more of activation of a cir-cuit. According to the scientific literature, activating neurons consis-tently over twenty-eight days allows them to begin to produce new proteins and internal structures. It took Jeri two months to be able to ride her bike and four for her vision to become completely normal; after her second accident, in December, her vision deteriorated, and it took four months until her optometrist could remove the prism from her prescription. It took Kathy three months to get normal speech back; Anna, who had Parkinson's, required three months on the device to get over the tremor in her right hand, and six months to get over those in her left.

The fourth kind of plasticity is *systemic neuroplasticity,* which takes many months to several years to occur. In this stage the patient no longer needs the device. It occurs only after all the previous plastic changes have stabilized, and the new networks have consolidated; the system is fully functioning and self-correcting—without the device. After Cheryl used the device for six months, she became aware that her residual effect was lasting all day every day, so she stopped using it. But within four weeks of stopping, her original symptoms all returned, meaning that the new neuroplastic changes had not yet stabilized. So she used the device again for a whole year, then stopped it a second time. This time she was fine for four months, then slowly declined. Only when she had used it for about two and a half years did she find that she was cured and didn't relapse when she went off it. She had achieved "systemic neuroplastic" change. She now had new self-sustaining networks, plus some recovered networks. Yuri often speaks of using the device for about two years without interruption to build a stable residual effect for a nonprogressive brain injury.

He speculates that the device may also get results by stimulating neuronal stem cells (baby cells in the brain and their precursors, the neuroprogenitor cells), which may help patch the damaged circuitry. Stem cells have been discovered in a fluid-filled cavity in the brain, directly adjacent to the pons in the brain stem, called the fourth ventricle. These new cells would also contribute to general cellular health.*

---

* Low-level lasers (see Chapter 4) and the PoNS both get energy to the brain, but they generally work at different biological levels. As low-level laser light passes through the skull, it bathes all the *individual cells* in its path and has effects on individual cells. Light unblocks chronic inflammation and energizes injured tissues preferentially. So the laser light chiefly works, as far as we now know, on the *general* neuronal and cellular health throughout a brain region. The PoNS, by contrast, works on existing functional networks that are "wired together" and related to one another. It thus chiefly improves the *specific network functions* of neurons. Because the PoNS and low-level lasers work at different levels of the brain, some people, as I have seen, benefit from both. If the problem involves inflammation—as in a brain injury, postsurgery, stroke, meningitis, possibly MS, and some kinds of depression—it might make sense to try low-level lasers first, to normalize the brain's cellular environment, and then the PoNS to normalize the network.

That said, I do think some homeostatic correction happens with lasers as well. Gaby's hypersensitivity to sound improved drastically, for instance, which is a homeostatic effect. That

With the PoNS, one can divide the intervention into the stages of healing I have proposed. The *neurostimulation* leads to improved homeostasis, or *neuromodulation,* which balances the network. The neuromodulation quickly decreases the patients' supersensitivities and appears to reset the brain stem's reticular activating system that regulates arousal level, restoring a normal sleep cycle. This leads to *neurorelaxation,* allowing the circuits to rest and restore their energy. Ongoing *neurostimulation,* combined with the patients' restored energy, allows them to turn on dormant circuits by engaging in mental and physical exercise, which is now increasingly possible. Only when homeostasis is corrected, and the brain is modulated, rested, and sufficient energy is resupplied so that brain rhythms can be restored, can a patient have a chance of overcoming the learned nonuse that I argue sets in with most brain injuries and diseases. Finally, the patients are ready for learning and *neurodifferentiation.* All these phases combined foster the optimal amount of neuroplastic change.

How long a person will have to use the device depends upon the illness or symptom. To treat a progressive disease, such as progressive types of MS or Parkinson's, will require long-term use, perhaps even for life, because the disease causes new damage every day. As Yuri puts it, "MS doesn't rest." Patients with a progressive illness find that if they interrupt the program before connections are consolidated (because, for instance, they have to travel and leave the device at home), they may stop making progress or their symptoms may return. Ron Husmann, the singer who had MS—an autoimmune inflammatory condition—developed serious arthritis, which also has inflammatory components; he went for multiple operations to replace both his knee and shoulder joints. Overwhelmed by all the time he spent going to surgeons, and supporting his wife through her own surgery, he found little time to use the PoNS, and his voice regressed. The PoNS helped his *symptoms* while he used it, resetting his noisy networks, but because the underlying inflammatory *pathology* and

---

may have occurred spontaneously after her damaged cells recovered, because while undergoing laser therapy, she was doing all kinds of mental and physical rehabilitation to activate her networks. It is possible the light activated damaged interneuron systems in its path, healing them, so they could neuromodulate damaged functional systems.

the *pathogenic* factors (which caused his MS-associated inflammation) could not be addressed, his brain reverted to its noisy state when he couldn't use the PoNS. This is why it is important, wherever possible, to address the brain's *general* cellular health as well as the *specific* wiring issues.*

The reasons the PoNS improves some symptoms but not others are not yet altogether clear. For noisy networks, the effects are dramatic and quick. Jeri, Kathy, Mary, and Ron all experienced remarkable improvements in disabling symptoms that had been in place for a very long time. I do not at this point claim that the device is generally eliminating the underlying progressive illness any more than our current medications do. What it is doing is eliminating many disabling symptoms that medication cannot, and without any known side effects. It teaches us, too, that many of our worst neurological illnesses and injuries progress not simply because the underlying illness has progressed but because the original illness has disturbed the person's nervous system enough for "noise" and learned nonuse to set in.

Norman Mailer, the abrasive novelist, wrote in *Advertisements for Myself*, "Every moment of one's existence one is growing into more or retreating into less. One is always living a little more or dying a little bit." I suspect something like that occurs in the brain. Absence of healthy activity in a noisy neural network does not simply lead the network to grow dormant; it leads to network disintegration and chaos. (Also, noisy networks, because they are dysfunctional, likely can't be taken over by other mental functions, as happens in a healthy brain network.) The upside is that if we can restore homeostasis to noisy neural networks, we can slow symptom progression that we think of as mercilessly progressive.

In problems that are not progressive, it appears possible to build up a residual effect over time, to the point where the device is no longer needed. But for progressive illness, it may be required for long periods, or life—it's too early to say. (And some illnesses that we have not thought

* Approaches to MS that modify the diet, or remove toxins from the body, are attempts to address the *general* cellular problems that might give rise to inflammation throughout the body.

to be progressive actually are, as we've recently learned is the case with some concussions.) Other cases are like that of Sue Voiles, for whom a huge proportion of the brain stem was removed to save her life. Sue's improvement has been slow. Her balance has improved so she can stand unassisted—in church, she recently noticed, she didn't need to use the pew for support. But she still needs a walker when moving, though recently, to her surprise, she walked out into her driveway without it. Sue, another former athlete, has been using the device daily for almost two years.

New Frontiers

"You can't imagine what mess we are in," says Yuri, exasperated at the mounting work, "with every patient giving us something new!" The team is finding that the device works for problems they never dreamed it would, and they feel the burden of having to research them all. It's not so easy to have an all-purpose brain stem homeostasis corrector.

Having published their pilot study of MS, and with the Omaha MS study in progress, they are gearing up for a study on stroke, Parkinson's, and TBI. The U.S. military recently began a study of soldiers with TBI and the device; a second study in Omaha is assessing the device to help children with acquired brain injury after neurosurgery for brain cancer; in Vancouver, a study is to commence using the device on spinal cord injuries; and groups in Russia are studying it for Parkinson's disease, stroke, cerebral palsy, tinnitus (ringing in the ears), and hearing loss. The team has seen anecdotal improvements in people with migraines related to balance disorders, nystagmus (an eye tracking problem), brain damage after chemotherapy, neuropathic pain (including trigeminal neuralgia), dystonia, oscillopsia (a vision disturbance where objects seem to oscillate), dysphagia (trouble swallowing), spinocerebellar ataxia (a progressive illness in which the cerebellum wastes away, and the patient loses control of his movement), Mal de Debarquement syndrome (in which people get seasick and, back on land, find that a persistent sense of motion stays with them), and general balance problems. They think the device may help improve functioning for autistic spectrum disorders (where the cerebellum is often affected, and where balance and sensory integration problems are prominent), neuropathies, epilepsy, essential tremor, cerebral palsy, sleep disorders, some learning disorders, possibly neurodegenerative diseases other than Parkinson's including Alzheimer's, and age-related balance loss.

This isn't to say the inventors think it's a panacea. However, a device that can tune detuned brain networks—or rather, help them tune themselves—and then neuroplastically reinforce vital homeostatic circuits may well have wide applicability. The device may be especially effective in MS because it also turns off chronic inflammation, a newly discovered effect of electricity on the brain. Scientists have discovered a *neuroinflammatory reflex* that is housed in the vagus nerve (which the PoNS stimulates directly) and have recently used electrical stimulation of the vagus to cure rheumatoid arthritis, an autoimmune illness like MS, in a man for whom all medications had failed. The details of the neuroinflammatory reflex, and how it works to turn off an overactive immune system almost immediately, are discussed in detail in the endnotes.

WHAT MAKES SOME PHYSICIANS SKEPTICAL when they hear about the PoNS device is its seeming nonspecificity—its ability to affect so many brain and body systems. In recent centuries, Western physicians have tried to understand the body by breaking it down into smaller and smaller elements—organs, then cells, then genes, then molecules, and so on—believing that the smaller the unit, the more likely it is to carry the explanation of diseases and clues to their cures. In neurology, this approach has led to the seeming victory of the chemists and the geneticists over the electrophysiologists, who generally deal with huge waves of activity spread throughout the brain. It has led to a belief that each illness is best treated by a unique chemical or magic bullet to target the microscopic defect.

A device that appears to stimulate a huge network of the brain's own self-regulating, homeostatic system may appear too diffuse to be of use for brain diseases. We want our diseases to have a discrete address.

Hence the idea of an all-purpose intervention helping large networks rebalance themselves immediately is easily dismissed as quackery or a placebo cure. For several millennia the vitalists, who believe that the body functions as a whole and must be addressed as a whole, and the materialist-localizationists, who believe illness is a problem afflicting a part, have been battling it out. The localizationists are ascendant at the moment, but in truth, both schools have had important insights. The device, though it summons so much of the brain, is after all the product of a very focal analysis of the specificities and frequencies that some very small entities—receptors, neurons, and synapses of the tongue—respond to.

And yet it uses these very Western scientific ideas and methods to help the body help itself in a holistic and very Eastern way: to engage homeostasis and to encourage self-regulation as part of the process of healing. In this respect, it seems like a very natural way to harness science to heal. For homeostatic self-regulation isn't just one thing among others that living things do. Self-regulation, maintaining order within chaos, is the essence of life. It is what distinguishes the smallest living thing in its thin envelope from the harsh inanimate chaos that surrounds it. And it is what distinguishes us, insofar as we are animated, from the chaos that awaits us when we lose that ability to maintain order. Our bodies revert to chaos and become inanimate. Thus, self-regulation—the cure through finding homeostasis—is so welcome, so familiar, and so appealing because it is not something we can do only sometimes; it is, as long as we are healthy and alive, what we are always doing.

Chapter 8

A Bridge of Sound

The Special Connection Between Music and the Brain

> SOCRATES: And therefore, I said, Glaucon, musical training is a
> more potent instrument than any other, because rhythm and
> harmony find their way into the inward places of the soul, on
> which they mightily fasten.
>
> Plato, *The Republic*

I. A Dyslexic Boy Reverses His Misfortune

One day in the spring of 2008, I got a telephone call from a woman I had never met, to tell me about Paul Madaule, the man who had saved her son. At the age of three, her son, whom I'll call "Simon," was showing disturbing signs. He wouldn't respond to his name or answer back; if a ball was rolled to him, he wouldn't roll it back. He crawled and walked late and was clumsy and developmentally delayed. His mother, whom I'll call "Natalie," told me that the psychologist she took him to said he *might* be on the autistic spectrum. Another clinician said he displayed some "autistic-like symptoms," though Natalie doubted this diagnosis. His occupational therapist suggested that Natalie take him to Paul Madaule.

Madaule said Simon had the "peripheral" symptoms of autism; he agreed that he had major developmental problems, but Simon did *not* have what some saw as the core autistic symptom: the inability to imagine the minds of other people. Natalie told me that working with Madaule changed her son completely. Once withdrawn, he could now start up interactions with others, his movements and speech became fluid, and he was able to have "his first real conversation with me, ever."

But Madaule's techniques were so unusual, she confessed, that when she spoke of them to mainstream practitioners and parents of children with similar problems, they seemed not to believe her story: they were either skeptical or showed no curiosity about how a boy with autistic-like symptoms had lost them.

When I asked her what precisely Madaule had done, I could hear her preparing to tell me something she knew would sound far-fetched. Madaule, she said, had used music—usually Mozart, but modified in a strange way, together with modified recordings of her own voice—to rewire her son's brain. It had radically improved his ability not only to listen and relate, but also to perform, for the first time, many mental activities that had nothing to do with sound. This was music medicine: using sound energy to form a bridge into the brain, to speak its language.

Now, five years later, Natalie said, her son was "at the top of his class academically, has more friends than I can schedule in his calendar, is kind, empathetic, and hyperaware of social currency." His motor problems were gone, and he was a competitive swimmer, a soccer and cricket player, and a gold medalist in karate. "The work that Paul and his staff did has changed our lives in so many ways, and so profoundly. I don't know what I would have done if I hadn't come across it." She hesitated, then said, "I don't like to think about it."

PAUL MADAULE, I DISCOVERED, ACTUALLY lived on my street in Toronto, in an old Victorian house from the 1880s, hidden far back from the sidewalk, off an alley, behind a wooden fence, surrounded by a botanical garden the size of a small park. He had bought the property when it was a run-down, dilapidated, termite-infested rooming house with open sewage pipes; its lot had been used as a local dumping ground.

He quietly moved into one of the rooms. Whenever a tenant moved out, he and a friend would reconstruct and resurrect that space. By supporting himself on the rents from his remaining tenants, he was able to fix up the place one room at a time. Over the years, with the help of his wife, Lyn, he brought the vacant lot back to life, cultivating it into a hidden paradise. He had a way of rescuing treasures no one else could—both in his work with children and in his personal life.

Madaule, a handsome, dark-haired Frenchman, has huge, receptive brown eyes, symmetrical Gallic features, and facial bones that suggest the appearance of a Mediterranean artist. He is a humble, sensitive, and unintrusive clinician (an essential trait in those who help developmentally disordered, hypersensitive children). His soft, slow, nonmechanical way of moving has a calming effect on any room. His strong presence neither dominates nor advertises itself. After spending some time with him, you can feel the quality and reach of his attention; it is indeed the focus of an artist. Even if he is observing you, you don't feel disturbed or imposed upon, but rather that he is immersing his humanity in yours. But what is most striking about him is his deep and beautiful, assured, sonorous, calming voice.

It was not always so.

Paul was born with a devastating learning disorder, in 1949 in Castres, a small, isolated town in the south of France, a time and place that had little understanding of children's brain problems. Paul's parents took him to every known kind of specialist available in France in the 1960s: psychologists, psychiatrists, and *orthophonistes*—speech therapists—because he mumbled in an incomprehensible monotone. He always had to ask people to repeat themselves (even though conventional hearing tests reported his ears worked fine). He failed four grades in school (and, he says, passed a few that he didn't deserve to). He was diagnosed with "dyslexia," a word he could neither pronounce nor understand, used to describe the commonest learning disorder, involving difficulties in learning to read. Like many dyslexics, he reversed the letters *b* and *d*, and *p* and *q*, and the numbers 6 and 9 when printing them.

But his dyslexia affected much more than his reading. He walked, he said, like a duck. He walked into posts because of his poor sense of space and absentmindedness. Like many children with learning disorders, he was teased by his peers and even his teachers for his clumsiness; his own physical education teacher picked up on the mockery and called him *une oie grasse*—a fat goose. This was his welcome to the world of dyslexia.

I HAVE BEFORE ME A little peach-colored booklet, four by five inches, entitled, in French, *Carnet de Notes Hebdomadaires, Petit Séminaire de Castres,* which is Paul's weekly book of marks for grade ten. At the end of each week, his teacher wrote his grade in each of his subjects in a column, followed by his class ranking for the week. As I go through the booklet, two things are apparent. His grade for conduct and effort was always a pass. His grade for all of his courses was failing—and he was rarely close to passing. In the first week, Math 1/20; Language 3/20; Spanish 4/20; English 8/20. The booklet also gives his class ranking: he was twenty-fifth out of twenty-five students and held last place for every week of the year. The worst part for him was the weekly devastation he felt when he had to bring that report card home for his parents to sign. As is true for many learning-disabled children, his uncomprehending parents thought him lazy, so every report card day was unbearable, resulting in screaming matches, slammed doors, yelling, and crying; as he would later write, "It was hell for everybody."

Paul grew up plagued with self-doubt, which became worse as each year he fell further behind in school. He wondered if he might go to vocational school, but he was so clumsy he couldn't even turn a screwdriver. In social situations, though his thoughts came quickly, he either couldn't put them into words or he stammered. As a teen, he retreated to his bedroom and listened to the same songs over and over for hours. The one form of expression he enjoyed was drawing, and he loved the art of the modern masters.

He failed grade ten, having failed every single subject that year. Because he had failed four grades in a row, and was three years older than his classmates, he wasn't allowed to take the grade ten examinations again. Finally he gave up and dropped out.

A Chance Encounter at the Abbaye d'En Calcat

Suddenly at eighteen, he was isolated, without school or a job. With endless time on his hands, he often visited a Benedictine monastery, a ten-mile bike ride from his home. He was drawn there because there were artists there, and he hoped that maybe he could become one, art being the one activity that he could see himself doing. At the abbey, called Abbaye d'En Calcat, he found peace. One day Father Marie, a monk who had taken an interest in Paul, told him that a physician was visiting the monastery and had happened to give a lecture on dyslexia. Father Marie said the doctor had described symptoms very much like Paul's.

The physician, Dr. Alfred Tomatis, had been invited to the monastery to make a house call under peculiar circumstances. Most of the monks had fallen ill and were struggling with exhaustion and symptoms that nobody had been able to explain. Seventy of the ninety once-hardy monks, who had often gotten by on about four hours' sleep, were now listless all day long, slumping in their rooms. A procession of physicians had been brought through the monastery, each dispensing recommendations. Some advised more sleep, but the more the monks slept, the more tired they became. Specialists in digestion recommended that the monks—vegetarians since the twelfth century—begin eating meat. They got worse.

The last physician to arrive was Tomatis, which seemed absurd, because he was an otolaryngologist, an ear, nose, and throat specialist. But he was known to be a genius at diagnosis and had an interest in mind-body medicine. Tomatis set up equipment in a small room in the monastery and trained a monk to administer tests to his ailing brothers. He also consented to see Paul, but first he had to be tested.

When Paul arrived in the monk's room, it was filled with electronic machines, which looked like they were for hearing tests. He put on headphones and was told to raise his right hand as fast as he could when he heard a beep in his right ear, and to raise his left if the beep was in the left ear. Then he listened to pairs of beeps and was instructed to tell the monk which sound was higher and which lower. It seemed to Paul much like the hearing tests he had already had.

But Tomatis did not do hearing tests. He did *listening* tests. He saw hearing as a passive experience involving the ear; "listening" was active and was about what the brain could extract and decode from what came in through the ear. At the end of the test, the monk gave Paul some graphs and told him to go meet the doctor in the monastery park.

"Tomatis," said Dr. Tomatis, introducing himself. He was forty-seven years old and stood very straight, a posture developed from years of yoga practice. He had a broad expansive chest, a shaven head (rare in those days), and funny pointed ears. He was an intimidating figure. But when he spoke, his voice was calming, soft, and warm, with a soothing murmur. He had a twinkle in his eye that made Paul feel he really cared. His voice was one, Paul said, "*qui vous met en confiance*—that made you feel confident in yourself, confident enough to confide to another person, so I felt at ease, right away."

After Dr. Tomatis looked over the test results, he took Paul on a walk in the park and asked him many questions about art, his home life, his sexuality, his religion, his hopes and dreams. He raised every topic except Paul's horrendous difficulties at school. He freely differed with Paul, yet always made him feel his own views counted.

Finally Tomatis explained to Paul the meaning of his lifelong symptoms—his "*petite misères*," annoying little problems, in a way that made Paul understand, for the first time in his life, his difficulties reading and expressing himself, his extreme shyness, temper tantrums, anxiety, clumsiness, insomnia, and fear of the future. He explained too how these problems fit together, which seemed incredible, given that he had tested only Paul's listening. Paul thought, "He is the first person who ever talked to *me*; others talked to someone they saw." Tomatis invited Paul to come for treatment at his clinic in Paris, then inexplicably asked that he bring a recording of his mother's voice.

IN PARIS, IN TOMATIS'S OFFICE, Paul was again asked to put on headphones and told that the treatment would begin with listening, every day for several weeks. At first, he heard only scratchy, indecipherable static with bits of a tinny-sounding, electronically manipulated Mozart.

Tomatis told Paul he could do whatever he wanted while he listened, so he chose to draw and paint. Every week or so he was given another listening test, then met with Tomatis.

Days passed, and slowly he made out isolated words behind some of the scratchy sounds. The words seemed far away, from a distant world. Then a phrase, or even a sentence, might pop out. Several weeks into the experience, he noticed that his listening was improving—he was getting better at understanding sounds—and his symptoms were beginning to decline. One day he suddenly realized that all this time, in some of the screechy recordings, he had been listening to his mother's voice.

At the end of four weeks, he was a different person. It would require years of study to understand how this transformation had occurred: how "mere" energy—the energy and information of sound waves—had helped him rewire his brain.

A Compressed History of Young Alfred Tomatis

Alfred Tomatis was born in France at the end of December 1919, two and a half months premature, weighing just under three pounds. Today doctors pride themselves on being able to keep "preemies" alive. But the preemie has the arduous task of surviving, thrust from the protected natural paradise of the warm watery womb into an outside world of booming, buzzing confusion—of artificial incubators, machine noises, and hospital lights, with shiny metals and tubes threaded in and out of its three-pound body. In Tomatis's case, it happened two and a half months before his brain was sufficiently developed to process, filter, and buffer all these intrusive sensations. Nature's developmental clock is precise, and many sensory functions reach a state of readiness for external reality two weeks before the average expected date of delivery. The ear, however, is an exception: its parts reach full size and become operational halfway through pregnancy.

"I have an unshakable intuition," Tomatis wrote, "that my work and speculations are deeply bound up with the conditions and events, feelings and sensations, conscious and subconscious thoughts, basic needs, and secret desires which surround my entry into the world and then put an indelible mark on my infancy." The circumstances of Tomatis's prematurity were to haunt him for his whole life. His father, Umberto Dante, from Piedmont, Italy, age twenty when Alfred was born, was a charismatic opera singer and would become one of Europe's finest voices; his mother was a teenager. "My arrival in the world," Tomatis wrote,

> does not seem to have been expected, much less hoped for, by my sixteen-year-old mother.... The birth seemed to pose a problem for everyone in the family, and no doubt they were eager to get rid of this unexpected baby quickly and with little fuss. Remarkable compression efforts were used to prevent this pregnancy from being noticed; the corsets of that past age, so strongly supported by unbending whalebones, readily helped.

These attempts to hide the pregnancy, Tomatis came to believe, triggered his premature birth and left him with a very strange post-traumatic tendency.

> The compression also apparently influenced my need during the first forty years of life to live tightly swathed in clothes, with a body belt that cut me in two, and restricted also by narrow confining shoes. At night, I did not sleep unless eight blankets were piled upon me. Though I was not cold, I needed to experience this pressure of the world around me to reproduce the vital conditions I had known in my mother's womb.

This symptom may seem idiosyncratically neurotic, but it is not unheard of in people born premature or on the autistic spectrum. The author Temple Grandin, herself autistic, found that deep pressure on her body settled her, and invented a "squeeze machine" to calm herself. Though Tomatis was not autistic, he was in tune with some of the more atypical cravings that autistic and premature people experience. But once he finally understood the origin of his cravings for pressure, he lost the need for it.

Communication with his mother, Tomatis felt, was "never easy. All my attempts at intimacy were repulsed." The family lived in Nice, although Tomatis's singer father was often on the road six months of the year. Young Alfred, from birth on, was in constant ill health, suffering from digestive disorders. A doctor came by and couldn't understand Alfred's symptoms but said, "I must search for the answer." This so moved Alfred that he resolved to become a doctor himself.

Young Alfred idealized his father, Umberto, but from a distance, because he was so often away. One day Umberto said to Alfred, "I have thought this over carefully. My boy, if you really want to become a doctor—and a good doctor—you must go to Paris. We don't know anyone there, so you'll have to manage all by yourself, but you'll learn what life is all about, and that will certainly be of some use to you."

Alfred was only eleven, but thinking this plan would give his father pleasure, he went. He boarded at a school, experiencing years of great loneliness. After failures at school, he noticed that he learned his lessons best if he read them out loud. He studied feverishly, going to bed late and waking at four a.m., imitating in this respect his workaholic father. He often worked to the sound of Mozart.

In his third year at school, he won nearly all the academic prizes in his grade. In high school, the philosopher Jean-Paul Sartre was his teacher. Then Alfred completed two certificates in sciences, finishing first in both, including one at the Sorbonne. Just as he was beginning medical school, World War II broke out, and he was drafted. Early in the war, his entire unit was taken prisoner by German and Italian troops. He helped organize a successful escape and joined the French Resistance as a courier. By day, he helped a physician in a labor camp. After the Allies landed in Normandy, he was assigned to the French Air Corps and began to study ear, nose, and throat medicine (ENT, or otolaryngology), still under the influence of his father, who so loved music and sound.

The First Law of Tomatis

Young Tomatis had demonstrated academic brilliance and an uncompromising work ethic; in this next period, he began to show genius. As the war ended, he completed his medical degree and worked as a consultant to the air corps, where he made important observations using an audiometer, a machine that showed that aircraft factory workers were going deaf in a certain range of their hearing, at 4,000 Hz. He was one of the first to demonstrate the occupational health hazard of noise. He noticed also that deafness caused by jet engines, gunfire, and explosions led to movement and psychological problems. The ear had a relationship to the body, it seemed, that had not been observed.

At roughly the same time, in his medical practice, he began treating opera singers, often friends of his father's who had developed trouble controlling their voices. Singers were referred to otolaryngologists then, because orthodox medical opinion believed that their problems occurred because they strained their voices, damaging their vocal cords, which are part of the larynx. The conventional treatment was to give the patient strychnine (a poison) to tighten the muscles of the vocal cords. When one of Europe's leading baritones, who had been told his vocal cords had become stretched and too slack, was referred to Tomatis, he decided to give him the same test he had given the aircraft workers—and discovered a similar hearing loss, in the range of 4,000 Hz. Tomatis began to suspect that the accepted theory that the larynx was the essential organ for singing was wrong; it was, he would prove, the ear.

He began testing the volume of the sound produced by the opera singers in his practice, using a machine to measure it in decibels. Typically, when singing at half strength, the singers produced 80 to 90 decibels. At full strength, they could achieve up to 130 or 140 decibels. He calculated that because his sound equipment, a meter away from the singer, was detecting 130 decibels, the volume within the singer's skull, directly affecting the ear, was 150 decibels. (By comparison, the volume of a French Caravelle jet engine—a sound level he had measured in the air corps—was 132 decibels.) At certain frequencies, because of the intensity of the sound they produced inside their heads, singers were singing themselves into deafness; they sang poorly because they heard poorly.

In the late 1940s Tomatis continued to attack the conventional wisdom that the larynx is the key organ for singing. He showed that contrary to conventional wisdom, singers with bass voices did not have larger larynxes than those with higher voices. Human beings aren't constructed like pipe organs, in which larger tubes produce lower sounds. Powerful tenors sing at frequencies from 800 Hz up to 4,000 Hz, but so do baritones and basses; the only difference is that the baritones and basses can add lower notes, because they can hear lower notes. He summed it up by saying provocatively "One sings with one's ear," a statement that caused much laughter.

But when scientists at the Sorbonne presented their studies of his work to the National Academy of Medicine and the French Academy of Sciences, they concluded that "the voice can only contain the frequencies that the ear can hear." The idea came to be called "the Tomatis effect" and became the first of what would be his laws.

His next project was to discover the difference between the "good" singing voices and "bad" ("good" being those widely considered the great singers of the day). He built a machine, which he called the sonic analyzer, that could display a picture of all the different frequencies in a person's voice. Using this device on singers, he made discoveries that laid the groundwork for healing children with disabilities.

This project began in an unlikely way. While Tomatis was working with opera singers, he gathered all the recordings he could find—old wax phonograph cylinders for gramophones, records, and master recordings—of the world's most famous opera singer, Enrico Caruso, who had died in 1921. He studied them in detail with his sonic analyzer, expecting to find that Caruso's singing voice would go as high as the human speaking voice, which can produce sounds up to 15,000 Hz. To his surprise, Tomatis found that Caruso's voice went only to 8,000 Hz. (Most fine singers' voices, he would later discover, go only to 7,000 Hz.) Caruso's voice had had two periods. The first lasted from 1896 to 1902, when it was very fine; the second was the "spectacularly beautiful" period, lasting from 1903 until his health declined, when it was even better. Tomatis found that in the second period, his voice was objectively *less rich* in terms of frequencies and for *all* the sound frequencies below 2,000 Hz. During the second period, he hypothesized, Caruso couldn't hear low frequencies well.

Further research showed that in early 1902 Caruso had had an operation on the right side of his face, which probably affected his Eustachian tubes (which connect the middle ear to the back of the throat). Tomatis had noticed that people with blocked Eustachian tubes had the same drop in frequencies that Caruso had. The operation, he concluded, had made Caruso partially deaf so that, ironically, he could hear only in his new singing range and thus could not produce the sounds of lesser quality below it. "It was as if Caruso," Tomatis wrote, "had benefited from a sort of filter which allowed him to hear essential, high frequency sounds rich in harmonics as opposed to low frequency fundamental sounds." Unable to hear, and thus produce lower tones (which normally interfere with perception of higher tones), Caruso had a richer perception of his superhigh overtones. Tomatis used to joke that Caruso was condemned to sing beautifully, and there was nothing he could do about it.

Tomatis's Second and Third Laws

Next, Tomatis invented a new instrument to help singers with damaged voices. He called it the Electronic Ear and it became the basis of all Tomatis's treatments. It consisted of a microphone, a system of amplifiers and filters to block out some frequencies and emphasize others, and headphones. A performer would sing or speak into the microphone and hear his or her own filtered voice through the headphones.

When he assessed his struggling singers, he found that they were not hearing high frequencies well. So he set up the filters on the Electronic Ear so that they *could hear themselves with Caruso's ears*—that is, with the lower frequencies blocked—allowing them to hear the higher tones better. When singers sang into Tomatis's machine, their voices improved radically. This led him to formulate his second law: "If one brings to the compromised ear the possibility of hearing the lost or compromised frequencies correctly, these are instantly and unconsciously restored in the vocal emission." Put simply, hearing, if "fixed," can heal the voice. He had singers train several hours a day over several weeks, listening to themselves through "Caruso's ears." With training, their new ability to listen and sing well lasted even after they stopped using the machine. And so he formulated his third law, the Law of Retention, which was that training the ear by exposing it to the proper frequencies can lead to a *permanent* effect on listening (and hence the brain) and the voice. Tomatis knew that this was a form of brain training: "the sensory apparatus we know as the ear is simply an external attribute of the cerebral cortex." (In Chapter 7 I called this permanent effect of brain training the residual effect; it is a result of neurons firing together and wiring together, making lasting changes in the brain.)

Tomatis also made observations on the energizing effect of good listening. He noticed that when he used the Electronic Ear, especially on singers with imperfect voices, "all, without exception, felt an increased sense of well-being. Even among those who were not singers, many confided in me that they felt like singing." When they unblocked their high frequencies, clients would puff up their chests like opera singers. They stood straighter, breathed more deeply, felt they had more energy and vitality, and listened to themselves better—all quite involuntarily. With blocked high frequencies, they would speak in lifeless, de-energized voices, and they would slouch; their voices would become hard to take, monotonous, and even draining on the listener.

Tomatis also observed that the ear is intimately connected not only with balance but also with posture. There is a distinct *listening posture,* often seen when people listen to classical music: the right ear in most people is a bit forward, as is the head. This listening posture, he observed, is tied into the overall tonus of the body: the person looks spry, and alert. Just as neurons are never totally off, so too in a healthy person, relaxed muscles are never totally slack. Tomatis argued that input from the ear has an impact on the verticality and tonus of the entire body—and of course certain kinds of music make people feel they must *get up* and dance. His observation that good listening is energizing suggested to him that higher frequencies energize the brain, and he summarized it by proposing that "the ear is a battery to the brain."

The Auditory Zoom

Tomatis kept making discoveries at a feverish pace. He noticed that when subjects listened with the Electronic Ear, filtered so they heard like Caruso, they pronounced the letter *r* with a distinctly Neapolitan accent. Knowing that Caruso was from Naples gave Tomatis an idea. Perhaps accents, too, are a function of the frequencies people hear. Testing, he soon found that the French, for instance, hear in two ranges, 100 to 300 Hz and 1,000 to 2,000 Hz. Speakers of British English hear in one higher range, from 2,000 to 12,000 Hz, which makes it hard for French people to learn English in England. But North American English involves frequencies from 800 to 3,000, a range closer to the French ear, making it easier for the French to learn.

Soon Tomatis was able to help people learn second languages by setting up the filters that reflected those of a native speaker. These "different ears," he argued, were probably based on different "acoustic geographies." Whether a speaker is raised in a forest, on an open plain, on mountains, or by the sea has a major impact on the sounds he hears, because certain frequencies are muffled or amplified by different environments. When he set the Electronic Ear's filters to "British ear" and put it on French children who were studying British English, their English improved, and for some reason, their grades in other subjects did too. So Tomatis increasingly turned his attention to the relationship between these "different ears" and language, learning, and severe learning problems.

Arguably his most important discovery was that the ear is not a passive organ but has the equivalent of a zoom lens that allows it to focus on particular noises and filter others out. He called it the auditory zoom. When people first walk into a party, they hear a jumble of noises, until they zoom in on particular conversations, each occurring at slightly different sound frequencies. Once a person forms a conscious intention to listen to a particular conversation, the listening, from a physiological perspective, is never passive, because two muscles within the middle ear allow it to focus on particular frequencies and protect it from sudden loud sounds. In most people, most of the time, this muscular adjustment, which makes the auditory zoom possible, occurs automatically and unconsciously. When loud sounds occur, the zoom shuts them down reflexively. However, the zoom can sometimes come under partial conscious control, as when we attempt to tune in to an important conversation in a very noisy room or learn a second language.

The first of the two muscles is the stapedius. When it tenses, it increases the perception and discrimination of the medium-high-frequency sounds of language, while muting the lower tones that overwhelm higher frequencies, allowing the listener to extract speech sounds from the environment. The second muscle is the tensor tympani, which modifies the tension of the tympanic membrane (the eardrum). It complements the stapedius, and when it tenses, it decreases the perception of low-frequency sounds in background noise. Both of these middle ear muscles contract when we speak, so that we don't injure our ears with the sound of our own voices. This happens not only with opera singers; a child screaming is about as loud as a passing train. Tomatis also observed that when these muscles do not work well, because they are weak, as is the case with many children, they receive too much of the low frequencies (and thus too much background noise) and not enough of the higher frequencies of speech.

These muscles of the middle ear, which tune in on speech, are regulated by the brain. As studies by the neuroscientist Jonathan Fritz and his colleagues from the University of Maryland show, when particular frequencies carry important information (in an experiment, it might be a tone indicating that a shock will soon follow), the brain map areas for those frequencies in the auditory cortex grow within minutes, to better tune in on them. When the frequencies stop, the brain map areas may revert to their previous size or, sometimes, persist. Thus the auditory zoom has a neuroplastic component.

Many children who have had chronic ear infections have hypotonia (generalized low muscle tonus) of the ear muscles. Hypotonia *throughout the body* is common in children with developmental delays. This overall low muscle tonus also affects their ear muscles, so they cannot focus on specific sound frequencies. Thus they only hear *nondifferentiated* noise, muffled sounds, or too many sounds at once, so their auditory cortices never get clear signals and can't develop normally. That was what happened to Paul: because everything he heard was muffled, everything he said was mumbled, and his auditory brain maps were poorly differentiated. Many children on the autistic spectrum have problems with the auditory zoom as well.

Tomatis realized he could use the Electronic Ear to exercise the auditory zoom by manipulating sounds. For people with nondifferentiated auditory maps, he played sound frequencies that would alternately stimulate and relax the slack ear muscles and the brain circuits involved, to give them a workout. People listening to his modified music were being trained to make more *differentiated* brain maps, and with them, they could start to differentiate speech from background noise.

Speaking Out of One Side of Our Mouths

Tomatis made yet another major clinical discovery—something we all look at every day of our lives, but never see. He discovered that almost every human being talks primarily out of one side of the mouth. People with good listening skills overwhelmingly speak with the *right* side of the mouth, and the sound of their speech enters their right ear. The right ear and its circuits are also important for singing. All the professionally successful singers that Tomatis examined—with one exception—were "right-eared"; when he played noise into their right ear, so they couldn't hear their voices on the right, their singing voice deteriorated.

The left hemisphere is the area where most people—be they right- or left-handed—process important verbal elements of speech. However, each brain hemisphere gets most of its sound input from the ear on the *opposite* side of the body.* Hence most of the nerve fibers supplying the left hemisphere come from the right ear. Thus the fastest, most

---

* According to Tomatis, the right ear sends three-fifths of the fibers of its auditory nerve to the left hemisphere, and two-fifths go to the right hemisphere. Similarly, the left ear sends three-fifths of its nerve fibers to the right hemisphere and two-fifths to the left.

direct nerve pathway to the left hemisphere's language area, for most people, is via the right ear. There are a few exceptions, in some left-handed people.*

The day Tomatis and Paul met, as they walked outside the monastery, Tomatis saw that there was more animation on the left side of Paul's face, and more movement on the left side of his lips and mouth when he talked, and that his left side—and left ear—leaned into the conversation. This behavior meant that Paul was hearing speech with his left ear. Sound signals had to take the roundabout, less efficient path to get to his left-hemisphere language area: they had to pass from his left ear to his right hemisphere, *then back across, through the middle of his brain,* to his left hemisphere. The resulting delay, up to 0.4 second, contributed to Paul's inability to process the speech of others in real time, causing a time lapse whenever he tried to put his thoughts into words and contributed to his tendency to lose his train of thought. This is because, over time, speaking on the left side of the mouth and listening with the left ear can lead to disorganization in a developing brain, contribute to learning disorders that seem unrelated to listening, and give rise to stammering and stuttering.

Most people do certain activities with their right hemisphere, and certain activities with their left. For instance, most right-handers write with their right hand, use a baseball bat on the right side, and use the right hand for activities that require strength, coordination, and control. Their right hand is dominant, and is controlled by the left hemisphere. But Paul, Tomatis observed, used his left hand for some activities, and his right for others, a pattern called mixed dominance, which is typical of people with dyslexia who are left-ear listeners, and which can,

---

* Some left-handed people who speak well, such as President Bill Clinton, use both sides of the mouth to speak, meaning that they listen on both sides equally. Ninety-five percent of healthy right-handers process key elements of verbal language in their left hemisphere; the remaining 5 percent process them in their right. Seventy percent of left-handers process key aspects of verbal language in the left hemisphere, 15 percent in the right, and 15 percent bilaterally. Since only about 10 percent of people are left-handed, the overwhelming majority of people process language activities on the left. For the small number of left-handed people who have the relevant speech area in the right hemisphere, modern Tomatis practitioners do not train right-ear listening. See S. P. Springer and G. Deutsch, *Left Brain Right Brain: Perspectives from Cognitive Neuroscience* (New York: W. H. Freeman, 1999), p. 22.

thought Tomatis, indicate a brain problem. Because of his mixed dominance, Paul was unable to differentiate brain areas for his right and left hands or to use his hands to do different tasks simultaneously, such as playing the guitar, where one hand strums and the other is on the fingerboard. Such mixed dominance contributed to his overall clumsiness and poor handwriting and even affected his eye tracking when he was reading. Instead of reading from left to right in a systematic way, frequently his eyes strayed back to the midline of a sentence or jumped around the page. To make Paul a right-eared listener and correct his mixed dominance, Tomatis set the Electronic Ear to stimulate Paul's right ear and its circuitry by decreasing the volume to the left.

Paul was not just a slow listener. He often missed what people were saying, Tomatis realized, because he heard *too much in the low frequencies* and not enough in the higher ones. The reasons were several: First, Paul had visibly low muscle tonus throughout his body, which led to his poor posture, clumsiness, and dislike of fast movements. This bodily hypotonia affected and weakened Paul's ear muscles and auditory zoom, so it couldn't differentiate the frequencies of human speech. Second, Paul listened mostly with his left ear. Tomatis had found that the right ear and its brain circuit generally hear more of the higher speech frequencies than the left. Thus Paul often heard more background noise and hum than clear speech. Since the right ear and its auditory cortex normally process the higher frequencies, stimulating the right side also trained Paul's brain to process speech more clearly.

Training the Brain by Stimulating the Ear

Tomatis divided his listening program into two phases. The first, the passive phase, usually lasts fifteen days. It is called passive because the client needs only to hear the modified music, without concentrating on it. (In fact, it's best if he doesn't pay too close attention to the music, because that activity can trigger the old listening habits that the therapist is trying to overcome.)

Mozart's music is usually modified with the filters emphasizing high frequencies, so it often has a whistling, hisslike sound. With children adolescents, the mother's voice, filtered to accentuate the higher frequencies, is also added. In the early stages of the listening, the mother's voice is so filtered that it is very hard to identify and sounds more like a squeaky whistle, from another world. When the mother's voice is not available, the music alone will suffice. (In the passive phase, the microphone attached to the Electronic Ear is not used. The child simply listens to the music or the mother's voice through headphones.)

The Electronic Ear, defined by Tomatis as a "simulator of proper listening," is composed of two audio channels. One channel feeds the client music that is filtered to emphasize higher treble frequencies and deemphasize lower frequencies. (The higher frequencies are the frequencies of human speech.) The channel with the lower frequencies replicates the hearing that a poor listening ear, with poor muscle tone, experiences. When this channel is played to people with listening problems, their ear muscles "relax," and they replicate their usual listening habits. The filter is always switching between the high-frequency channel and the lower-frequency one, with the volume of the music triggering this switch between channels. When the volume is low, the low-frequency channel is heard; when it gets up to certain decibels, the high-frequency channel kicks in. Each time it switches to the high-frequency channel, the ear muscles and high-frequency listening are exercised; when it switches back to the lower frequency, the muscles and the neurons related to those frequencies can rest. These cycles of exercise make up the passive phase of the listening training.

This switching back and forth between channels triggered by the music's changing its volume (called gating by electronic engineers) injects a sense of novelty into the listening, and novelty is a powerful way to engage brain plasticity. Having a novel sensory experience awakens the brain's attention processors, and new connections are more easily made between neurons. It secretes dopamine (and other brain chemicals) to consolidate the connections between the neurons that recorded the event. This transaction is the brain's way of saying "Save that one!" Over the years Tomatis made sure that the gating, or switching back and forth, was *not* predictable, because surprise is key to brain change. He found that prerecorded tapes lacking random changes were not nearly as effective.

The passive phase ends when the filtering, which gradually decreases over time, is completely eliminated from the Mozart and the mother's voice.

Typically a rest period of four to six weeks is scheduled between the end of the passive phase and the beginning of the active phase, so that the client can consolidate, integrate, and practice his listening gains. At this phase in Paul's training, he was listening better and with less effort. All his previous teachers and tutors had told him he had to try harder. Now that his brain was getting the right information, he discovered he needn't work harder to do better, because there was "flow" to his listening.

When the passive phase ended, Tomatis surprised Paul with the suggestion he go to England, instead of returning home. He told him it was so he could learn English—a daunting task for anyone with listening problems. Tomatis wisely orchestrated Paul's adventure so that he could test his new skills away from Castres, the environment that had been so undermining for him. Paul was ecstatic, but also puzzled. Twice before he had tried to learn English in England, failed, and given up. But now he went and was able to make himself understood, connect with people, and enjoy exploring the London of the 1960s. "Everything," he wrote, "seemed surprisingly easy, even the English language."

On Paul's return, Tomatis's next surprise, to reinforce the idea of a new start, was to suggest that Paul enroll in a boarding school near Paris, though Paul had never successfully completed grade ten. He was intimidated, but Tomatis insisted that Paul aim to get the high school diploma—required for university admission—in two years, and he reassured him that if he put as much effort into school as he had put into his listening training and having fun in England, he'd succeed. Going to school near Paris would allow him to continue the next phase of treatment, which would focus on his difficulties expressing himself.

THE ACTIVE PHASE CAME NEXT. To learn to express himself better in speech, Paul, wearing headphones, spoke into a microphone and listened to his own voice through the Electronic Ear. Because his auditory processing had so improved, he could now for the first time really *listen* to his voice, and use his own voice to improve his auditory processing—and to energize himself. He began to pronounce words with close attention, moving his lips and other muscles, while feeling the vibrations of his lips, throat, and facial and other bones that occurred when he spoke. As he sounded out various words, he developed a more fully differentiated proprioceptive awareness—an awareness of the exact position of his lips, tongue, and other body parts. As in a Feldenkrais lesson, he was using awareness to differentiate his brain maps.

Tomatis now encouraged Paul, who mumbled and spoke in a monotone, to hum, pronounce vowels, and repeat sentences to improve his speech flow. Though a speech therapist might have done this work, Paul did it while using the Electronic Ear, with filtered feedback through his headphones. That enriched the medium- and high-range frequencies of his voice, making it more vibrant, stronger, more expressive, and richer in timbre. Tomatis, influenced by his own yoga practice, trained Paul to sit ramrod straight and breathe properly. And one day, to Paul's surprise, he went into a bookstore and realized, as he was leafing through a book to look at the pictures, that he was actually reading and understanding it.

To improve Paul's reading, writing, and spelling, Tomatis asked him to read aloud, while consciously tracking the words with his eyes and listening through the Electronic Ear. To reinforce the newly established neural pathways, Paul also read aloud without the Electronic Ear for thirty minutes a day while making a fist with his right hand and pretending it was a microphone, and reading into it. That simple technique bounced sound off Paul's fist and back to his right ear, reinforcing right-sided listening and the dominance of higher frequencies.

At the boarding school, Paul, despite his fear, made friends quickly and no longer felt like a lost soul. Each weekend he bused into Paris to work on his listening skills. That first year he took and passed his driver's test—the first test he had ever passed. As the school year unfolded, he found that school went from being impossible to being merely difficult. Each day he did his Tomatis homework assignments, reading aloud. As the world of words opened up to him, he found that in his spare time he had switched from drawing to writing poetry. Humiliated that he was twenty years old and still in high school, he buckled down and passed his graduation exam, which in France most students fail on the first try. Now Tomatis asked him about his plans. Paul said his new goal was to help others as he had been helped: he wanted to become a psychologist and study with Tomatis.

A long apprenticeship began, with Paul living in the Tomatis home (where Tomatis's office was) from age twenty to twenty-three. By day, Paul's room was an office for a psychologist; by night, it was his bedroom. Paul began university and helped at Tomatis's clinic, learning how to filter music, record mothers' voices, and assist learning-disabled clients. Eventually he became a senior member of Tomatis's team. Tomatis brought Paul into his personal life and invited him to dine with the family and guests—opera singers, musicians, artists, scientists, psychoanalysts, philosophers, and religious figures from all over the world—making university seem dull by comparison. Paul completed his psychology degree at the University of Paris, at the prestigious Sorbonne, and became licensed in 1972.

Paul's first assignment from Tomatis was to start a listening center in Montpellier, in the south of France, and then another one in South Africa. After Tomatis had a heart attack in 1976, Paul came back to Paris to help train practitioners and coteach with Tomatis. Together they traveled throughout Europe and Canada. In addition, during this period, Tomatis wrote *La nuit utérine* (The Prenatal Night), a book about the prenatal roots of human language development, and the brain circuits involved in listening. Even though neuroplasticity was not yet accepted in neuroscience, Tomatis began to declare, "*Le cerveau est malléable*"—the brain is malleable.

Paul, who as a young boy could barely communicate, was now lecturing in several languages, eloquent in both English and French. With his new "ear," he was able to learn Spanish quickly. The boy who once could barely organize himself helped set up thirty centers in Mexico, Central America, Europe, South Africa, the United States, and Canada. From 1979 to 1982, Tomatis came to live in Toronto for six months a year, and helped set up the Listening Centre there, with Paul and the psychologist

Tim Gilmor as codirectors. Paul found Toronto a welcoming city and settled there, where he would take what he learned in France to new levels, to help some of the most challenging cases of arrested brain development.

II. A Mother's Voice

Born Halfway Down the Stairs

A thirty-four-year-old British solicitor, a woman I'll call "Liz," was awakened from sleep with a pang. Only twenty-nine and a half weeks pregnant, she was going into premature labor. Within seconds, her husband was on the phone to the ambulance. She tried to get down the stairs, but halfway down the baby's head came out. As she made it to the bottom, she delivered him herself. The entire labor lasted fifteen minutes. The baby was hypothermic—very cold, a blue-gray color—and too young to breathe properly by himself. She thought she would lose him. The ambulance got them to the hospital, where he was put on a ventilator machine to help him breathe. On his second day, his parents were told he wouldn't survive the night. They stood vigil by his incubator.

He did survive, but children born that prematurely are likely to have many complications. "Will," as I'll call him, had suffered oxygen deprivation, which can cause brain damage. Over 60 percent of the first two years of his life were spent in the hospital. At three months he had surgery for a hernia, then became unable to urinate, so he needed a second operation. He developed convulsions, requiring two admissions for suspected meningitis. He lost a kidney caused by infections. He suffered from pneumonia and swine flu. He was on antibiotics permanently (a burden on the gastrointestinal tract, because antibiotics kill the healthy organisms necessary for digestion). Instead of the blissful peace of the womb, and the gentle sleep and endless embraces of infancy, Will endured constant discomfort, invasions of his body, and brushes with death, while his parents watched helplessly.

WILL BECAME A FUSSY BABY, waking every night around one in the morning, staying up for four to five hours a night, disconsolate. Liz and her husband, "Frederick," lived for two and a half years on two to three hours of sleep. Will didn't like food, or even textures in his mouth, or any kind of sticky substance on his hands. He flapped his arms, as do many children with developmental disorders. He spent most of his days under a table or a sofa, maneuvering himself to feel pressure on his middle. When he went to bed, he had the same peculiar longing for a heavy weight of blankets on him that Tomatis had had.

Will's language development was delayed. His first word was "Dada" at ten months, but he never used it to identify his father. He would repeat the word for five minutes at a time. At fifteen months, he had a handful of words but never used them for communication—he used them to make "noises." He seemed deaf, because he didn't respond to his name. He didn't crawl or walk. And yet his parents could see that despite his problems, given the slightest relief from his torment, he was an affectionate baby.

At fifteen months, Will's doctors said he should get the measles, mumps, and rubella vaccine (MMR); because his immune system was so weak, if anyone was likely to get these illnesses, it would be him. Three weeks later he developed a fever of 105 and slipped into unconsciousness. The emergency room doctors suspected meningitis, and as they attempted to insert an intravenous needle, he became conscious. He struggled so hard, it took eight people thirty minutes to pin him down. Liz looked into his eyes as he was being pinned. To her they were saying "Why do you let them do this to me?"

After that he was terrified of needles and any kind of restraint.

AT THIS POINT, HE STOPPED speaking. From sixteen months on, Will didn't utter a single word. His personality changed—he withdrew. It was difficult to know which of the many stresses had caused his silence.

"At eighteen months," Liz says, "he wouldn't play with any toys. He was very autistic-like. He would turn a car over and spin the wheels—but would never play with it for its intended purpose. He was obsessive beyond comprehension, opening and closing every door for hours." He would run around furniture, as though he were trying to see the front, the side, and the back at the same time. He would put a piece of paper on the table, then run around the table. Out of his regular environment, at a mall, he would be unable to process all the new stimuli. At the park, he wouldn't go on the slide or the swing. All he did was run up and down along the fence railings.

He was unable to read his own bodily needs, didn't know if he was hungry or thirsty, never went to the cupboard to get food or tried to get a drink. He walked on tiptoes, an action seen in children with developmental problems—the persistence of a primitive "plantar" reflex. (The plantar reflex occurs when a physician strokes the bottom of the foot and the person's big toe turns up reflexively; it is present in young infants. It should disappear, but if it doesn't, that signals a brain problem.) He was so uncoordinated from low muscle tonus, he couldn't hold a crayon or a spoon.

Unable to speak yet so often overwhelmed, he had a horrible way of discharging his emotions. When he went into a meltdown, he would bite his hand or arms, and because of his exceptionally low muscle tonus, could bend forward and bite his own stomach, drawing blood. Afterward "he became calmer, like it was a release," says Liz. "As we look back at videos of him, the hurt in his eyes is unbelievable."

The family was referred to a developmental specialist. "On the day that changed my life forever," Liz says, "I was told by a very experienced pediatrician that he had *very severe cognitive impairment based on brain damage,* and was the mental age of six months, though he was already two years two months. The consultant spent an hour with Will. She got out a tea set and asked him to make tea. All he did was stack the cups, and knock them down. She also did the U.K. autism test, and it didn't show signs of autism. And she said he was *not* going to get better, and that by the time he was thirteen, he would probably have the mental age of a two-year-old."

Liz questioned how the doctors could be so sure of Will's prognosis, earning a reputation as a "neurotic mother" with the staff of the National Health Service. She read fiendishly about premature babies and in January 2011 found descriptions of children who seemed like Will in a book by Sally Goddard Blythe, called *Reflexes, Learning and Behavior.* Liz sent a long description of Will to Goddard's Institute for Neuro-Physiological Psychology, and Peter Blythe, the neuropsychologist who had set up the institute, contacted Liz and asked her to bring films of Will since birth. Liz asked him if there was anyone in England who could help, "and he said, 'No. There's only one man who can help Will. And that man is in Toronto.'"

"WE ARRIVED IN CANADA. IT was a heavy snow in March," says Liz. Will was nearly three and hadn't said a word for eighteen months. He couldn't sleep, walked on his tiptoes, was constantly frustrated, and in perpetual motion.

Paul Madaule examined Will and was confident his problems were chiefly neurological, mostly related to the vestibular or balance apparatus in the ear (introduced in Chapter 7) and how it related to the relevant brain areas that process balance.

Tomatis had emphasized that ears have two different functions. The cochlea, or "ear of hearing," as Tomatis called it, processes audible sound. It detects the sound spectrum from 20 to 20,000 Hz. The vestibular apparatus, or "ear of the body," as Tomatis called it, normally detects frequencies under 20 Hz. People experience the lower range of these vibrations, 16 Hz and slower, as "rhythmic" because they are slow enough for a listener to perceive *the intervals between* the individual waves. These frequencies often induce body movement.

Tomatis called the vestibular apparatus the "ear of the body" because the semicircular canals within it function as the body's compass, detecting its position in three-dimensional space and how gravity affects it. One canal detects movement in the horizontal plane, another in the vertical plane, and another when we are moving forward or backward. The canals contain little hairs in a fluid bath. When we move our heads, the fluid stirs the hairs, which send a signal to our brains telling us that we have increased our velocity in a particular direction. The signals from the vestibular apparatus travel along a nerve to a specialized clump of neurons in the brain stem, called the vestibular nuclei, which process the signals and send commands to the muscles to adjust themselves, to maintain balance. The "ear of the body" allows infants to switch from being mainly horizontal, crawling creatures with big heads to standing erect on narrow feet and walking without falling.

The specialists in England had assumed that the reason Will ran around furniture and other objects was that he couldn't see things in three dimensions, so he circled them to detect their depth. Paul had a different take. He thought Will's brain was "starved" for vestibular stimulation, because of a vestibular problem. By running around things, he was trying to stimulate his balance sense, which normally integrates input from the semicircular canals of the ear, the bottom of the feet, and the eyes, all of which give important sensory input about orientation in space.

Normally, when a child turns his head to look at something while walking, his vestibular sense tells him that he, and not what he is looking at, is moving. But when Will moved his head, he saw what he was looking at as moving, and it fascinated and energized him, so he could keep moving for hours without tiring. And because Will had a vestibular problem, he felt unstable in his own body and always felt as though he were in a rocking boat, always moving, and because his world was moving, he had to move with it.

One reason Will wanted heavy objects on him was that he could not tell where his body was *in space,* a consequence of his poor vestibular function. The balance system gives a person the sense of being grounded, rooted, and bounded, so necessary for having a settled, stable sense of self. Children born prematurely miss out on the allotted time nature usually provides for feeling enclosed in the protective comfort of the womb; they are born before their brain can filter out unnecessary sensations, so they feel assaulted by stimulation. Paul believed Will wanted pressure on his body as part of his attempt to integrate all his sensations and experiences as part of a single self—a way of "pulling himself together." Nurses working with premature babies often swaddle them tightly in blankets, which settles them. Will was swaddling himself.

Will's nonverbal, two-way communication with others told Paul that he appreciated that other people had minds; that realization meant, by the common definition, that Will was not autistic. But Will had what Paul called "the peripheral symptoms of autism," such as tiptoe walking and hypersensitivities. Ten weeks of prematurity, followed by two brutally traumatic years, had led to what Paul called "missteps in development." And Will suffered from "the discomfort and fear which comes from being close to death, which adults can verbalize and kids cannot, but which I am sure has an impact on little kids." Paul's feeling was that the British diagnosis was true as far as it went—parts of Will's brain may have been "unrepairable"—but that diagnosis left out the possibility that Will may not have developed normally because he hadn't received the kind of stimulation he needed, at the time he needed it, to awaken normal development. Paul couldn't know which of Will's symptoms were based on brain cell death, and which on global developmental delays. But because he knew the brain is neuroplastic, his approach was "Let's stimulate Will's brain and see what happens."

THE FIRST FIFTEEN DAYS OF Will's treatment were devoted to the passive phase. For ninety minutes, Will listened through headphones to Mozart, and to his mother's voice reading nursery rhymes, both filtered. After that, Paul played Will unfiltered Gregorian chants, sung by a choir of male voices. These Gregorian frequencies were to relax him, after intense sound stimulation. The rhythm of the chant matched the breathing and heartbeat of a calm, relaxed listener. To Liz, it seemed Will knew, almost immediately, that this process was helping him. Each morning he was more eager than the last to get out of his stroller, get up the steps, burst through the doors, and start.

Paul told Liz that Will might sleep a lot while listening to the music, and he did. Paul also predicted that near the end of the first week, Will would probably start sleeping better. On the sixth night, Will slept through the night for the first time in his life.

"It was absolutely unbelievable," says Liz, crying. "When someone says something like that is going to happen—and it will change your son's life—these are things you hold them to."

The first time Will listened to his mother's highly filtered voice—so filtered Liz couldn't recognize it—he started to look at her more and connected more deeply to her. He wanted more interaction and would sit close to her and try to join her in activities, or he would pull her toward him. His frustration and anger toward her eased. "It felt like he knew it was me," she says. Yet this was intriguing because he had, after all, heard her unfiltered voice all his life. Though children don't consciously identify their mother's voice with the whistling sound, Paul and his staff constantly see children who have shown no connection, or who show a limited or ambivalent one, spontaneously hug their mothers and for the very first time make eye contact and show signs of tenderness. Hyper children become calmer; goody-two-shoes children begin to act out in a healthy spirited way; and most become better listeners and talkers. Paul wrote, "It is as if the filtered sound of the mother's voice increases the child's desire to be born to a world where sound and language are a means of communication." Some autistic children start babbling, then for a few days scream high-pitched sounds, then begin to speak and make eye contact. Adults who do the training with the mother's voice may find they are less tense, sleep better, express more emotion (both pleasant and unpleasant), and become more energized.

Paul also made a prediction about Will's language. "He was very specific," says Liz. "He said, 'Expect to see language changes on day four.'" And on day four Will said his first word. He was on the floor, listening to filtered music, when he said "lion" while placing a picture of a lion into a jigsaw puzzle. It was the first word he had ever used in context. The next day, as he put the number eight into a puzzle, he said "eight." He added one new word a day, always while listening to the filtered music. On their last day in Toronto, Darlah Dunford, one of Will's therapists, put him on a swing and said, "Ready, steady, go!" and swung him several times. Then she said, "Ready, steady . . ." but didn't release the swing until he spoke the final word. He completed her sentence, saying "Go!" and she swung him.

After fifteen days, Will had ten words, was using them in context, was sleeping through the night, and was playing appropriately with toys for the first time. He was no longer always moving. And he stopped biting his stomach and drawing blood.

THE MOTHER'S VOICE PLAYS A special role in the treatment of premature children—it is one of the strangest aspects of Paul's technique, but it seemed even stranger when Tomatis first developed it. It is now established that a fetus can recognize its mother's voice, but when Tomatis first proclaimed that the maturing fetus—curled up in the womb, oddly enough, in the shape of an ear—could hear sounds and recognize the mother's voice, medical schools were teaching that fetuses, and even newborns, were not capable of awareness. The argument—routinely made as recently as the 1980s—was that the infant's nervous system was not sufficiently complete. The unborn child was a witless tadpole.

In the early 1980s, scientists (and especially the Toronto psychiatrist Thomas Verny) gathered studies proving that the fetus has experiences in the womb. Until then, only some mothers (who believed it made sense to sing to their fetuses) and a few psychoanalysts (including D. W. Winnicott) argued that the unborn child perceived and had feelings. Freud and Otto Rank, who believed that birth could be traumatic, agreed with these ideas. Tomatis read about the unborn child's alertness in the work of the neonatal neurologist André Thomas, who demonstrated that newborns, surrounded by conversing adults, turn only to their mother's voice. Tomatis wrote that this action must indicate recognition of "the only voice of which he or she was aware while still in the fetal stage."

"My own experience as a premature baby often stirred up and guided my *libido sciendi*," or desire to know, wrote Tomatis. In the 1950s, eager to better understand the origins of listening, he wondered what it would be like for an infant to hear the mother's voice in utero—from within her body. To find out, he built an artificial womb and filled it with fluid, designed to replicate the sounds of the intrauterine environment. He equipped the "womb" with waterproof microphones, and from inside it he played sound recordings from the bellies of pregnant women. As he listened, he heard deeply soothing sounds: from the intestines, the brooklike gurgling of fluids; the rhythm of the mother's breathing, ebbing and flowing like the surf; her heartbeat; and in the distant background, the faint sounds of her voice. He saw premature birth as emotional trauma that the infant experienced, in part, because of the sudden loss of all these sounds. He suggested that the mother's voice be piped into incubators to soothe premature infants, a practice that was taken up in parts of Europe. And to help people who had had auditory problems since infancy, he began to use the mother's voice in the Electronic Ear, filtered so it sounded as it did in the womb.

By 1964, scientists had demonstrated that the eardrum and the inner bones of the ear are already *adult size* halfway through pregnancy; that the acoustic nerve is mature by then and can conduct signals; and that the temporal lobe, which processes sound, is also largely functioning. Eventually 3-D ultrasounds and methods of monitoring the fetal heart and brain waves showed that fetuses respond to voices. Recent studies confirm that the fetus can differentiate its mother's voice from other voices. Barbara Kisilevsky and her colleagues, working with sixty pregnant mothers (on average 38.2 weeks pregnant), played a recording of each mother's voice, ten centimeters above her abdomen; they found that the heart rate of the fetus increased, but not when they played strangers' voices. Recent studies have replicated André Thomas's findings that newborns prefer their mother's voice to that of strangers and prefer stories that were read to them by their mothers in the last six weeks of pregnancy to new stories. Immediately after birth, newborns can distinguish the "mother tongue"—the language the mother spoke while they were in the womb—from another language, and newborns have neural networks sensitive to native speech before birth.

Tomatis believed that all unborn children, during the four and a half months that their ears are functioning within the womb, grow "attached" to the sole voice they hear murmuring a language they do not understand. Some argued, "But isn't the contact between child and mother primarily a physical one?" to which he answered, "Language, too, possesses a physical dimension. By causing vibrations in the surrounding air, language becomes a sort of invisible arm by which we 'touch' the person listening to us in every sense of the term."

Paul puts it this way: "We don't relate to people directly; we relate through our voice. *It is a medium.* The brain is a tool user, and the voice is a tool." The unborn child in the womb hears many lower-frequency sounds (like the heartbeat and breathing), and then the mother's voice, which has low but also higher frequencies of speech, occasionally breaks through.

Paul continues, "We can imagine the unborn child making a first attempt to 'connect' with the more agreeable sound of the voice of her mother. But unlike a radio, the voice is not always 'on' and the fetus cannot control it. She has to wait until it comes on to enjoy it. Thus the first motivation to reach out is born. This is followed by the first gratification—the pleasure of hearing this sound again. This initial silent 'dialogue' gives birth to listening. . . . Many mothers sense and respond to their unborn child's silent quest for dialogue. They sing the same songs over and over again. . . . The unborn child does not understand the meaning of the messages sent by the mother's voice. What he 'understands' is the emotional charge of those messages."

WILL RESPONDED PROFOUNDLY TO THE listening therapy: he slept better, spoke, formed closer emotional connections, and was able to regulate his emotions. At that point he had finished his fifteen-day passive phase. Paul said that Will would need six weeks for his brain to consolidate his gains. His development would continue, but as he started to communicate for the first time, he would also develop new frustrations. Paradoxically, this change would be a sign of progress.

When the family returned to Britain, Will continued to develop. He got up to twenty-two words, his sleep was now "fantastic," his appetite improved, and many of his unusual symptoms vanished. He was no longer squashing himself underneath weights, running around tables, looking at objects from different angles, or opening and closing doors. Toys he had never played with were now being used appropriately.

Six weeks later, in May 2011, they returned to Toronto for a second fifteen-day visit, to begin the active phase. Will listened to filtered music again, but also to his own filtered voice while he spoke or sang. Over the fifteen days his vocabulary grew, he was able to communicate better, and he became calmer. Because he could communicate his emotions and thoughts, he didn't rage or bite himself when frustrated, and Liz could now reason with him. He progressed to role-playing and pretend play, and his imagination flourished. Sound stimulation had so awakened his brain that he developed a sense of smell for the first time.

But as Paul had predicted, he was often frustrated. Two to three days into his second treatment phase, having begun communicating, he suddenly expressed intense annoyance and threw tantrums whenever his parents couldn't immediately understand him. Having tasted communication, he wanted as much as possible. Then after a month, his frustration diminished as quickly as it had begun.

"Paul said he would be speaking in sentences by Christmas," says Frederick, "and literally a week before Christmas, he did."

Paul had developed a portable Electronic Ear, called the LiFT (for Listening Fitness Trainer), and he gave Liz one to take home to England. Paul kept in touch by Skype, modifying Will's program as needed. In late 2012 speech and language therapists in England declared Will's language, speech, and comprehension to be age appropriate for a four-year-old. In eighteen months, with Paul's help, he had moved through more than four years of language development, because in fact, at four, he read and comprehended at a six-year-old's level. Frederick marveled the day Will read the word *scientist*, thinking, "Two years ago he couldn't speak!" In September the pediatric consultant in the U.K. apologized, saying that she had "got it totally wrong," and she admitted that Will's progress completely blew her away and that she would now direct other children like Will to listening therapy.

THE PEDIATRIC CONSULTANT'S ORIGINAL ASSESSMENT—that Will would not progress—no doubt had its source in the doctrine of the unchanging brain as she had been taught it and as it was still being applied to premature infants. While many premature lives are saved, the long-term statistics are that between 25 and 50 percent of such infants (who have not had listening therapy) have cognitive and learning disabilities, attention problems, social interaction difficulties—and often cerebral palsy. The view of mainstream physicians has been that such catastrophic deficits must be caused by brain cell death.

But a 2013 study by Justin Dean and Stephen Back shows that when fetal lambs in the womb sustain even a catastrophe as deadly as lack of oxygen to the brain, it does not necessarily kill all brain cells, though it may decrease the number of neuronal branches and synaptic connections between the neurons. These oxygen-deprived fetuses have a smaller brain volume than normal, but it is *not* caused by an overall loss of neurons. Rather, the smaller brain volume is caused by the lack of connections between the neurons. The neurons have fewer dendritic branches to receive signals from other neurons, and the branches they have are shorter, and there are fewer synapses between neurons. The neurons hadn't matured properly. Dean and his colleagues concluded, "Our findings question current assumptions that the cognitive and learning disabilities in preterm survivors arise principally from irreversible brain injury resulting from neuronal degeneration."

Prematurity, even without oxygen deprivation, contributes to fewer connections between neurons because a rapid increase in the branching of fetal neurons normally occurs in the last third of pregnancy—the period when most premature babies are extruded from the womb. The problem is that mainstream physicians have no training in using mental activity or sensory stimulation to "hook up" disconnected neurons and help them mature, training that would take advantage of the fact that "neurons that fire together wire together." It took experts like Alfred Tomatis and Paul Madaule to devise ways of stimulating neurons to fire and wire to connect, because everyday experience—of which Will had plenty—is insufficient to do so. Before he could make use of everyday experience to mature, he had to pass through the steps I have described: in the first few days he required appropriate *neurostimulation,* which turned on the parts of his brain that *neuromodulate* arousal. He got the neurostimulation and began to sleep properly. This state of *neurorelaxation* allowed him to accumulate energy so that he was soon able to make huge leaps in language development and sensory discrimination, a sign of *neurodifferentiation*.

It's June 2013, and Will is back at the Listening Centre for his third visit. We are in the sensory room, filled with swings, hammocks, and toys with different textures. Will is listening to filtered music with the headphones wrapped around his thick blond hair. He has cherubic cheeks and is a charming, disarming chatterbox.

"Hallo!" he says immediately to me with great warmth, making good eye contact. Darlah stands over a mirror on the floor, holding a tube of lotion, and asks Will, "How many squirts do we do?"

"Seven!" he answers joyfully. "Can I skate on it?"

"Yes," says Darlah, helping him pull off his socks and putting seven squirts on the mirror. Will stands on the slippery surface and moves his feet around on it. He falls, emits peals of laughter, and plays with the lotion, which is all over him. This is the boy who couldn't tolerate gooey or sticky textures. He gets up and runs in place.

Will is learning to integrate sensory input, motor movement, balance, and coordination. That he had had problems integrating sensory input could be seen in his hypersensitivities to sound and tactile sensations, his need for constant movement, and his lack of coordination.

When Paul works with children who can't speak or who have immature or delayed speech, he often finds that moving them on a swing while they are wearing the Electronic Ear stimulates their speech, showing the interplay of the vestibular apparatus and the cochlea. Movement naturally induces speech, he has observed, and mothers, by bouncing their tots on their laps, are stimulating their children's vestibular system, preparing the way for speech.

Tomatis emphasized that we have two ways of picking up sound. First, *air* conducts sound waves through the ear canal to the cochlea; this is called air conduction. Second, sound waves vibrate directly against the *bones* of the skull, which conduct sound to the cochlea and the vestibular apparatus. This is called bone conduction. Tomatis found that he could best influence the vestibular apparatus through bone conduction because it conducts lower frequencies especially well. So he attached a small vibrating device to the headphones of the Electronic Ear, to sit directly against the skull. Will's headphones were thus equipped with a bone conduction vibrator. Its impact on his vestibular system brought about a radical decrease in his need to "move around" when he looked at objects because he was no longer starved of vestibular stimulation. The stimulation to his poorly functioning vestibular apparatus (which had left him feeling he was always moving) fixed it and left him feeling more at home in his body, less clumsy, and more grounded.

The Listening Centre used objective measures to monitor Will's vestibular functioning. When a person with a healthy vestibular apparatus is seated in a rotating chair and is then spun rapidly and stopped suddenly, his eyes will quickly jerk, many times, in the direction opposite to his spinning. This normal reflex, called postrotary nystagmus, is a sign that the vestibular apparatus is detecting body movement and sending signals to the eyes to readjust where they look. But many developmentally delayed children, and children on the autistic spectrum, don't have postrotary nystagmus. When Darlah first spun Will and stopped him, his eyes stayed still. But a couple of days ago, when Darlah spun Will, he said, "I feel funny," and his eyes showed nystagmus for the first time—a sign his vestibular apparatus was kicking in. When she got him to explain what "feeling funny" meant, it turned out he was dizzy, a new experience for him.

JUST BEFORE WILL'S LATEST VISIT, he had to have his adenoids removed. Since every operation triggers the unresolved traumas of his previous surgeries, Will regressed a bit in his skills and behavior. "Yesterday," says Liz, "he tripped and fell and said to me, 'Why did *you* let me trip?'"

"If anything goes wrong, he blames his mom. He doesn't blame me," says Frederick, puzzled.

"I hear that all the time," says Paul. "From the standpoint of the suffering child, Mom is the cause of all his pain. The one who gave me life, gives me all the problems of life. And that makes mothers feel very guilty—inappropriately so. We do everything we can to remove that with counseling, but another way to settle that child down is to use *her* voice, the mother's voice, which can be very soothing in this situation." To help out, Paul played Will the recording of Liz's voice, and it calmed him quickly. Such is the rectifying power of the filtered voice, sounding just as it did in the sanctuary of the womb, before his life's troubles began.

Two days later it's Will's fifth birthday at the Listening Centre. Will is not simply talking—his vocabulary is downright sophisticated. When Darlah brings in two bags of birthday presents—toys he's grown to love in the sensory room—he says, "I wasn't expecting *that!*" and gives Paul a big hug. Then he takes a drink from the water fountain and goes to throw out his cup. Seeing two wastebaskets side by side, he reads a sign over one out loud, "'Recycling drinking cups go here.'"

The cake comes out, and he smiles and yells, "Hip, hip, hooray! A big hooray!" in his little-boy English accent, and he dances. "It's a white cake!" he exclaims, and blows out the candles. "Are we going to share it?" he asks Liz, subtly instructing her to begin cutting the cake.

Liz says, "Last night he said to me, 'Mom, will I be bigger in the morning?' And I said, 'Well, you'll have to look in the mirror.' And he did, and said, 'Look, my neck's longer!'" He's a happy boy—he jokes—and though Liz, Frederick, Paul, and I have talked about his eventually needing to work through the terrible traumas of the first few years of his life—episodes he never brings up—for now, as long as no one tries to restrict him physically, he displays the most pleasant, outgoing, endearing of temperaments, overflowing with affection.

Will goes to a regular public school now.

Paul, feeling so happy for Will, leans over to me and says, "I agree that neuroplasticity is the ability of the brain to change at any time and any age. But when you have the opportunity to use it early—as we got to do with Will—there is so much more you can do. Had we waited another ten years, he would have been so damaged by then. We could have helped him, but we would have had a child who had years of struggle, was completely lost in his senses, was unable to put a sentence together, unable to express his feelings and needs, and all those experiences would have accumulated, leaving him locked within himself."

Liz, Frederick, Will, and his baby sister return to England tonight. Will's extended family back home is incredulous. "They can't comprehend," says Liz, "that Will listened to filtered Mozart, Gregorian chant, and his mother's voice, and it changed his life. It's surreal."

Frederick pipes in, "It was like a miracle for us. But it's all true. All the specialists and consultants—all but Peter Blythe—said he was brain-damaged and would be an eighteen-month-old forever. And most people would accept that. But she"—he points a trembling finger at Liz, holding their one-year-old daughter—"wouldn't believe it."

I look over at Liz, bouncing her healthy baby girl on her lap. Liz has blond hair and earnest eyes; she is wearing stylishly torn jeans and looks for just this moment like an ordinary mother, at her son's happy but otherwise unremarkable fifth birthday.

III. Rebuilding the Brain from the Bottom Up

Autism, Attention Deficits, and Sensory Processing Disorder

For over a hundred years, most neuroscientists have thought of the brain as having a "top" and a "bottom." While scientists would disagree about exactly where to draw the line between top and bottom, almost everyone agreed that the frontal part of the thin outer layer of the brain, called the frontal cortex, was "topmost." This frontal cortical area was thought to process the "higher" human attributes, such as the ability to reason, plan, control impulses, concentrate for long periods, use abstract thought, make decisions, and imagine what others are thinking and feeling. This idea took hold, originally, because damage to those top regions led to problems with all those mental functions.

Since many psychiatric disorders of childhood affect those "higher" abilities, treatments for these problems were designed to target the frontal cortical structures. But those treatments are not especially effective. They generally aim to control or diminish symptoms, and none heal the brain or remove the problems permanently. In this chapter I take a different approach and show that sound therapy works initially from the bottom up; that it can rewire the brain for the better; and that these results are often permanent.

One reason sound therapy has not attracted more attention is that the structure of the brain that it has a major impact on—the subcortical brain—has been poorly understood. It is "sub" because it sits underneath the thin top layer of the brain, the cortex. So it is anatomically lower, or toward the bottom.

Unfortunately, the subcortical brain has at times also been treated as far less sophisticated than it really is. The reasons are several. First, because it is buried deeper in the brain, the subcortical brain was often difficult to access with the technologies that were available through much of the twentieth century. Thus it was hard to observe and to appreciate its full role. Second, the subcortical brain is the only brain structure in many simpler animals, and because these animals don't have the "sophisticated" thinking abilities of human beings, it was assumed that the subcortical brain is a simpler brain. As evolution proceeded, a thin outer layer of cortex developed, surrounding the subcortex, and was seen as "added on" to the subcortical brain. Since these more recently evolved animals, equipped with a cortex, appeared to be more intelligent, it was assumed that their higher intelligence came from the cortex, the crowning achievement of evolution. Human beings have the most cortex of all. Given the rigid localizationism of the time, it was assumed that all higher thinking abilities took place solely in the cortex. If a person had a problem performing a complex thinking activity, its cause must be in the cortex.

The fallacy in this reasoning is that it presumes that when a new structure developed in evolution, it was simply added on to the older structure and that it now works independently of it. But what really happened was that as a new structure was added, the older ones adapted; the presence of a new structure modified the old, and old and new now *work together* holistically. Recent studies in animals and humans have demonstrated this phenomenon beautifully: they show that as the cortex evolved and increased in size, the subcortical structures grew massively and were modified. Once again the lesson is that localization, while instructive, can be taken too far and often is. Our cortico-centric view has failed to take into sufficient account the contributions of the subcortical brain. Its relevance is demonstrated by the fact that when it is stimulated by sound, such stimulation can lead to astonishing improvements in the "higher" mental capacities of children with the common psychiatric disorders of childhood.

Autistic Recoveries

Some observers might have thought that Will's many different developmental problems meant that he had autism. But he did not suffer from what many clinicians now argue is the central clinical feature of autism, an inability to appreciate that other people have minds, leading them to have little interest in relating to others. Will, no matter how troubled he was, always sought connection to others. In some children, the absence of interest in connecting to others becomes especially obvious when it was present early in life but was then lost.

Jordan Rosen was a healthy, bright child who appeared to be developing fairly normally, much like his two siblings. His parents' only concern, and it was slight, was that at a time when most children have half a dozen simple words, he was still in the babbling phase. Perhaps it was a coincidence, but at eighteen months, one week after he was vaccinated, he got a bad stomach flu. Then he stopped all eye contact with people, ceased responding to his name, and seemed no longer able to read facial expressions. He also stopped playing and lost all ability to connect to others emotionally. His mother, Darlene, noticed that he didn't seem to understand that other people had minds and feelings, and that he treated them as though they were things. When he got a bit older, if he wanted a drink, he would pull her hand to the fridge, as though her hand were a tool to open doors. He became aloof, and when he was in a room with his parents, he acted as though no one was there. When he heard particular songs, he would run around the house holding his hands over his ears, screaming. He was enraged, unmanageable, and inconsolable; he would bang his head against the floor and wall and against Darlene throughout the day. He was eventually kicked out of day care for biting others. When the doctors couldn't believe how long and violent his tantrums were, Darlene filmed them. At three he still had no language, speech therapy didn't help, and the doctors said he might never talk. A developmental pediatrician and a child psychiatrist specializing in autism, affiliated with Toronto's Clarke Institute of Psychiatry, diagnosed autism.

One of the physicians wrote that "Jordan has severe impairments in verbal and non-verbal communication as well as reciprocal social interaction." These are core symptoms of autism. He also had "a markedly restricted repertoire of activities and interests including some obsessive behaviors," meaning he would do the same thing over and over again and not much else—another core feature of autism. Jordan repeatedly collected and lined up toy blocks or cutlery. He became so obsessed with certain videos that his mother had to buy a second machine to rewind the one he had just seen, because he would scream if one of his favorites wasn't playing constantly.

His parents were told that nothing could be done, and that they might have to institutionalize him permanently. As I looked over pictures of him before eighteen months, I saw a happy child with a sparkle in his eye; in all the pictures afterward, his eyes were blank or wary.

A support group for parents of autistic children reinforced the message of no hope. Someone mentioned Paul's Listening Centre, only to dismiss it as a pipe dream. "So," says Darlene, who is a spirited person, "I looked into it." After all, her son didn't listen and couldn't speak, and like many autistic children, he was hypersensitive to incoming sensation, most often sound.

When he was three, Jordan started working with Paul, who saw that the boy had no real language: he used the few "words" he did have as noises, out of context, without intention of communicating. After listening therapy, including the mother's voice, he started talking, and his behavior normalized. He then got boosts every six months over several years. He eventually developed friendships, went to a normal school, graduated with honors, and went to university in Halifax.

In December 2013 I caught up with Jordan to find out what had happened to him over the long term. Paul hadn't seen him since the mid-1990s, when he last treated him. Jordan is now a well-spoken, handsome twenty-three-year-old. His eyes sparkle, and he jokes with me, teasing. He's engaging. He recently completed a bachelor of management and globalization degree. He tells me that university, for him, "was the best time ever. Meeting people from different places and cultures—but mostly partying." He smiles. His relationships mean a lot to him, he tells me, and he keeps in touch with his circle of friends from Halifax, and has made new ones since moving back home to Toronto. "I keep my family close to me, too," he adds. His language is well developed, apt, and gently witty.

Jordan has a job in logistics, getting products from one country to another, and deals with people from all walks of life, from all over the world. It requires diplomacy and skill with people. I ask him if he has to deal with "difficult people." He explains that if he has to give criticism, he will protect the person's self-esteem by complimenting him or her. When dealing with someone who is particularly challenging, he first tries to find a nice way to handle that person. "You can always get angry as a last resort." This from the boy who was constantly—literally—banging his head against the wall. He clearly knows all about other people's minds.

The Listening Centre was the only treatment Jordan had for his autism, apart from the speech therapy, which didn't help him. When he was sixteen, he wrote a poem that included the lines:

> The doctors said I was autistic
> And it was as if I locked my mind up in a shell
> They said there was not a solution
> But to lock me up in a mental institution.

Instead, Jordan has become one of a growing number of children who have had life-transforming improvements in their autism. In his case, the word *cure* would be appropriate. Paul doesn't claim to perform such wonders with all autistic children. But he has found that most of the autistic patients who he thinks will benefit from listening therapy do improve significantly, though many will still have remnants of the condition.*

A boy I'll call "Timothy" is a more typical case. He has made huge improvements but still has some remnants of autism. Like Jordan, he was at first generally healthy, but then, at eighteen months, he had an autistic regression. His initially normal mental, emotional, and language development regressed. He seemed to lose interest in relationships with people: he stopped speaking or responding to his name, stopped making eye contact, stopped normal play, and began to have rages. As he approached three, he was stuck in his own world, and his mother, "Sandra," and her husband felt the acute loss of their son: "We just want to have a relationship with him." He had all the core symptoms of autism and was diagnosed by several expert physicians as having severe autism. Sandra told me that she and her husband were told that "he would not have a normal life, would never go to a normal school, or train for a job."

At the Listening Centre, Timothy immediately settled down. On day one of the program he stopped his constant movement; on day two he slept for ten hours, the longest since his autistic regression. On the third day, his mother told me, "He seemed like a different person. Then my husband comes home, and Timothy goes over and hugs him for the first time since we lost him to autism." Timothy's progress was slow and steady and took a number of years. He came to see Paul once a year, for ten hours of listening and working on expressive speech, and for help in dealing with the new issues that arose at every stage of growing up, especially puberty. Listening therapy is not simply hooking a person up to a machine. It requires a therapist like Paul who understands how to

---

* Paul Madaule has found that listening therapy can help about two-thirds of children with autism who come to the Listening Centre. "Help" means improvements ranging from a Jordan-like outcome (not frequent) to a Timothy-like outcome (more typical) to a more modest but very welcome improvement that permits the child to make better use of existing therapies, and to participate more in school and in social and family life, in such a way that he or she is far more regulated, self-aware, and independent. Generally, the younger the child with autism is when therapy begins, the better. Ongoing yearly "boosts" are helpful, and often the children themselves ask to go back to the center, saying, as did one child, "I need the music again, to calm down inside."

connect to the mind and heart of someone with autistic or other learning problems.

Timothy went from needing educational assistants in class to being on his own. By seventeen, he had become an A student, even in English—a stunning accomplishment for a boy who had lost his speech. He has a steady friend and is moving toward being more independent from his family. He has gone from severe to mild autism, and he is on track to graduate from a normal school with his peers and to get a job. His parents, who had only wanted to "have a relationship with him," now have one.

Though autism has been thought to be incurable, Martha Herbert, M.D., Ph.D., a pediatric neurologist and researcher at Harvard Medical School, and author of *The Autism Revolution,* also documents cases of children with autism who have made life-changing improvements. "For decades, most doctors told parents that autism was a genetic problem in their children's brain," she writes, "and that . . . they should expect their toddler's troubles would be with him/her forever." But autism, she demonstrates, is frequently a *dynamic process.* It is *not* only genetic, *not* only a brain problem, *not* caused by any one thing, and is *not always* beyond help, especially if the therapy is begun when the child is very young.

In some cases, autism is present at birth or soon after; but in "regressive autism," the child's mental development at first seems fairly normal, and then, typically between the second and third year of life, the symptoms begin.

Autism rates are now skyrocketing. Fifty years ago, one in 5,000 people had it. In 2008 the Centers for Disease Control had the rate at one in 88. In 2010 it rose to one in 68 (and one in 42 for boys). While some of the increase may be caused by a heightened awareness among physicians, so that they diagnose it more frequently, many clinicians who treat it believe that more children are developing the disorder. Certainly, the rise is happening too quickly to be explained by genetic factors, which take generations to unfold. As Herbert points out, "Hundreds of genes are now associated with autism. Most of them are not of major effect. In most cases they probably create modest vulnerability. . . . Even genes that cause autism in a strong way . . . will only affect a fraction of a percent of the total number of people with autism . . . and some with that gene don't get autism."

Genes put a child at risk of autism, but environmental factors are generally required to turn that risk into an illness. Many of these factors turn on the child's immune system, causing it to release antibodies and produce chronic inflammation that affects the brain. Many autistic children have immune system abnormalities and overactive immune systems. They have high rates of gastrointestinal infections and inflammation, food sensitivities (often to grains, gluten, dairy, and sugar), asthma (which involves inflammation), and inflammation of the skin. Anti-inflammatory drugs are known to decrease autistic symptoms. True, there are other noninflammatory factors, too, such as chemical deficiencies, but inflammation is emerging as a key factor. Herbert gives many examples of children who made radical improvements when inflammation was addressed. Caleb, a boy who had many signs of inflammation and many infections, then developed regressive autism, but his autism went away at age ten, when his mother eliminated gluten from his diet.

Another stressor is toxins, which also can irritate the brain and cause inflammation. Today's babies are exposed to toxins in the womb, and they are born prepolluted. Children at birth have on average two hundred major toxic chemicals in their umbilical cord blood, including some that were banned thirty years ago. Many are direct neurotoxins. Toxic chemicals, because foreign to the body, trigger immune reactions.

The Inflamed Brain Is One in Which Neurons Don't Connect

Autism is not only, as was once thought, a brain disease. Herbert shows it is an expression of *a whole body disease* that affects the brain's health, too. Chronic inflammation in the body can have an impact on all the organs, including the brain. In 2005 a team from Johns Hopkins University School of Medicine showed that autistic brains are frequently inflamed. Autopsies found inflammation in the cortex (the outer layer of the brain) and the brain axons; the inflammation was "particularly striking in the cerebellum"—the subcortical area with close links to the vestibular system (which is targeted by sound therapy). Recall, as I discussed in Chapters 4 and 5, that the cerebellum fine-tunes thought and movement; it is also stimulated by newer versions of sound therapy.

Since 2008 five studies have shown that a significant number of autistic children have antibodies coming from their mothers that targeted their brain cells while they were still in the womb. One study found that 23 percent of mothers of autistic children had such antibodies. By comparison, only 1 percent of mothers of children without autism had these antibodies. Scientists don't understand what triggers the antibodies, but likely the mother was exposed to an infection or toxin that altered *her* immune system. When this kind of antibody was injected into pregnant monkeys, their offspring showed behaviors similar to those of autistic children. Autistic children also have high levels of antibodies in their blood. (Whether vaccinations, designed to trigger antibodies, can trigger problematic inflammation in a *subgroup* of children is controversial and is dealt with in the endnotes.) Herbert's theory is that all these stresses and inflammation affect the brain and damage the neurons.*

Chronic inflammation disturbs developing neuronal circuits. Brain scans show that many neuronal networks of autistic children are "underconnected" and that neurons at the front of the brain (which deals with goals and intentions) are poorly connected with those neurons at the back (which process sensation). Other brain areas show "overconnectivity," a problem that can lead to seizures, also common in autistic children. Underconnection and overconnection combined may make it hard

---

* Herbert's theory is that when "demands are placed on the whole body by a combination of poor food, toxins, bugs, and stress, likely with genetic vulnerabilities in the mix," the brain's support system is overwhelmed. Herbert and Weintraub, *The Autism Revolution* (New York: Ballantine Books), p. 119. Inflammation produces a lot of waste. The brain, like the rest of the body, always has to clear away waste products and dead cells, then rebuild and resupply new nutrients to the neurons. The brain's glial cells perform this task. When glial cells are overwhelmed, they swell and can't adequately support their neurons; the blood supply to the neurons is decreased, and their mitochondria (the energy generators in the cell, discussed in Chapter 4) are stressed. Eventually some neurons, no longer properly supported by their glial cells, start "idling" and stop performing their normal signaling functions. As I have emphasized, when neurons are dysfunctional or injured, they still fire, producing "noise," or they become overexcited or dysregulated. When the glial and neuronal system is overwhelmed, Herbert points out, a brain chemical, glutamate, which normally excites neurons, is released in large quantities. This contributes to neurons becoming too excitable and may lead to hypersensitivities and, in my terms, a noisy brain.

for the brain to synchronize its activities between areas. In summary, autism is the product of genetic risk factors and many environmental triggers, which can sometimes affect the child before birth, sometimes after, and immune reactions and inflammation are prominent. These combined factors overwhelm the developing brain, so that neurons don't connect properly and can't communicate well with one another.

Neuroscientists have recently learned more about "wiring issues" in autism, which help explain how listening is affected by the condition. In July 2013 Stanford University scientists led by Daniel A. Abrams and Vinod Menon showed that in autistic children, the area of the auditory cortex that processes the human voice is underconnected to the brain's subcortical reward center. When a person accomplishes a task, the reward center fires and secretes dopamine, triggering a good feeling and reinforcing the motivation to repeat that task. The study, which used a special MRI that shows linkages among brain areas, found that speech areas in the left hemisphere (which process the more symbolic parts of speech) and speech areas in the right hemisphere (which process the musical and emotional components of speech called prosody) were underconnected to the brain's reward center. The outcome? A child who can't connect the brain areas that process the voice with the reward center will be unable to experience speech as pleasurable.

How Listening Therapy Helps Autism

This loss of the pleasure of speech, I believe, has a devastating impact on a child's ability to bond with his or her parents or with anyone else. Leo Kanner, who in 1943 first described autism, noticed that these children seemed indifferent to the human voice and made no attempt to speak; one of his patients "did not register any change of expression when spoken to." It is now clearer that the voice plays a role in parent-child bonding, and that indifference to it has implications for the bond. A 2010 study revealed that when a nonautistic child is stressed, then hears his or her mother's voice, oxytocin is secreted in his brain. Oxytocin is a brain chemical that induces a calm, warm mood and increases tender feelings and trust, allowing parents and children to bond with each other. The parents' voices soothe the child and promote the development of communication. But oxytocin levels are significantly lower in people with autism. (The cause of the lower oxytocin is not yet worked out, but I suspect it is often secondary: as I will describe shortly, in many children it may be a result of auditory sensitivities making listening painful, leading to an underconnectivity between the auditory areas and the brain's reward center.) Whatever the cause, no "vocal bonding," to coin a phrase, occurs.

While many autistic children are indifferent to the pleasure of the voice, they are not indifferent to sound. Most are hypersensitive to sounds, which is why they so often cover their ears in great distress, and their nervous systems go into fight-or-flight mode. To understand why this reaction occurs, and how music can help bond a mother and an autistic child, I wish to emphasize a few key points about evolution.

The neuroscientist Stephen Porges has shown that specific sound frequency ranges are tied to our sense of safety or danger. Each species has different predators, and the sounds made by those predators turn on the prey's fight-or-flight reaction. A direct link exists between the auditory cortex and the threat systems in the brain, which is why unexpected, startling noise can trigger immense, immediate anxiety. Species also evolved to communicate in sound frequencies that their predators are unable to hear. (Reptiles, which have preyed on medium-size mammals such as humans for millions of years, cannot detect the frequencies of human speech.)

When people feel safe, the parasympathetic nervous system *turns off* the fight-or-flight reaction. As Porges has brilliantly demonstrated, the parasympathetic system also *turns on* a "social engagement system," as well as the muscles of the middle ear, allowing people to listen to, communicate with, and connect with others. The parasympathetic system helps us connect with others precisely because it regulates the brain areas that control the middle ear muscles, which are used to tune in to the higher frequencies of human speech and also turn on the muscles used for vocal and facial expression. Being in "parasympathetic mode" is about being calm, collected, *and* connected.

Tomatis showed that many children with autism, learning disabilities, and speech and language delays—and also those who have had multiple ear infections—cannot tune in to the frequencies of human speech because they cannot use their middle ear muscles to dampen the lower frequencies. When lower frequencies are at full volume, they mask the higher sounds of speech, leaving autistic children hypersensitive to sound, especially continuous sound, such as vacuum cleaners, and alarms. In humans low-frequency sounds also trigger anxiety because they remind us of predators. Battered by sound, these children remain in fight-or-flight and cannot turn on the social engagement system. Training the circuit that controls the middle ear muscles can decrease hypersensitivity and increase social engagement (as Tomatis said) so that attachment to others can become pleasurable.*

The findings of Porges, Tomatis, and others, I believe, mean that it is time to rethink the theory that the core feature of autism is an inability to empathize and apprehend the existence of other minds. This may not always be the case. Children who are constantly battered by their sensations, and who are in constant fight-or-flight, cannot turn on or develop their social engagement systems or be aware of other minds. Their inability to be aware of other minds may often be secondary to the brain's sensory processing problems. As Paul puts it, the purpose of our sensory systems is "both to *reach out* to the world, but also *protect us* from the world of sensation. But if you are too sensitive, you develop mechanisms to cut the world off."

Learning Disorders, Social Engagement, and Depression

One of Tomatis's students was a physician who was skeptical that sound could correct learning problems. That attitude changed when his own daughter's life was hanging in the balance. Ron Minson had been chief of psychiatry at Presbyterian Medical Center in Denver and head of the

---

* Porges points out that one can tell when children are hypersensitive to sound by looking at them. The "facial nerve," which regulates the middle ear muscle, the stapedius, also regulates the muscles that lift the eyelids and control facial expression. When we are interested in what a person is saying, our middle ear muscles contract, allowing us to tune in on the person's speech frequencies and keep our eyelids open wide. We look interested. By reading facial expressions, an experienced teacher can tell whether a student is listening in class or whether the lesson is falling on deaf ears. In many autistic children, this circuit isn't working, so they look vacant: their facial muscles are flat and unexpressive.

Behavioral Sciences Center at Mercy Medical Center, where he taught before he went into private practice.

After losing a child to crib death, he and his wife, Nancy, adopted a delightful infant, Erica. A happy toddler, in grade one she had trouble sounding out letters, reversed them, and couldn't spell or do math. Her voice was flat, she struggled to understand others, and she couldn't tell if they were joking, angry, or being insistent. She failed first grade, and as each school year passed, she experienced a steady diet of failure.

An astute colleague of Ron's thought she might have dyslexia, so they tried all the conventional approaches—private tutors, speech and language pathologists, and special education—but to no avail. Ritalin-like stimulants for her poor attention just made her feel "hyped up." Erica became a sullen, depressed, rebellious adolescent warrior. Psychological testing concluded that "she lived in a fantasy world, much of the time, characterized by magical thinking." Antidepressants gave her side effects that made her feel worse than being depressed. In high school, her reading was still at fifth-grade level, and she fought every attempt her parents made to help her. Her school gave up on her, and by the time she reached eleventh grade, she was so filled with despair, she dropped out and worked as a chambermaid, at a car wash, and at a fast-food restaurant, but was routinely fired for a bad attitude or for not showing up. At eighteen, when her peers were talking about their GPAs and heading to college, she was looking at her future and couldn't see her life working out. Like so many young people with learning disorders, she gave up on herself. She became suicidal. Ron was an adept psychiatrist, and yet with the person he wanted to help most, it seemed he could do nothing.

One day when she was nineteen, she slipped into a warm bath with a razor blade to slit her wrists. Just then, her cat came into the room, jumped up on the bath ledge, and licked her shoulder. Erica changed her mind.

Around this time, another colleague of Ron's went to a conference and heard Paul Madaule tell how Tomatis had helped him. Ron says he "blew it off" because it sounded too weird. But as Erica's depression worsened, he did a literature search on Tomatis and discovered the one paper on the subject in English, Paul Madaule's "The Dyslexified World."

"I read it and I cried," said Ron. "I realized that I finally had an idea of what it was to be caught in that world."

"The Dyslexified World" (or *"L'univers dyslexié,"* as Paul originally called it) was written when he was only twenty-eight years old, yet remains one of the more remarkable papers on a clinical subject that I have read. It is an understated clinical masterpiece. Psychiatry gives learning disorders short shrift. *The Diagnostic and Statistical Manual of Psychiatry* (DSM-IV-TR) offers only impoverished categories with titles such as "reading disorder." To meet the criteria, you must be unable to read, as measured on standardized tests, implying that dyslexia is only an academic problem.

Paul's paper blasted this idea apart. It begins:

In the eyes of many, dyslexia might appear to exist only in the classroom, since it is the label which designates the child with reading problems. . . . Here my purpose is to focus on the dyslexic youngster himself, on the person hidden behind the phenomenon known as "dyslexia" precisely because the dyslexic child lives with his dyslexia all of the time: at recess, at home, with his friends, alone, asleep and in his dreams. The dyslexic is dyslexic every second of his life. . . . The dyslexic child is difficult to grasp because he does not have a grip on himself. He disorients others because he himself is disoriented. In fact, he projects onto others his own inner world, which we will describe as "dyslexified."

Paul then describes how psychotherapists often feel helpless with adolescent dyslexics, unable to handle them, and how dyslexics themselves seemed to be "playing a role with no clear idea of what they wanted," and how "a direct and open relationship with them was often impossible." Here was an explanation of how a teacher and a school system, otherwise helpful, could write a child off; how parents were so often at a loss; how a diagnostic system could, through the hollowness of its description of dyslexia, practically ignore this condition. Dyslexia was disorienting to everyone concerned.

Even conscientious teachers got "dyslexified" by these youngsters, becoming "disoriented" and "battle-weary" and ascribing to dyslexic youngsters all manner of vices, labeling them "idle, lazy, stupid, rude, inattentive, 'out of it,' having a bad influence." And "because these students transmit their inner malaise to those around them, they often serve as scapegoats for their peers."

Paul compared being dyslexic to visiting a foreign country, where the language is always unfamiliar:

> The foreigner knows what he wants to say, but is able to express it only in an incomplete or imperfect way. The inadequate vocabulary and poorly constructed sentences he uses to express his thoughts are only approximations. Nuance is impossible.... [He] acts on his partial comprehension rather than the actual meaning of the other person's words.... [T]he effort of searching for the right words and trying to understand what the others are saying requires so much concentration that the foreigner soon loses the thread of his ideas and quickly feels tired and worn-out.

His self-confidence is shattered; he dreads new surroundings; he feels chronically homesick for he knows not what and finally withdraws.

Then the paper added something else new: that even though dyslexia is supposedly about a problem with words,

> [m]any dyslexics live with a virtually constant feeling of uneasiness within their body, this instrument they can neither control nor master.... Dyslexics are dyslexified throughout their entire body. They are often awkward in their physical movements and seem hampered or constricted by their bodies.... They do not know what to do with their legs and arms, and particularly their hands. Their posture, whether it is slumped or tense, lacks flexibility and naturalness.

The psychological effect of it all is a wish to escape to a place "where language is not necessary." But "for the dyslexic, however, there is no native land to return to." With classmates, he cannot keep up with the repartee. On vacation, the dyslexic cannot enjoy socializing with other children, games, or sports. To escape reality, he withdraws into an imaginary world of dreams, reveries, fantasy, and absentmindedness. He is immature and in adolescence becomes vulnerable to alcohol and drugs. He can fall into fringe movements, into the hands of dream merchants, con artists, and manipulators. With all these problems, the dyslexic soon becomes neurotic or deeply depressed and suicidal. Psychotherapists, Paul explained, are at a loss with dyslexics because the principal tool of psychotherapists is verbal communication. The dyslexic cannot translate his disability into language; introspection, without a way of fixing the problem, only opens up old wounds.

In 1989 Ron told Erica that he had heard of a program, involving music, that might help her, and he told her he would do the entire program with her. He took her to the Sound Listening and Learning Center in Phoenix, run by Billie Thompson, a center Paul had often visited, to help guide its development. Though Erica was acutely suicidal, a psychiatrist decided she didn't have to be hospitalized if her father was constantly with her. "So we stayed together," Ron says, "in the hotel, for the next three weeks, for the fifteen listening sessions. My hope was that she would learn how to read and overcome her dyslexia, *and then eventually* her depression would lift."

To his surprise, her dark depression lifted almost *immediately.* Her all-day sleeping disappeared. Her mental and physical energy began to blossom within four or five days, and she brightened. The biggest difference was that she immediately became able to express what she was thinking and feeling. (In my terms, neurostimulation of the centers that energize the brain, the reticular activating system, led to a neuromodulation of her sleep-wake cycle, and to neurorelaxation, which resulted in her being reenergized.) Now she could regulate her mood, learn, and differentiate. The neurorelaxation stage also involved the activation of her parasympathetic system, which turned on social engagement. Now she could relate to others. Ron observed how articulate Erica was; he had never heard her speak so directly. Stunned and delighted at the speed of her changes and her new openness, he asked, one night in the hotel, why she had resisted her parents' previous attempts to help her. She answered, "'Everything you did with the therapies showed me what I couldn't do. So I shut down. I felt I was supposed to be on another planet, and I didn't belong here. I was waiting to die.'"

"Hearing her talk about the anguish," Ron told me, "and not feeling any hope, I said, 'Erica, I'm so sorry. I'm so sorry. I just didn't know.' And she said, 'That's okay, Pop, you didn't understand.'"

Telling me about that conversation from so many years ago, Ron wept. "I still feel it. I had wanted so much to help my daughter, and I was helpless and scared and angry at her for not trying. I just didn't get it. When I learned how miserable she was inside and how my best attempts to help her just made it worse, we bonded as never before."

ERICA IS AS FRANK AS her father. "I was a very angry child. When I hurt myself, I didn't cry, I got angry. I felt I didn't fit anywhere." She told me how close she was to killing herself. But now her once-atonal voice is rich, warm, energetic, engaging, and expressive. She remembers those transformative days when she first put on the headphones and heard the screechy music. "A couple of days into it, I was able to sit down in the hotel and talk to Pop about what I was feeling." She told her father she felt listened to and truly heard for the first time, and that never, in her life, had she felt so connected to a human being.

It might be tempting to describe Erica's breakthrough as triggered by her realizing how much her father loved her, as demonstrated by his willingness to go through the therapy with her. But that wouldn't do justice to what happened. Erica told me she always remembered "feeling 100 percent loved by my parents," even during the worst periods. She and her father had tried and failed to connect many times before: "Before I felt like he was talking at me, not with me, because my brain was not registering sound as others did. I just didn't understand. After Tomatis, I understood what he was saying. Within three to four days in Phoenix, I woke feeling happier, bouncier, with more energy. One day I was able to add up the bill for lunch, while it was upside down. And math had always been hardest, along with spelling."

After the active phase, her confidence shot up. She got her first steady job as a receptionist at a hair salon and soon worked her way up to manager. She got her high school diploma through correspondence. Eventually she got a job at a bank, where she stayed for fifteen years, managing millions of dollars daily. She's held steady jobs for years. She reads voraciously now, and the only remnant of her dyslexia is that she sometimes reverses letters when tired.

Totally unanticipated for Ron was a change in his own sleep patterns. Now he could be wide awake after only four or five hours' sleep and feel refreshed. He was more relaxed and more in touch with his emotions. He found he could release pent-up hurts. A knot of tension that had been lodged in his stomach for thirty years vanished. It could be argued that this surge in well-being was the relief of a father who had seen his daughter's suffering end, but it was more than relief, because the changes have lasted decades. Everything he saw with Erica, he would later write, "flew in the face of all my clinical experience as a psychiatrist. What's more, it was happening without medications." Ron Minson began studying French and left for Europe to study with Tomatis.

Attention Deficit Disorder and Attention Deficit Hyperactivity Disorder

On his return, Ron Minson found that he was able to take hundreds of people off antidepressants and stimulants like Ritalin used to treat attention deficit disorder (ADD), and use sound therapy instead. A colleague, Randall Redfield, began working with Ron and Kate O'Brien Minson to make a version of the Tomatis equipment that, much like Paul's LiFT, was portable and small enough to fit on a person's belt. This allowed the program to integrate movement, balance, and visual exercises with listening, to train a person to process input from multiple sensory systems at once, stimulating the brain all the more. They called the program Integrated Listening Systems, or iLs.

Ron reports that over the years he's helped 80 percent of his clients with ADD get better and never again need medication, with its side effects. Of people who have attention deficit hyperactivity disorder (ADHD), a disorder in which people are highly distractible *and* impulsive and hyperactive, about half get better. The rest are helped with a neuroplastic treatment called neurofeedback (described in Appendix 3).*

Sound therapy works with ADD for a number of reasons. As Paul points out, a good auditory "attention span" is in large part the ability to listen well for a long time, without being distracted by new, irrelevant external stimuli; concentration, he says, is "the ability to cut out parasitic information in order to 'listen to oneself thinking.'" About 50 percent of the children he has treated have attention deficit disorders, though many *also* have auditory processing problems, learning disorder problems, and hypersensitivities to sound, all of which make it still harder to pay attention. In psychiatry texts, these disorders are always separate, but in the real world, they often come together.

"Gregory," a boy with classic ADHD who came from extremely deprived circumstances, was helped with iLs. His biological parents were homeless crystal meth addicts, and his mother drank vodka during her pregnancy. Gregory was put into state custody, then adopted by a woman I will call "Chloe" and her husband. When Gregory turned three, Chloe observed he was hyperactive. "He was impulsive. He didn't appreciate personal space. If he ran up to a child, he would be right in their face, talking very loud, and would walk into doors, knock his head on tables, had black eyes, and accident after accident." He would also do risky things, fidget, couldn't stay in his seat at school, and disrupted others. He blurted out answers to questions before they were finished, interrupted others, and couldn't play quietly. By the time he was four, his teacher complained daily that "Gregory is out of control." He had symptoms of distractibility, didn't listen to others, didn't finish what he started, because something else caught his attention, and was always losing things. He had *all* the behavioral symptoms of ADHD and was diagnosed by several physicians, experts in ADHD; he was prescribed the stimulant Adderall.

---

* There are many children who are mistakenly labeled as having ADD or ADHD in the classroom. This includes children with psychological traumas who are emotionally preoccupied; highly playful children; highly creative and intelligent children who are bored; underexercised children, especially males who require more "rough and tumble play" to learn to control their impulses; children with a sensory processing disorder (discussed below); those with an auditory processing disorder; and "pseudo-ADD" caused by too much time spent using computer devices, as described in *The Brain That Changes Itself*.

But Chloe was loath to put a child with a developing brain on a stimulant medication. Ritalin given to very young animals appears to lead to depression-like symptoms over the long term. Because these medications don't train a child to focus, the problems return when medication is discontinued.

Instead of filling the prescription, Chloe looked for alternatives. She learned about Kids Kount, a treatment center for children with developmental problems of all kinds. Founded by speech-language pathologist Andrea Pointer, with occupational therapist Shannon Morris, Kids Kount has treated two hundred children using iLs. Gregory underwent iLS twice a week for three months. His ADHD improved. His listening treatment was tailored to his problems. First he was exposed to low frequencies and bone conduction, to stimulate his vestibular apparatus and calm and "ground" him by turning on his parasympathetic nervous system.

"Adding the movement, balance and visual components of iLS while he listened made a huge difference in his ability to pay attention," says Pointer. "The movement triggers dopamine, which is key for motivation and attention. So we were giving him a natural chemical response that medication gives."

I asked Chloe what she noticed. "The calm! I think we saw the calm, after about two and a half weeks. The main difference was his ability to sit still in class, to listen, to follow instructions. It was huge. The overall effect is a lot less impulsivity. Stopping to think about what he is going to do, before he does it."

Getting Gregory to do iLs was not the only change Chloe made. She noticed that he had extraordinary sensitivities to foods with gluten and sugar: "Giving my son sugar is like giving him crack." It made him more hyperactive. A 2013 Harvard study shows that very-high-sugar foods—typically processed foods—actually turn on a part of the brain that is affected by crack and cocaine. He needed to be off sugar, to boost his general brain cell health, but also needed iLs to stimulate and train his attention circuits.

"The difference in my son with iLs, and watching what he eats, is night and day," says Chloe. It was easy to distinguish between the help he was getting from the iLs and his dietary changes. When he went off his diet, the setback was almost immediate. The iLs improvements were slow and steady, and the more Gregory used it, the longer he could go without regular use. Now he is functioning well in school and no longer needs iLs on a regular basis, except for the occasional boost once or twice a year.

Chloe says, "The notes home from school now say, 'Gregory had another great day!'"

New Contributions as to How Sound Therapy Works

One of Ron Minson's most important contributions has been to update Alfred Tomatis's theories and resolve some important confusion about how sound therapy works, especially with respect to attention. Most brain scientists have thought of attention as a "higher cortical function," meaning that it is processed in the thin outer layer of the brain. It has long been known that the frontal lobes—at the "top" of the brain—help people form goals, stay on task, and perform more abstract kinds of thought; they are required for maintaining attention. Neuroscientists assumed that attention difficulties were caused by frontal lobe problems. Supporting that assumption was the fact that, on brain scans, people with ADHD have smaller frontal lobes than their more attentive peers.

The confusion that Minson has helped resolve is this. Signals from sound therapy don't go directly to the frontal lobes; rather, they go to various subcortical areas, beneath the cortex, that are involved in processing incoming sensory input. So how can they help improve attention?

Sound therapy can correct attention problems by stimulating all the subcortical areas illustrated in the figure on page 338.

All these subcortical areas in the figure are stimulated initially by sound therapy, especially when combined with movement. Recent brain scan studies have shown that people with ADHD also have decreased brain volume in the cerebellum (which, again, fine-tunes the *timing* of thoughts and movements, and balance). As a person's ADHD gets worse, the cerebellum decreases further in size. As patients get better, however, the cerebellum increases. Children with ADD who can't wait their turn or blurt out answers are sometimes having trouble *timing* their

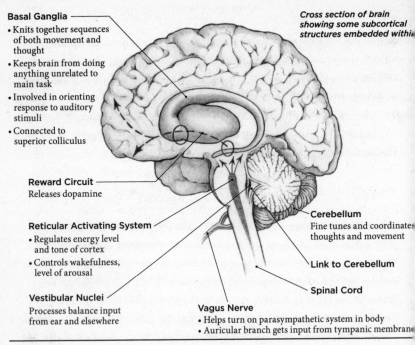

Basal Ganglia
- Knits together sequences of both movement and thought
- Keeps brain from doing anything unrelated to main task
- Involved in orienting response to auditory stimuli
- Connected to superior colliculus

Cross section of brain showing some subcortical structures embedded withi

Reward Circuit
Releases dopamine

Reticular Activating System
- Regulates energy level and tone of cortex
- Controls wakefulness, level of arousal

Cerebellum
Fine tunes and coordinates thoughts and movement

Link to Cerebellum

Spinal Cord

Vestibular Nuclei
Processes balance input from ear and elsewhere

Vagus Nerve
- Helps turn on parasympathetic system in body
- Auricular branch gets input from tympanic membran

Areas of the subcortical brain that are modulated by sound therapies in ADD and ADHD

actions. Tomatis's listening therapy and iLs have an impact on the cerebellum, as well as a huge impact on the vestibular system, which is linked to the cerebellum. Adding balance exercises, which iLs does, further stimulates the cerebellum.

The music in sound therapy turns on and enhances the connection between brain areas that process positive reward (which give us a feeling of pleasure when we accomplish something) and the insula, a cortical area of the brain that is involved in *paying attention*. This was shown only in 2005, by the neuroscientists Vinod Menon and Daniel Levitin, using fMRI scans.

Stimulating the vestibular system with music and movement therapy causes it to send signals to another subcortical area, the basal ganglia, which is also part of the attention circuit. People with ADHD have smaller basal ganglia. Normally, the basal ganglia contribute to staying focused by inhibiting the brain from doing anything unrelated to the main task. To pay attention to one thing requires inhibiting the temptation to attend to something else. Also, when the basal ganglia are underactive, people will tend to leap before they look, which can show up as hyperactivity and distractibility.

There is a direct link between the ear and the sensory pathways of the vagus nerve. Sound therapy, as Minson and Pointer explain, stimulates the sensory vagus, which supplies the ear canal and tympanic membrane. Stephen Porges has shown that the vagus system has many branches. We've discussed how it turns on the parasympathetic nervous system, to calm a person down. This is especially important in children with attentional and other developmental problems, because they are often very anxious, and in fight-or-flight reactions. But there is another aspect to the vagal system, which Porges calls the "smart vagus"; it allows a person to pay close attention, communicate, and get ready to learn. Stimulating the vagus with the right kind of sound therapy can put a person into a calm focused state, as many who love music know.

Another subcortical area that is stimulated by music is the reticular activating system (see Chapter 3). *Reticular* means "netlike" or "networklike," and its neurons have short connections with one another, so it resembles a net. This activating system is nestled in the brain stem. It receives input from all the senses and processes the information to determine how awake or aroused and attentive a person should be. When an alarm clock goes off in the morning, it rouses the activating system to awaken the cortex. When turned on "high," the activating system will wake an underaroused person—such as many people with ADD, who are often in a dreamy state. It powers up the cortex from below.

The subcortical brain areas are the first to receive signals from the ear. In people who have subcortical problems and can't handle incoming sensation, the auditory cortex does not get the strong clear signals it needs to do its job. However, argues Minson, they can compensate, to some degree, if they work much harder at paying attention. (We have seen this use of the cortex to perform subcortical activities before: John Pepper used his frontal lobes to do the work of the basal ganglia, when he did his conscious walking technique.) The problem is that this process is exhausting. Ron puts it this way: "If there is poor subcortical organization, you have to use all your cortical resources to perform those subcortical functions. What we are doing, by targeting the sub-cortex, is improving brain organization from the bottom up." This huge insight applies not only to people with ADD and ADHD but to many children with learning problems and sensory problems, and to children on the autistic spectrum, all of whom have subcortical problems.

The Disorder That Isn't: Sensory Processing Disorder

"Tammy," as I'll call her, was a month old when she became extremely fussy and refused to breast-feed. On the rare occasion when she tried to feed, she gagged, had difficulty swallowing, and started choking. She cried constantly, never fell asleep after a feed, couldn't nap, and was never calm. She couldn't gain weight and couldn't stand being touched.

Tammy's pediatricians jumped to the conclusion she must have re-flux, meaning that when she swallowed food, instead of passing from the stomach into the intestines, it would mix with the stomach acid, then go back up the esophagus, causing an acid burn. The doctors gave her medications, which failed, so she was hospitalized and given many invasive tests. A tube with a tiny scissors in it was passed through her mouth down her digestive tract; the doctor snipped off pieces of her esophagus, stomach, and small intestine. All tests came back normal. So they inserted a nasogastric feeding tube into her nose and down into her stomach, but the tube caused great distress. Tammy kept ripping it out. The gastroenterologist told her mother, "If she can't keep the NG tube in, or do bottle feeding, the only alternative is to surgically implant a tube through the front of her abdomen, into her stomach." Surgery was scheduled.

Tammy actually had sensory processing disorder (SPD), not a gas-trointestinal problem. Such children feel many sensations too intensely (as though they lack a volume control for incoming sensations), and the brain can't integrate sensations from different senses. Many children with eating problems, including some colicky babies, actually have sensory processing problems, which make them picky eaters. These sen-sory problems were perfectly summarized in Edgar Allan Poe's 1839 story "The Fall of the House of Usher," wherein the narrator recounts how Roderick Usher described the condition:

> He [Roderick] entered, at some length, into what he conceived to be the nature of his malady. It was, he said, a constitutional and a family evil. . . . He suffered much from a morbid acuteness of the senses; the most insipid food was alone endurable; he could wear only garments of certain texture; the odors of all flowers were oppressive; his eyes were tortured by even a faint light; and there were but peculiar sounds, and these from stringed instruments, which did not inspire him with horror.

Note that Roderick could tolerate some *peculiar sounds,* a point to which we shall return.

One reason Tammy's physicians missed her diagnosis is that a sensory problem is one in which the symptoms are subjective—and babies don't have words to convey their experiences. Sensory problems show up as feeding problems because feeding is about taking in not only food but also *sensory information.* First the infant sees the breast, looming large, a visual sensation; then she smells the distinct odor of the lactating mother's body; with her touch sense, she feels the engorged nipple in her mouth and the breast on her cheek; then the milk's texture; and finally its sweet taste, and she experiences the warmth of the milk moving into the stomach. An infant must process all these sensations simultaneously, with a developing brain doing this complex integration for the first time! Once this mysterious fluid goes inside, it gives rise to satisfaction, gastrointestinal contractions, and sudden cramps as gas builds up like a ball of internal pressure expanding from within, only relieved when discharged.

A child with a sensory processing disorder experiences all these sensations as an overwhelming barrage from within and without. As Jean Ayres wrote in her 1979 classic describing sensory integration problems, "You can think of sensations as 'food for the brain'; they provide the knowledge needed to direct the body and mind. . . . Food nourishes your body, but it must be digested to do so. . . . But without well-organized

sensory processes, sensations cannot be digested and nourish the brain."
To use Paul Madaule's language, the poorly organized sensory process
cannot adequately *protect us* from the world.

Now imagine the experience of a hypersensitive child—who can't tolerate suckling at her mother's breast—being sent to the hospital and sub-
jected to many surgical procedures, invaded with needles and tubes. The
hypersensitive SPD child like Tammy may well get more tests than the
child who has a gastrointestinal problem, because the SPD child's tests
will always come back negative—triggering more tests. Could any result
be more macabre, terrifying, and traumatizing for such a sensitive child?

And yet her physicians didn't think of it, because, unfortunately,
this very real diagnosis is one that hasn't been included in the psychiatric or medical diagnostic manuals.

TAMMY WAS SEVEN MONTHS OLD when she began treatment in Denver
at Dr. Lucy Miller's STAR Center. STAR stands for Sensory Therapies
and Research. Working with Ron Minson, the clinic started her on
twenty sessions of sound, with lots of bone conduction and traditional
occupational therapy that used movement and sensation, such as brush-
ing her skin to give her tactile stimulation, or gently compressing her
joints so she could get a better sense of where her limbs were in space.
Three times a week she listened to the iLs music while moving in a small
Lycra swing. It was hoped that with this proper "sensory diet" of controlled sound, movement, and balance input that Tammy would learn
to integrate them. Sensory integration of simultaneous sensory input
occurs in the superior colliculus, a clump of neurons in the brain stem.

She had never liked swinging, "but with headphones on, her body
would relax, and she would sit and look up at you calmly," says her
mother. "Often she would go to sleep, which was amazing, because she
never simply dropped off to sleep.

"Within two and a half weeks we saw dramatic improvement,"
she says. Tammy's feedings became more frequent, and her behavior
changed. She began to regulate and calm herself. Now she is in first
grade. "Today she is an absolute joy. Tammy is outgoing, cuddly, smart,

and reads two levels above her grade. Her improvement has been drastic and lasting. She has a large repertoire of foods she will accept, and textures don't seem to be a problem. She is comfortable in her own skin." She will not grow up to be like Poe's overexcited, raw, isolated Roderick Usher. She is, as far as I know, the youngest person in the world ever to have undergone a neuroplastic therapy.

IV. Solving the Mystery at the Abbey

How Music Raises Our Spirits and Energy

There remains one piece of unfinished business, the matter of the languishing monks of the Abbaye d'En Calcat, whose mysterious illness brought Alfred Tomatis to the monastery in the same weeks that eighteen-year-old Paul Madaule sought solace there. When Tomatis arrived, he found seventy dispirited men, who were, he said, "slumping in their cells like wet dishrags." When he examined them, he found the cause was not an infectious outbreak but a theological event. The Second Vatican Council of 1962–65, called Vatican II, had instituted new ways for the Church to respond to changes in the modern world. The monastery had just been taken over by a zealous young abbot who, though Vatican II did not forbid Gregorian chant, decided that the singing the monks did from six to eight hours a day served no useful purpose, and he ended it. A collective nervous breakdown ensued.

Monks often take vows of silence; now with chanting eliminated, they had no stimulation from the human voice, neither their brethren's nor their own. They were starved not for meat, vitamins, or sleep, but for the energy of sound. Tomatis reestablished the chanting, then saw that many were too depressed to sing. So in June 1967 he asked them to sing into Electronic Ears and listen to their own voices, through a filter adjusted to emphasize the higher, energizing frequencies of speech.

Their slumping posture changed almost immediately, and they became more upright. By November, almost all were restored, and they returned, reenergized, to their Benedictine work schedules of long workdays and only a few hours of sleep a night. The Benedictines, Tomatis said, "had been chanting in order to 'charge' themselves, but hadn't realized what they were doing."

Chanting, in many traditions, is known to energize the chanter. Tomatis himself chanted, to keep charged through the day. "There are sounds which are as good as two cups of coffee," he said. He was so energetic that he slept only four hours a night.

Just as some voices energize and "charge" both the speaker and the listener, making both more alert, other voices "discharge" or sap the energy of whoever produces them—or hears them. (Some teachers who might otherwise be stimulating have voices that drone on and put their students to sleep because they produce enervating sounds, owing to their own listening problem.)

For a chant to be effective, the chanter must produce high frequencies, which stimulate the cochlea, which has many receptors for these frequencies. When sung properly, Tibetan Buddhist chants of "om"—often perceived as deep and low—actually produce many high overtones, or harmonics, which is why they sound so rich. "It is the high frequencies," says Paul, "that give life to the sound. You can have a low voice that is lively . . . rich in harmonics that are high frequency. Or, you can have a voice that is high but narrow and poor in overtones, which will be unattractive. Anyone can produce a low-toned 'om,' but it will be flat without the highs." It can take decades for a monk to perfect this sound, which is so filled with harmonics (higher sounds), it is actually a chord. A solitary monk, listening to himself singing in a resonating stone monastery or medieval church with vaulted ceilings that amplify his voice's higher frequencies, might as well be sitting inside a huge Electronic Ear, because the effect is the same.

GREGORIAN CHANT DOES NOT ONLY energize; it is also effective in calming the spirit at the same time, which is why Paul often ends his clients' listening sessions with it. The Gregorian music that he plays is modified to quickly alternate between emphasizing the higher and the lower frequencies, so it also has a training effect on the middle ear system; but the chant still covers the full spectrum of sound, which strengthens the calming, grounding effect.

The rhythm of the chant often corresponds to the respiration of a calm, unstressed person, and it has an immediate calming effect— probably by entrainment. Entrainment is a process in which one rhythmic frequency influences another, until they synchronize, or approach synchronization, or have a strong influence on each other. In a somewhat different way, waves of water influence one another when they intersect.*

Brain scan studies show that when the brain is stimulated by music, its neurons begin to fire in perfect synchrony with it, entraining with the music it hears. This happens because the brain evolved to reach out into the world, and the ear works as a transducer. Transducers transform energy from one form into another. For instance, a loudspeaker transforms electrical energy into sound. The cochlea inside our ear transforms patterns of sound energy from the external world into patterns of electrical energy that the brain can use internally. Even though the form of the energy changes, the information carried by the wave patterns is often preserved.

Since neurons fire in unison to music, *music is a way to change the rhythms of the brain*. An expert in the neuroplasticity of sound, Dr. Nina Kraus of Northwestern University, and her lab colleagues recorded the sound waves given off by a Mozart serenade. They also placed an electrical sensor on a person's scalp to record his brain's waves as he listened to the Mozart. (Brain waves are the electrical waves produced by millions of neurons working together in time.) Then they played back

---

*Entrainment was discovered in 1665 by the Dutch physicist Christiaan Huygens, who was also the first scientist to propose that light was made of waves. He observed that two swinging pendulums mounted together—out of sync—will over time begin a synchronized swing, in what he called an "odd sympathy." This occurs because moving pendulums create waves of vibration that influence each other. Similarly, striking one tuning fork in the proximity of another of the same frequency will start the second one vibrating—giving off a sound—even if the two forks are not touching, because as a tuning fork vibrates, it creates pressure waves in the air, which is a medium that can conduct these waves.

the patterns of the brain waves firing. Amazingly, they found that the sound waves from the Mozart piece and the brain waves that they triggered looked the same. They even found that the brain waves in the brain stem sounded the same as the music that triggered them!*

Neurons can be entrained by a variety of nonelectrical stimuli, including light and sound; these effects can be demonstrated using an EEG. Many kinds of sensory stimulation can radically alter the frequency of brain waves. For example, in a hyperexcitable brain, as in some cases of photosensitive epilepsy, strobe lights (flashing at about ten times a second) can cause large numbers of neurons to fire synchronously; a victim may have a seizure, lose consciousness, and start writhing out of control. Music can cause seizures as well.†

Entrainment is so graphic that when people are hooked up to EEGs and asked to listen to a waltz rhythm of 2.4 beats a second, their brain waves' dominant frequency spikes at 2.4 beats per second. No wonder people move to the beat of a song—much of the brain, including the motor cortex, is entrained to that beat. But entrainment also happens between people. When musicians jam, their dominant brain waves begin to entrain with one another. In 2009 the psychologist Ulman Lindenberger and his colleagues hooked nine pairs of guitarists up to EEGs, while they played jazz together. The brain waves of each pair began to entrain together, to synchronize their dominant neuronal firing rates. No doubt this is part of what musicians' "getting into a groove" is all about. But the study also showed that entrainment didn't occur only between the musicians. Different regions of individual musicians' brains synchronized as well, so that overall, many more areas of the brain showed the dominant frequency. Not only were the musicians playing

---

* You can hear and see the brain responding to music by going to the lab's Web site at www.soc.northwestern.edu/brainvolts/demonstration.php. Kraus and her colleagues were able to hear the "sound" of the brain waves by recording them on an electroencephalogram (EEG), which uses electrical sensors placed on the scalp to measure the electrical waves produced by the brain, then amplifying them. They then resampled the EEG recording of waves as a .wav file (much like the files people use to listen to music on MP3 players or iTunes).

† Oliver Sacks describes a case from the scientific literature of a man who had a seizure at 8:59 every evening. It was found to be caused by the sound of the church bells preceding the BBC nine o'clock news. No other sound caused the seizure, only the sounds of that specific frequency. O. Sacks, *Musicophilia: Tales of Music and the Brain* (New York: Alfred A. Knopf, 2007), p. 24n.

together in an ensemble; the coordinated ensembles of the neurons within each player's brain were playing together with the ensembles of neurons in their fellow musicians' brains.

Because so many brain disorders are caused when the brain loses its rhythm and fires in an offbeat or "dysrhythmic" way, music therapy is especially promising for these conditions. The rhythms of music medicine can provide a noninvasive way to get the brain back "on beat." Kraus and others have shown that the subcortical brain areas, which were once thought to lack plasticity, are in fact quite neuroplastic.

Different rhythms of neuronal activity correspond to different mental states. When a person is sleeping, for instance, the dominant rhythm—that is, the brain waves with the highest amplitude—on an EEG are those that are firing 1 to 3 brain waves per second (or 1 to 3 Hz). When a person is awake and in a calm, focused state, the brain wave frequency is faster, about 12 to 15 Hz; as she concentrates on a problem, the 15 to 18 Hz waves are dominant; and when she is worrying about a problem and anxious, the waves increase to 20 Hz. Normally our brain rhythms are set by a combination of factors: external stimulation, our level of arousal, and our conscious intentions (say, to focus on a problem, or to go to sleep). Within the brain are multiple "pacemakers" that, like a conductor, generate the timing of these rhythms. But with neuroplastic training, we can develop some control over our brain rhythms. Neurofeedback (see Appendix 3) trains a person whose brain rhythms are off to control them. So it is excellent for people with attention or sleep problems, or a noisy brain in general.

But it is not a sound therapy. One that is, and which focuses directly on rhythm, is called Interactive Metronome, and I have seen some remarkable results with it. The brain has its own internal clock or timekeeper that is offbeat in some children. Some children's clocks run too fast and they become "early responders" to sensory stimuli. They interrupt other people, and seem impulsive, irritable, or inconsiderate, but their problems are really with timing. Other children may seem unmotivated and "slow" socially and intellectually, but, again, their problem is timing—an internal clock that is too slow. Training that clock—by learning to listen to and react to sounds—so that one is "on beat" can be transformative for these children. Suddenly, they seem more alert, and present.

•••

"THE EAR IS A BATTERY to the brain" was one of the aphorisms Tomatis used to sum up its power to "charge" the cortex. He attempted to explain how this might be possible, using the science of his day, and was largely speculative. In the model I propose, the neurostimulation of therapeutic music resets the reticular activating system, which is why people often sleep in the first stages of listening, then emerge reenergized. But another reason music can lift the spirits, as Daniel Levitin and Vinod Menon have demonstrated, is that it turns on the reward centers of the brain, which increases the production of dopamine, which in turn increases feelings of pleasure and motivation. As Levitin writes, "The rewarding and reinforcing aspects of listening to music seem . . . to be mediated by increasing dopamine levels. . . . Current neuropsychological theories associate positive mood and affect with increased dopamine levels, one of the reasons that many of the newer antidepressants act on the dopaminergic system. Music is clearly a means for improving people's moods."

I hypothesize that another reason sound stimulation lifts spirits in people with brain problems is that they so often have desynchronized neuronal firing throughout poorly connected areas (as we saw in autism, for instance). As I see it, the desynchronized brain is a noisy brain, firing random signals, always wasting energy; it is an overactive brain that gets little done, exhausting its owner. Music resynchronizes the brain by entrainment and gets neurons firing together, so that the brain is much more efficient.

ALFRED TOMATIS, WHO WAS ALSO devoted to yoga, believed that good listening, speaking, and being energized all have an intimate relationship to upright posture. When people feel energized, they generally assume a more upright posture: they puff up their chests, allowing themselves to breathe more deeply. We see this move to verticality in animals, too; dogs, when they are excited, perk up, looking more erect. They also may perk up their ears, in a posture of active listening.

Music's generally stimulating effects on posture are visible in Down syndrome children, who are born with low muscle tonus and are diagnosed as "floppy babies." Low tonus contributes to poor posture, as well as speech difficulties, even a tendency to drool. By training the brain circuits for their hypotonic middle ear muscles, using passive listening, Paul has helped many Down children not only improve their listening but also develop better muscle tonus throughout their bodies, thus improving their posture and hence their breathing, which allows them to pass more oxygen to the brain. Their drooling improves or stops, and their speech gets better. All these effects lead them to become more focused, alert, and visibly uplifted.

Kim Barthel, an expert on treating fetal alcohol syndrome (a childhood disorder typified by brain damage and mental retardation, caused when a mother abuses alcohol while pregnant), uses recorded modified music, partially inspired by Tomatis, called Therapeutic Listening. It has helped these children improve their energy, level of arousal, language processing, memory, attention, and auditory sensitivities.

In one remarkable case, using the stimulant effects of music, Tomatis helped a boy whose left hemisphere had been entirely removed, by the famous neurosurgeon Wilder Penfield, to stop life-threatening epileptic seizures. After the operation, the boy was barely able to speak and was paralyzed on the right side of his body. When the boy was thirteen, he was brought to see Tomatis. Despite years of speech therapy, the boy spoke very slowly with great difficulty, and his attention span was so short, it impaired his school performance. Tomatis hooked the boy up to the Electronic Ear and stimulated his sole hemisphere with sound. "A few weeks after the music," Tomatis wrote, "activity on the right side of his body had become efficient and was permanently established. His speech regained its qualities of timbre and rhythm. The child now expressed himself normally, with a well-modulated voice, which strongly contrasted with the dull and lifeless voice he had at the beginning of the treatment.... Our patient had become calm, open, and cheerful." Sound therapy, Tomatis believed, had awakened the remaining hemisphere.

Sound can sometimes help people with severe traumatic brain injury, who are chronically fatigued, reenergize and regain lost mental abilities. A twenty-nine-year-old woman I'll call "Mirabelle" was driving down a mountain near Denver. As she circled under an overpass, an eighteen-wheeler tractor-trailer, descending at high speed, lost its brakes, flew off the bridge, and landed on her car, leaving her with a serious TBI. She was disabled and lost her job, and after trying all conventional approaches and medications, she still suffered from cognitive deficits and hypersensitivities. She could no longer read and had a terrible memory, headaches, depression, and, above all, unrelenting fatigue. Says Mirabelle, "I was told by my neurologist that the first three months of my recuperation would be the crucial part of it, and there would be no significant healing after that." Four years passed with no progress. By chance she heard Ron Minson give a lecture. He had realized that brain-injured patients, like children with developmental disorders, have energy, sleep, attention, sensory, and cognitive problems. In her first month using iLs, Mirabelle slept most of the time she listened to the music, but within a month she became reenergized and her cognitive skills returned. She was able to go to university, retrain in the sciences, and get into a very competitive program in speech and language pathology.

INEVITABLY, THE QUESTION ARISES, "WHY MOZART?"

Some practitioners use other composers and forms of music, but most Tomatis practitioners stick to Mozart, especially compositions with violins, because it is the instrument richest in higher frequencies and can produce continuous sounds that are easy on the ear. Tomatis also favored Mozart's more youthful compositions, which are simpler in structure and more appropriate for children. "Originally," says Paul, "Tomatis didn't use only Mozart. He was using Paganini, Vivaldi, Telemann, Haydn. But little by little, by natural selection, we finished up with just Mozart. It seemed like Mozart was working with everybody, and had the effect of both charging, stimulating, and relaxing and calming. Which means, to me, regulating them.

"Mozart, more than any other composer, prepared the path, primed the nervous system, primed the brain—wired the brain—and gave it the rhythms, melodies, flow, and movement required for the acquisition of language. Mozart himself started playing music extremely young, and by the time he was five was already writing surprisingly sophisticated compositions. He had wired the language of music into his brain so early that it was not much influenced by the rhythms of his own language, German. For Tomatis, that was the reason the music of Mozart is so universal. It doesn't have the strong imprint of a specific language, the way Ravel has a French imprint, and Vivaldi an Italian imprint. It is a music which goes beyond cultural or linguistic rhythms."

Mozart, continues Paul, "is the best pre-language material we have been able to find. It has nothing to do with making children more intelligent, as some think. It has to do with helping the prosody—the musical part of language, and the emotional flow of language—to come out more easily. That is why Mozart is such a good mother! Because the mother's voice does the same, is more personalized. Mozart is more universal, for all ages, races, social groups, as ethnomusicological studies have shown."*

TOMATIS WAS SO FAR AHEAD of his medical colleagues that he was all too often depicted as a quack who dishonored his profession by performing "nonmedical acts" with mere sound. His dumbfounded peers insisted that a physician can't cure a brain problem by passing sound into the ear. Instead of being cowed, he would shoot back a Tomatisism, saying that in fact the brain was a mere appendage of the ear and not the other way around. And he was, technically, quite correct: the primitive vestibular apparatus (the statocyst) actually evolved in animals long before the brain did.

---

* The modified Mozart used by Tomatis, Paul, iLs, and others over time in an individualized therapy must be distinguished from claims made in the media in the 1990s that mothers could raise the IQ of their children by having them briefly listen to unfiltered Mozart. This claim was based on a study not of mothers and babies but of college students who listened to Mozart ten minutes a day and improved IQ scores on spatial reasoning tests—an effect that lasted only ten to fifteen minutes! Hype aside, different studies by Gottfried Schlaug, Christo Pantev, Laurel Trainor, Sylvain Moreno, and Glenn Schellenberg have shown that sustained music training, such as learning to play an instrument, can lead to brain change, enhance verbal and math skills, and even modestly increase IQ.

Alfred Tomatis died on Christmas Day 2001. He did not live to see the explosion of understanding about the subcortical brain that we are now witnessing, which helps clarify how he achieved his astonishing results. Perhaps his critical peers should not be judged too harshly, either. The incredulity that attaches to "cures by instrumental music" may stem from our habit of linking music to beauty and leisure, and illness to pain and suffering. It also surely relates to music's uniqueness as an art form: as Eduard Hanslick wrote in 1854, in *On the Musically Beautiful,* instrumental music is the one art in which form and content are indistinguishable. We cannot ever say, with total confidence, what a particular musical phrase is "about," because the "musical idea" (as Hanslick calls the melody and rhythm) is not "about" anything. A Manet painting of a picnic is *about* the picnic. The beauty of instrumental music seems to come not from outside itself but from within.

And yet though utterly intangible, this invisible art reaches places in the heart and mind that nothing else can touch. It is indeed a very mysterious medicine, especially for those who want concrete explanations of how things work, in a culture that often favors the visual over the acoustic, and where "seeing is believing." What is heard is often suspect; the voice is transitory; people speak dismissively of "hearsay" and scoff that "talk is cheap." Sound exists momentarily in the ether, while for many, "the real," "truths," and "lasting proofs" are what can be seen physically, concretely. We like our proofs visible, like those of geometry, which literally demonstrates its truths pictorially.

And yet regardless of the culture we are born into, we all begin life in darkness, and we do our most substantial growth within it. Our first contact with existence is enclosed within the vibrations of our mother's heartbeat, the tide of her breathing, and the music of her voice, its melody and rhythm, even without our knowing the meaning of her words. Such longing as this engenders remains with us forever.

Afterword to the Paperback Edition

SINCE THE PUBLICATION OF THE hardcover edition of this book in early 2015, I have traveled to four continents to present its ideas and to learn about new clinical neuroplastic techniques, including some for traumatic brain injuries, spinal cord injuries, stroke, dystonias, Parkinson's, and learning disorders, among others that I will describe here.

But first I'd like to address perhaps the most common question I am asked: "If neuroplasticity is now accepted in neuroscience, why are these clinical approaches that make use of it not more widely available and mainstream?"

Part of the answer is that treatments, obviously, can't at the same time be *truly* cutting-edge and already mainstream. But at a deeper level, within neuroscience, "neuroplasticity" describes not just an area at the forefront of research; the very idea of "the neuroplastic brain" represents a revolutionary change in our fundamental understanding of how the brain works. Like all revolutionary ideas, it challenges the model it replaces and therefore faces obstacles, which will take time to overcome. Indeed, it took about two hundred years from the time that Michele Vincenzo Malacarne (1744–1816) conducted his first experiments demonstrating plasticity, until its widespread acceptance within neuroscience, and now it must overcome obstacles within medicine and health care.

The view of science and medicine that students get from textbooks is that developments occur through the steady accumulation of knowledge, but this textbook view, as Thomas Kuhn, the great historian of scientific revolutions, has shown, tends to obscure the tensions and differences within science, by presenting it as a unified whole. Kuhn brilliantly details how science often proceeds in great bursts. He argues that a scientific theory and its related laws and practices make up what he calls a "paradigm." No paradigm is perfect at describing the way the world is, and so, over time, some of the paradigm's inadequacies become apparent, and then a scientific revolution occurs and the existing paradigm is replaced by a new paradigm. During the revolution, there is great tension between advocates of the old paradigm and the new one.

Kuhn shows that when a scientific revolution is occurring, books describing the new paradigm are often addressed to anyone who may be interested. They tend to be clearly written and jargon free, like Darwin's *Origin of Species*. But once the revolution becomes mainstream, a new kind of scientist emerges. These scientists work on problems and puzzles *within* the new paradigm they inherit. They don't generally write books but rather journal articles, and because they communicate largely with one another, a specialized jargon develops so that even colleagues in adjacent fields cannot easily understand them. Eventually the new paradigm becomes the new status quo. The everyday activities of the scientists who defend the new status quo make up what Kuhn calls "normal science." Normal science assumes that the scientific community now, finally, "knows what the world is like," and the scientists "defend that assumption, if necessary at considerable cost. Normal science . . . often suppresses fundamental novelties, because they are necessarily subversive of its basic commitments."

Physicist and systems biologist Bruce West, Ph.D. (chief scientist in the Mathematical and Information Sciences Directorate at the Army Research Office, who worked with Nobel Prize winner Jonas Salk for many years), has categorized the different kinds of scientists in his book *Where Medicine Went Wrong*. First are the *leapers*, like Einstein and Newton, who create new paradigms and leap ahead of the rest. (As Schopenhauer put it, "Talent hits a target others miss. Genius hits a target no one sees.")

But most scientific activity involves normal science, working within paradigms, and is conducted by three types of scientists. There are the *creepers*, who investigate potential findings in areas that are predicted by the existing model but not yet established. There are the *sleepers*, usually teachers, who "mostly pass on to the next generation what they and others have previously learned" and spend time organizing and categorizing knowledge, and who "no longer participate in research that advances science." And finally there are *keepers*, who refine and redo experiments of well-understood phenomena, work on fine points within the existing paradigm, and who "as a group put forward all the objections to new theories and explain in extraordinary detail why this particular experiment must be wrong." They are "keepers of the *status quo*."

Keepers, sleepers, and creepers invest their lives in the existing paradigm and often draw their social status from its intellectual status. While keepers may serve science by coming up with good objections to a new paradigm, they are driven by a wish to defend the existing one, and not primarily by a quest for the truth. Versions of West's types also exist within medicine and influence how innovations are received.

IT IS SOMETIMES DIFFICULT FOR people not trained in medicine to apprehend the extent to which the paradigm of the unchanging brain penetrated medical practice. It influenced several generations' ideas of pathology and brain degeneration, diagnosis, and prognosis, determined the treatments that insurance would reimburse, in addition to the studies that major agencies would fund.

Clinically, the idea that the brain cannot change or heal tends to be self-perpetuating. If a clinician tells a patient who has had a stroke that he may make very minor progress for about six months (while the swelling and chemical changes in his brain are still resolving) but that he will "plateau" and not improve after that, the patient, if compliant, will not make attempts to improve, thinking more therapy pointless. His already damaged circuitry will likely atrophy even further, as it is a use-it-or-lose-it brain. Thus, the clinician's negative prognosis becomes a self-fulfilling prophecy.

While researching this book, I got to see the opposite: physicians dealing with patients who *were* getting better, and I observed a range of reactions by mainstream clinicians to the improvements brought about by the neuroplasticians. Most in the mainstream expressed great surprise and joy on their patient's behalf—spurring them on—and a deep curiosity about how the patient managed to improve. They began referring other patients to the neuroplastician who was so helpful. But distressingly often, I learned from some patients that their clinicians were indifferent, dismissive, and a few almost seemed disturbed by the very idea of these improvements. I recall one "keeper" physician who leapt to the conclusion that the diagnosis must have been wrong in the first place—even though (he was surprised to be reminded) he himself had made it and documented it extensively. I'm also reminded of the physician who told a patient nothing more could be done for her. Months later, that patient returned to the busy office, and reported she was improved by a new approach. She was reexamined by her skeptical physician using objective measures, which confirmed she was indeed radically improved. The physician seemed almost interested, but his eye caught the clock and he, knowing the waiting room was overfull, moved on to his next case without ever asking the patient who was leaving what cured her. It was as though the physician could not believe what he had just seen because he knew that "in theory" it could not happen.

ANOTHER OBSTACLE TO THE WIDER acceptance of these new approaches lies in the misuse of statistics and the underestimation of the importance of clinical case histories in neurological and psychiatric discoveries.

Whenever case histories of breakthroughs that were not supposed to occur are reported, it is a safe bet that someone will immediately cry out, "Anecdote, mere anecdote! Where are your randomized control trials!" This criticism confuses case histories with anecdotes. There is a time-honored distinction in medical writing between the anecdote and the case history. An anecdote is defined as a brief interesting report, often only a few sentences long. Anecdotes are stripped of many details, not unlike the subjects in group studies about whom we learn very little except their scores on a few measures. Case histories often contain hundreds of observations about a patient. They are the only place in medical reporting where we see, if not the whole patient, at least enough to get a picture of a living human being. As Oliver Sacks stated: in neurology, "all sorts of generalizations are made possible by dealing with populations [group studies]—but one needs the concrete, the particular, the personal too, and it is impossible to convey the nature and impact of any neurological condition *without* entering and describing the lives of individual patients." It is not possible to understand a person with a brain illness by describing them in bits and pieces. They must be made whole again, and not simply because the whole is the sum of the parts, but because with human beings, the whole is always *more* than the sum of the parts. Hence the need for case histories.

Even the shorter vignettes in this book are not simply "mere anecdotes" chosen for minor interest; they are anomalies, profoundly embarrassing to the doctrine of the unchanging brain. An "anomaly," according to Kuhn, is an observation that does not make sense within the framework of an existing scientific paradigm. Scientific revolutions and medical breakthroughs often begin by someone recognizing an anomaly. The Ptolemaic model of the universe, which still reigned in Galileo's time, argued that the sun, planets, and all the heavenly bodies orbited around the earth. When Galileo observed that Venus has phases (like our moon) that could be explained only by assuming Venus circled the sun, that observation was an *anomaly* that refuted the accepted view.

When people are told by clinicians at leading medical institutions that they will never get better, and then do manage to improve, they too are anomalies, and their significance resides not in their number but in their power to compel thoughtful clinicians to reexamine their basic premises. As the great neuroscientist and neurologist V. S. Ramachandran puts it: "Imagine I cart a pig into your living room and tell you that it can talk. You might say, 'Oh, really? Show me.' I then wave my wand and the pig starts talking. You might respond, 'My God! That's amazing!' You are not likely to say, 'Ah, but that's just one pig. Show me a few more and then I might believe you.'"

I principally use three kinds of evidence in this book to illustrate its core thesis—that the damaged or diseased brain can, at times, be improved if one understands that there are different stages of neuroplastic healing: detailed case histories, basic science (to show how these treatments work), and, where available, group studies of these approaches. In some cases, such as the scientific literature on light therapy, or exercise and the brain, there are thousands of studies; in others, far fewer. Putting together these three sources of knowledge is part of a sustained argument, to show that brain healing is possible. All three sources are needed because each has its strengths and weaknesses.

The case history is a time-honored method in psychiatry, neurology, and neuropsychology because it can reveal important concrete details that group studies with their average scores, and other abstract statistics, overlook. The yield has been extraordinary. As Ramachandran explains: "I think it's fair to say that, in neurology, most of the major discoveries that have withstood the test of time were, in fact, based initially on single case studies and demonstrations." From Phineas Gage, the railway worker who had a metal rod driven through his frontal lobes in an explosion, we learned about the function of those lobes. Gage survived the head injury but went from being a stable, courteous, hardworking person to an unreliable, lying, impulsive one. Thus we learned that the frontal lobes are involved in self-control, forming goals, and sticking to them. From the patient called HM, we learned about memory. HM had intractable epilepsy and so had two parts of his brain, called the hippocampi, cut out. After that he lost the ability to form short-term memories (though he retained all his long-term ones). We learned more about memory from HM than from decades of group studies. Ramachandran himself, working with a few cases, answered the riddle of the phantom limb—why people who lose limbs still feel they are present, and hurting—and how to cure them in some cases.

Case histories make hundreds of observations about a few people. Randomized control studies (RCT), and other group studies, make a few observations about many people—a population. RCTs are superior to case histories in particular kinds of situations, as when a public health official needs to know the number of people with pneumonia that penicillin will help compared to another new drug (say, 60 percent for penicillin,

30 percent for the new drug). RCTs tell us about the percentage of people likely to be helped in a population. But they can't tell a clinician, with an ill patient, the decisive thing he wants to know: "Will penicillin help the patient in front of me?"

RCTs have their limits. Attempts to replicate them often fail. John Ioannidis, M.D., and colleagues have shown that 35 percent of the conclusions of the finest RCTs cannot be replicated and that most published group studies in life sciences can't be replicated, leading to what the major journal *Nature* now calls "the replication crisis." There is less safety in numbers than we might wish.

The assumption underlying group studies and RCTs is that each person in the study has the *same* condition as the next, and that any other variation between the people in the group is relatively insignificant. But often this is not the case in brain problems. Two brain injuries may look the same, if not examined closely. But they are the same only in the way that two bombed-out cities look the same from thirty thousand feet. Both look like a pile of rubble. Seen close up, one city has lost its harbor, market, and train station, and the other its electrical grid, school, and hospital. Similarly, no two head injuries impact exactly the same areas of the brain. Experienced clinicians also know they don't simply treat "the disorder." They treat "the person with the disorder." Before the brain injury, one patient may have had many protective factors: exhibited a high IQ, been conscientious, exercised regularly, didn't drink or take drugs, and had no cardiovascular problems or previous head injuries. The second patient had a lower IQ, a learning disorder, was impulsive, an alcoholic, smoked, used cocaine, loved extreme sports, and had a number of previous concussions. A practitioner who concludes both had "moderate brain injuries" and assumes they have the same prognosis is clinically naïve.

TO THE PERSON WHO INSISTS that the idea that the brain can heal "all sounds too good to be true," one can only say, "Of course it *must*, if you accept the paradigm of the unchanging brain." Such critics often pose as skeptics, but are not skeptical enough of the paradigm they were taught. Unfortunately, behind this reaction is also an allegation that documenting cases that get better unexpectedly is to encourage false hope. For the true believer in the fixed brain paradigm, when it comes to recovery from a brain problem, any hope is false hope. So he does not hesitate to discourage patients and clinicians from exploring these treatments, even if he himself knows little about them.

As I make clear in the preface, to provide some hope where there was none is not to say every condition can always be helped; to say that the brain *can* heal is obviously not to say it *always* can. What I do claim is that the brain is more like the skin, bones, liver, and other organs that can heal than we appreciated. But to observe that the skin can heal does not mean it can recover from every burn. No treatment can help everyone.

My claim is that much can be learned by "reverse engineering" how the people in this book, who were told they could not improve, did so. (The documentary film of this book, to be released in 2016, will allow readers to see and hear many of these people, and make their own observations.) One reason for categorizing the stages of neuroplastic healing is that not all neuroplastic interventions work for all disorders. But now we can try to identify which stage of healing has been interrupted, and attempt to help the brain resume the healing process. As to exactly how many in a population can be helped by such approaches, it is simply too early in this new field to know. But it is not too early to notice the following transformation. In neurology, up to very recently, neurological nihilism was so prevalent for some conditions that the adage was "Diagnose and *adios*." The specialist was called in to diagnose the condition and give the patient the bad news, and because the patient was incurable, the two would never see each other again. What is exciting about this new era is that in many of these conditions there is a range of approaches we can try. Now we can sometimes say *au revoir*, see you again.

Thus, to those who only worry about raising false hope, I say, I wish that false hope was all we had to worry about. As I wrote earlier, we must also worry about false despair, a problem with no name. And, while false hope and false despair are like evil twins, each doing harm, they are not identical twins. The harm done by false hope is familiar, serious, but often *transient*, for when it comes to brain problems, if the treatment is ineffective, the patient is quickly brought back to cruel reality. But if the patient has a condition that might have been helped by one of these novel approaches, the damage caused by a clinician mistakenly telling a person nothing can be done risks condemning that person to a *permanent* loss of what would have been a fuller life.

Given the complexity of the brain and brain problems, and the tremendous variation caused by genetics and by how our different life experiences mold our neuroplastic brains in unique ways, there will often be some uncertainty about an individual's prognosis. It is precisely when there is uncertainty about important matters such as the outcome of an illness that our emotions, and our emotionally based attitudes, are most likely to prevail, and we swing, as the philosopher Spinoza observed, between hope and fear (and I would add despair). This tendency—this emotional contagion—can affect mainstream clinicians, researchers, and neuroplasticians alike, and of course, patients and their families. All may swing between their conviction a treatment will work and their despair that it is pointless to try.

For these reasons, there is often a temptation to declare to a patient, in advance, "This will definitely help you," or that "this will definitely not." A clinician's over-investment in his or her own remedies—something called *furor therapeuticus*—can be as dull-witted as neurological nihilism. What the patient usually needs is not a champion of a particular treatment but someone who is willing to be agnostic when matters are uncertain, and also relentless in exploring all available options.

Luckily, it is usually enough for a clinician to tell the patient the reasoning behind the technique that is being proposed and then say (if one thinks it possible that it will help), "I think this is worth a try, but there are no guarantees." For a person who has been told "nothing is worth a try," such a statement is often sufficient to mobilize them.

Now, let me briefly describe some new ways of initiating or unblocking some or all of the stages of neuroplastic healing, which I have begun to learn about in my travels.

SPINAL CORD INJURIES ARE A specialty at Neuroworx, an outpatient facility near Salt Lake City, Utah, where Dale Hull, an obstetrician, and Jan Black, a physiotherapist, are extending neuroplastic principles to the spine. When Dr. Hull was forty-four years old, he broke his neck doing a back flip on a trampoline and was left a quadriplegic, i.e., totally paralyzed and without sensation from the neck down and without bowel or bladder control. Victims of such an injury are told they will not recover and will need 24/7 care for the rest of their lives.

Dr. Hull, after working for three and a half years with Jan Black (who had been taught some Feldenkrais in her training), now walks, has nearly full movement of his arms and legs, though he still suffers from numbness, pain, and some bladder and bowel dysfunction. Learned nonuse affects the spinal cord, so Neuroworx prescribes intensive individually tailored exercise in doses far greater than most hospitals provide. The work done by Hull and Black conforms to the stages of neuroplastic healing, using neurostimulation as well as neuromodulation to correct imbalances in the damaged, "noisy" spinal cord. No two spinal injuries are identical, and not everyone progresses as far as Dr. Hull, but most go much further than they do with conventional treatment, and Neuroworx has helped other quadriplegic clients learn to walk.

DYSTONIAS ARE MOVEMENT DISORDERS THAT give rise to involuntary movements, spasms (sustained muscle contractions), tremors, and abnormal postures, affecting half a million North Americans. Dystonias are also very common in Parkinson's disease, stroke, and cerebral palsy. Joaquin Farias, Ph.D. (his Ph.D. is from a medical school and he has degrees in neuropsychological rehabilitation and sports medicine), has developed a neuroplastic therapy for dystonia and related neurological movement disorders. Now living in Toronto, he was born in Cartagena, Spain, where he became a precocious professional musician playing flute, piano, and harpsichord. By the age of twenty-one he began to have difficulty controlling the finger pressure he was applying to his instruments. He had a "focal" dystonia, which is often a career killer for musicians. Farias was told his disorder was genetically based and incurable. Yet he found a way to cure himself and then went on to help over five hundred others, including surgeons, physicians, neurologists, health-care workers, and more than three hundred musicians.

Dystonias take many forms. Some people have frequent, dramatic, disabling, and uncontrollable blinking and squinting, a dystonia called "blepharospasm." In patients with retrocollis, a cervical dystonia, the head involuntarily lurches back dangerously. When dystonias affect the voice box, they make it hard to speak. Generalized dystonias can involve the whole body: arms, legs, abdomen, larynx, and eyelids. The dystonias are poorly understood, though it is often claimed they have a chemical or genetic basis. Yet, the National Institutes of Neurological Disorders and Stroke Web site states there are "no medications to prevent dystonia or slow its progression." Treatments are often symptomatic, drastic, and invasive: implanting electrodes in the brain, cutting muscles, even stapling the eyelids of patients with blepharospasm to the bone so they can't blink. Most commonly, Botox is injected to weaken affected muscles so that they cannot contract.

Farias developed noninvasive treatments for a number of dystonias that yield dramatic and usually permanent improvements. He proposes that in dystonias, a "shock" occurs, affecting the brain's prefrontal cortex, an area that, in adults, controls and modulates our *primitive reflexes* (sometimes called neonatal reflexes) that are produced subcortically. A musician or surgeon, for instance, makes a movement that triggers an inappropriate primitive reflex in the hand, which makes it impossible to perform the intended movement. Meanwhile, appropriate circuits become dormant.

Newborns have a number of well-recognized "primitive" reflexes that occur automatically, in certain situations, but which fade as they age. For instance, the asymmetric tonic neck reflex (sometimes called "the fencing reflex") occurs when a baby is set down on its back. It sticks out one arm straight to the side and looks at it, while raising the other arm toward its ear. Primitive reflexes are fast responses. A baby, sensing it is falling from its mother's arms, will rapidly reach out to cling to her body. To do so quickly, the nervous system turns down the tonus of any "antagonist" muscles that would oppose the reflex.

Farias realized that each dystonia, when viewed closely, is an expression of one of the primitive reflexes that clinicians believed normally disappear as we age. Dystonias in different parts of the body release different primitive reflexes repetitively, neuroplastically reinforcing the pattern.

Dystonias also turn off a person's ability to properly sense movement. Farias was able to make these astute observations, in part because he has training in Eastern martial arts, yoga, qigong, and was influenced by the work of Feldenkrais.

He has developed many techniques to block a problematic reflex. He might block it by stimulating the antagonist muscles, or a more appropriate movement, or reflex, which competitively turns off the inappropriate primitive reflex. He turns off the reflexes with hands-on techniques, or music. Then he teaches the client to do so. A number of his dramatic cases can be seen on his Web site, fariastechnique.com.

Farias has started to work with Parkinson's patients, who often have tremors and dystonias. In just two sessions, I saw how one patient who has had Parkinson's for decades was able to discard her walker. I saw him rapidly decrease her tremor and several of her dystonias in her leg and abdomen, using his hands-on approach. This shows that some Parkinson's symptoms are not always the direct product of low dopamine but can be maladaptive, reversible reactions of the brain. This patient has more work to do, but two months after the initial session she told me, "I may deteriorate with my disease, but I have had two glorious months walking." My hope is that as she gets walking faster, it will trigger neurotrophic growth factors in her brain, as it did for John Pepper.

Farias has also noted that psychological trauma is in some way related to the dystonia. This is *not* to argue that dystonias are psychosomatic or hysterical symptoms. Psychological traumas can trigger reactions throughout the brain, turning off some circuits and turning on others. For instance, Farias realized that a client with a dystonia that made him look to one side was experiencing the reemergence of the asymmetrical neck reflex, in which babies turn their heads to one side. As Farias worked with him, he suddenly remembered that he had been physically attacked, and that during the attack he automatically looked away. In general, Farias believes that mental and physical traumas can trigger "brain shock" that turns off the prefrontal function, which regulates that primitive reflex and thus gives rise to the dystonia (which I would say is a form of poor neuromodulation) and which, over time, becomes neuroplastically reinforced, worsening. Farias undoes this with neurostimulation of brain areas that are in "shock" and suffering from learned nonuse. After this, the patient is sent home to practice and refine the appropriate movements, so neurodifferentiation can occur.*

Problems arising from persistent primitive reflexes also can exacerbate learning and sensory disorders, ADD, autism, brain injuries, and developmental delays. A number of techniques have been developed by clinicians in Australia, Russia, America, and Britain to undo persistent primitive reflexes in childhood conditions.

CONCUSSIONS AND TBIs, AS WE have seen, can be responsive to a number of neuroplastic approaches, and Cognitive FX is a clinic in Provo, Utah, that uses effective techniques to treat both, based on an approach developed by neuroscientist Mark Allen, Ph.D., and clinical neuropsychologist Alina Fong, Ph.D. Their first major successes were with NFL superstars such as Tom Brady and other athletes. Now they also help many other kinds of patients. The treatment takes only one week—a "boot camp" approach.

Allen and Fong use a modified functional magnetic resonance imaging (fMRI) scan, which they call Functional Neurocognitive Imaging (fNCI). A standard fMRI shows which brain areas are active when a person is performing a mental task but is not as helpful in locating the precise areas that are not working properly in a concussion or TBI. There are many fMRI studies of "normal" brains, but no study has systematically measured "normal" in quantitative terms. Allen and Fong's first unique contribution was to give to large numbers of people who had no psychiatric, drug abuse, or

---

* Collaborating with neurologists in Spain and elsewhere, Farias has followed over one hundred patients through various brain scans. But the scan of one of his patients was decisive for his theories because it examined the cortical *and* subcortical brain. Before and after fMRIs showed that while the dystonia was present, the prefrontal cortical areas were hypofunctioning, and the cerebellum (a subcortical area, often not thought to relate to dystonia) was hyperactive. With the training, the prefrontal cortex turned on again, and the cerebellar functioning normalized. These findings led Farias to propose that there is some kind of "shock" that turns off the prefrontal lobes, which normally inhibit primitive reflexes, causing them to emerge. These scans need to be repeated in other patients. We don't yet know what percentage of dystonias can be helped, but from the hundreds of people Farias has dealt with, we now know that many have a neuroplastic basis and can be improved.

neurological problems six well-validated neuropsychological tests during an fMRI scan. Though only six tests were used, each test assessed many different mental functions. (For example, a logic test can assess reading, memory, and abstract thinking.) These tests enabled Allen and Fong to develop a data-based picture of what a "normal" brain looks like while performing tests. Next they examined people with concussions and TBIs. Using their new fNCI scanning technique, they found that 99 percent of the subjects showed abnormalities in precise brain areas. Since standard scans are of limited use in most concussions, the fNCI represents a great leap forward.

Allen and Fong also discovered that when brain-injured subjects have difficulty performing everyday cognitive tasks, some brain areas are hypo-activated (underactive, or dormant), while others are hyperactivated. They have learned that the hyperactivated areas work harder—too hard—trying to take over, or compensate, for the areas that are not working properly, so the patient is easily exhausted and prone to error, and to headaches.

Consider that the brain often has several ways of performing a single cognitive function. Driving to a new address a person can either use a map (which involves visual-spatial brain processing) or look out for major landmarks before turns (which involves visual-shape recognition). If one system is injured, the other system can take over and compensate for it. People with brain injuries, brain fog after cancer chemotherapy, strokes, attention deficit disorders, learning disorders, and movement disorders all make use of compensations.

Knowing precisely which areas are underperforming allows Allen and Fong to use brain, movement, balance, vision, and other exercises to target the exact areas that are hypofunctioning, and avoid overstimulating the ones that are already hyperfunctioning (which might only make things worse).

Scans at the end of the "boot camp" week show that previously hypofunctioning areas become activated to normal levels while the hyperfunctioning areas deactivate and no longer have to work so hard. In most cases of concussion, the fNCIs normalize, coinciding with remarkable clinical improvement.

This fNCI-based approach is a wonderful demonstration of neuromodulation. These patients initially show learned nonuse in semidormant circuits that are hypofunctioning. Then they receive appropriately targeted neurostimulation, which turns on dormant circuitry, relieving the hyperfunctioning areas from working so hard. The brain then becomes neuromodulated. Sleep usually improves (a sign of neurorelaxation). EEGs before treatment often show a dysregulated, noisy brain, which responds to brain wave training.

The brain exercises that Allen and Fong use were developed by neuroscientist Michael Merzenich, Ph.D., and colleagues, and is called BrainHQ. The BrainHQ suite covers a number of major mental functions. A National Institutes of Health multicenter study of normal elderly adults showed that a short course of BrainHQ exercises produced improvements that lasted ten years and generalized to be useful in everyday life—the crucial test of the benefits of brain exercises.

Like the other treatments in this book, the effectiveness of the Cognitive FX approach is not attributed to the technology alone. Each treatment is clinically tailored to the individual client's needs. I referred a number of people with TBIs, one going back to early childhood, to the clinic. Almost all improved. In March 2015, I met a sixteen-year-old athlete who had had three witnessed concussions, the most recent occurring five months earlier. She was left with a post-concussion syndrome (or TBI) with ongoing headaches, balance problems, poor focus, memory problems, fatigue, hypersensitivity to sound, inability to multitask, and depression. By the end of her week at Cognitive FX, she told me, "[it] helped me get my life back. I feel I'm back to my normal self." Her mood got better, headaches disappeared, and her focus and cognition all improved. Her initial fNCI scan showed areas of hypoactivation and hyperactivation. After treatment, all the areas normalized. The majority of patients with her symptoms show similar improvements. Patients with more severe TBIs do not do as well. In addition, some patients with cognitive symptoms caused by MS, cerebral palsy, stroke, and some learning disorders have also seen those symptoms improve.

HIGH-QUALITY BRAIN EXERCISES CONTINUE to be developed. Cellfield is a computer-based program to treat dyslexia, developed in

Australia by inventor Dimitri Caplygin. Cellfield works to intensively neurostimulate the brain networks that process visual and auditory aspects of reading. On average, dyslexic students who fit the program profile advance the equivalent of two grade levels in their reading over the course of ten hours of the program. It is available in English and French versions. Another brain exercise approach has developed out of the tradition begun by the recently deceased Israeli developmental psychologist Reuven Feuerstein, Ph.D. Donalee Markus, Ph.D., a student of Feuerstein's, developed her own exercises for people with learning disorders and TBIs and also NASA's critical thinking program. She works one-on-one, developing a tailor-made exercise program for each individual. Her work is described in one of the most penetrating personal accounts of a TBI, and a recovery, ever written, called *The Ghost in My Brain*, by Clark Elliott, a professor of artificial intelligence at DePaul University in Chicago. Her brain exercises were critical for Professor Elliott's recovery.

OPTOMETRY CAN ALSO BE USED to rewire the brain. Most TBIs distort visual processing in some way (as we saw with Jeri Lake), and Donalee Markus works with a remarkably innovative optometrist, Dr. Deborah Zelinsky, at the Mind-Eye Connection, who applies the latest neuroscience to her field. The retina not only has two kinds of photosensitive cells, rods, and cones, but several kinds, all with different functions. I visited Dr. Zelinsky just north of Chicago, and she showed me how she can use optical lenses to alter sensory filtering, by directing light to different retinal cells and brain circuits. This can influence activity in the brain stem and hypothalamus (which, as we have seen in Chapter 4, has a link to the eye) to better regulate body chemistry, sensory integration, and even some auditory processing. Dr. Zelinsky also played a major role in Professor Elliott's recovery, and works frequently with patients with learning and cognitive disorders as well as TBIs.

I'D LIKE TO CONCLUDE BY describing two other related techniques that can help some patients with TBI. French-style osteopathy and cranial therapy are hands-on approaches that can involve the practitioner making very gentle movements of the patient's head. They appear to work in four ways. First, in almost all injuries where the head sustains a blow, there is some trauma to the neck, which they help. Second, as we shall see when we discuss Matrix Repatterning in Appendix 2, high-impact injuries often involve alterations in energy distribution in the head (sometimes called "energy cysts"), which can be resolved with these treatments. Third, they can turn on the parasympathetic system and neuromodulate the nervous system. Fourth, these approaches are often helpful in relieving the soft-tissue problems that are blocking normal circulation and drainage of waste products from the brain. These approaches can supplement the other approaches to TBI in this book and the appendices. Though these approaches are not new, I mention them because in 2015 it was discovered that the brain does in fact have a lymphatic system, adjacent to the skull, and so only now do we understand how these hands-on approaches might be helping in a fifth way, to promote better lymphatic circulation in the brain and restore the general cellular health of the neurons and glia by helping the brain to detoxify.

While I had the luxury of investigating the approaches in the main body of the book and appendices for sometimes as long as eight years, and have had less than a year to explore the ones I have just described, I find that they too are explicable in terms of the stages of neuroplastic healing. That they represent just a small selection of the many new approaches I encountered in that brief period suggests to me that we are in the midst of a great transformative moment in the science of healing: the birth of a new field, which we might call "clinical neuroplasticity."

Norman Doidge
Toronto, Canada
January 2016

Appendix 1

*A General Approach to
TBI and Brain Problems*

IN THIS BOOK, I HAVE sometimes linked one illness or disorder with one treatment. But as a rule the proper approach is to take into account the patient with the disorder, and the stage, or usually stages, of neuroplastic healing that would be best emphasized for that person. For instance, I have described many different approaches to stroke and brain injury throughout this book. For head injury alone, low-intensity lasers, the PoNS, and sound therapy all were helpful for some patients. The approaches described in Appendices 2 and 3, on Matrix Repatterning and neurofeedback, and those in the Afterword can also help people with traumatic brain injuries. The future of this new field will involve learning how to combine neuroplastic and other approaches to activate all the stages of neuroplastic healing in a way tailored to the individual person's needs, such as the pairing of physical and mental exercise and electrical stimulation with the PoNS in Chapter 7. In Chapter 4 Gaby's rehab integrated exercise (tai chi, which also has a mental component) and light therapy. The researcher Robin Green has shown that a combination of cognitive stimulation and physical and social stimulation reduces post-TBI brain shrinkage in some patients. Other preliminary work by her and her colleagues suggests that there may be a role for brain exercises in treating TBI, based on those developed by Michael

Merzenich. Edward Taub's group used biofeedback, followed by Constraint-Induced Therapy, to treat a tetraplegic woman with total paralysis following a spinal cord injury. Similarly, children with developmental disorders may benefit from many approaches: listening therapy, Feldenkrais work, neurofeedback, and psychotherapy. Since inflammation is so prominent in the autistic brain, and these children are hypersensitive, it is possible that low-intensity lasers and the PoNS may help them. Whenever a patient with cognitive problems has a partial response to one neuroplastic approach, it is useful to consider adding another one to see if it will help. I also think in terms of improving general brain health whenever possible. A quantitative EEG (QEEG) is a test that can indicate if a patient has a "noisy brain." This study is often done by advanced neurofeedback practitioners, and must be interpreted by an expert who has actually met with the patient, not simply run the information through a machine.

The recoveries I described used equipment designed by major contributors to the field, not knockoffs. But the results were brought about by irreplaceable clinicians, with vast experience. The family of treatments that I am describing makes up a new clinical discipline that has many tools at its disposal. This is fortunate because not everything works for everyone, of course. Ideally, it is best to work with a knowledgeable health-care provider who understands the individual patient's condition, and who, if several approaches are required, can guide the patient on which to try first. When it comes to rewiring the brain, patience is required, and sometimes improvements are incremental, so consult before abandoning one of the techniques. But know that neuroplasticians who have spent years mastering one approach are not always as familiar with others.

Additional new neuroplastic treatments and training techniques for stroke, pain, learning problems, mental decline, and other brain problems and psychiatric disorders are described in *The Brain That Changes Itself*. Readers looking for neuroplastic approaches for themselves or loved ones might consider examining both books, which, taken in combination, give a fuller description of the applications of neuroplasticity. Additional information is available on my Web site, normandoidge.com.

Appendix 2

Matrix Repatterning for TBI

MATRIX REPATTERNING IS A FORM of treatment developed by an extremely creative Canadian clinician, Dr. George Roth. This procedure can be very helpful for some people with TBI and other head injuries, even as a *first* intervention, before trying some of the other methods discussed in this book. It can sometimes remove problems that get in the way of the brain's undertaking its own spontaneous neuroplastic healing. Sometimes it seems sufficient to help a person with a persistent traumatic brain injury get better; at other times it works well combined with different approaches.

George Roth, a doctor of naturopathic medicine, a chiropractor, and a serious student of French osteopathy, made a number of important clinical discoveries about how energy transfers into the head, causing traumatic brain injuries.

All head blows involve an energy transfer into the body. When the blow occurs, the force will dissipate through the body, the brain, and the skull. The person needn't even have direct contact with an object for an energy transfer to occur. Shock waves from a bomb blast will transfer energy to damage the heart and brain. In car accidents, these energy transfers affect not only the skin and bones, but the fluid-filled organs of the body as well. Studies of bone and other tissues show that when they absorb the energy associated with these blows, they change both their structure and how they conduct electrical energy. A structure that changes its electrical conductivity when its shape is changed is called a piezoelectric structure. (In Greek, *piezo* means "I press" and is related to the concept of "pressure.") According to Roth, when the head absorbs a massive amount of energy in an injury, piezoelectric changes alter the electrical environment of the brain so that the neurons become less able to conduct signals. In electrical terms, the tissues around the brain, especially the bones and connective tissues, go from being good conductors of electricity to resistors that block flow. This, Roth believes, gives rise to many brain injury symptoms.

We have known since the 1840s that applying electric current or magnetic fields to fractured bones facilitates their healing. It has been common for Canadian orthopedic surgeons to use this practice when a broken bone is too damaged or the fractured ends are too separated to connect and heal by themselves. Worldwide about 100,000 fractures have been healed with the help of electric current. Magnetic fields can also heal injured tissues and are frequently used by physiotherapists. These treatments are believed to work because electric current—generated by the bones themselves—is normally part of the natural bone healing process.

Roth restores normal flow in two ways, using both piezoelectric pressure and magnetic fields.

Based on the original piezoelectric experiments that showed pressure on bone changes its electrical conduction, he has found that gently holding the bone, the shape of which has been distorted by an injury, is enough pressure to change its piezoelectric properties. This allows an injured bone to change from an electrical resistor to a conductor once again. I have witnessed this many times. After the gentle holding, the bone spontaneously returns to its normal shape (this is shown by measuring it, and with X-rays or photographs). Tender spots on the bone disappear.

Since the hand has also been shown to be a source of measurable electrical fields because of its nerves and muscle fibers, Roth uses it as a magnetic field. Or he increasingly uses an electromagnetic pulse generator near the injured tissue, while applying gentle pressure on it with his hands, to speed this process.

Over the years I have followed a number of his TBI patients on whom these techniques were applied: often, their long-standing headaches, mental fog, dizziness, sleep or multitasking problems, and other TBI symptoms were resolved partially or completely.

Roth has had many patients with multiple concussions. A typical case is that of José, a forty-four-year-old manager of a large government department. In August 2012 he was standing on a picnic table in the rain, trying to tie up a tarp, when he slipped and smashed his head on the wooden deck below. It was just one of five concussions he had suffered—others were in hockey and a car accident. He got the usual symptoms of headache, fatigue, dizziness, hypersensitivities, severe cognitive problems, and an inability to absorb information or multitask. He was sleeping up to sixteen hours a day.

Because his symptoms persisted, his neurologist diagnosed post-concussion syndrome. José was away from work, disabled for six months. He tried many treatments and medications. Finally, his neurologist told him that waiting it out was the only option left to try. José had waited out concussions before, but this time he was stuck and depressed. "This had gone on forever," he told me. "By the time I saw Dr. Roth I was desperate."

When Roth examined José physically, he found many neurological signs of head injury, including eye tracking problems, hearing impairment, and "hyper" reflexes in both his legs—a sign of injury to the neurons in the brain that regulate movement. I spoke to José after he had had six sessions with Roth over six weeks. He was able to go off his medication, discontinue his other treatments, and return to work. His brain fog disappeared, and his neurological signs improved. After one more session, his headache was gone.

"What is interesting," said José, "is that when Dr. Roth did touch my head, it was on the exact spot where there was piercing pain—without me telling him. In fact, he is the first person really to touch my head. My GP never did, my neurologist never did, my physiotherapist didn't."

My working hypothesis is that José, with his hypersensitivities and other symptoms, had a diffusely noisy brain from his injury, and that Roth was able, by his techniques, to allow José's brain to neuromodulate itself by restoring normal conduction. I saw a dramatic demonstration of Roth's ability to normalize neuronal firing when I met with an adolescent who had serious epilepsy. The cause was uncertain, but she had had a head injury as a child, which can cause epilepsy. Her epilepsy was so serious that she had a pacemaker implanted. The device was designed to interrupt seizure activity by sending signals to the brain. She could also turn the device on if she felt a seizure coming on. But it was only partially successful. After several sessions of Matrix Repatterning, the frequency of her seizures decreased radically.

The reason I think it is useful for some patients to undergo Matrix Repatterning before other treatments is that if the general flow of energy is blocked, the other treatments may not work nearly as well. Because we know that head injuries can also increase a person's risk for dementia, epilepsy, and some kinds of Parkinson's, I view it as prudent to have a Matrix assessment after a blow to the head. I have also seen Roth treat people who had acute head traumas right after the injury; they recovered much more rapidly than they might have if treatment had been delayed. Observing such cases has led me to hope that one day Matrix Repatterning will be routinely applied in hospital emergency departments.

Appendix 3

*Neurofeedback for ADD, ADHD,
Epilepsy, Anxiety, and TBI*

NEUROFEEDBACK IS A SOPHISTICATED FORM of biofeedback and an extremely versatile treatment that is useful for many of the conditions described in this book. It has recently been recognized by the American Academy of Pediatrics as a treatment for removing ADD and ADHD symptoms as effectively as medications. It rarely has side effects, as it is a form of brain training. It also has been approved for the treatment of certain kinds of epilepsy and is effective for many other conditions, including certain kinds of anxiety, post-traumatic stress conditions, learning disorders, brain injuries, migraines, and sensitivities that affect the autistic spectrum, to mention a few. It is a neuroplastic treatment but is not better known because it was pioneered before neuroplasticity was widely understood.

As we have seen, when neurons fire by the millions, they create brain waves. Brain waves, which have been measurable since the early to mid-twentieth century, are measured in waves per second. Different brain waves correlate with levels of conscious arousal and types of conscious experience. For instance, the EEG will show very slow waves when people are asleep (or have brain injuries); their brain waves get faster as they enter a dreamy, half-awake state, then a calm focused state with eyes open. They go still faster if the person is very anxious.

A series of accidental discoveries made by Barry Sterman, originally with cats, showed that animals hooked up to EEGs could learn to train their own brain waves. Early work that Sterman conducted for NASA used this "self-training" technique to prevent epilepsy in astronauts. In epilepsy, the brain fires too much. (The astronauts were getting epilepsy from their exposure to rocket fuel.)

A conventional neurofeedback session involves hooking a person up to an EEG, a noninvasive way to detect brain waves, then displaying the waves on a computer screen.

People with ADD or ADHD often have fewer of the calm, focused waves (called low beta waves) and more of the brain waves most of us have when we are falling asleep (theta waves). When a teacher looks over at a student who seems to be staring out of the window with a glazed look in his eyes, and says, "Johnny, are you listening or are you asleep?," Johnny—part of whose brain is producing high theta waves—is actually on the edge of sleep, and he can't easily help it. In a neurofeedback session for ADD, the person is trained to raise waves associated with calm focus and lower waves associated with sleepiness and impulsivity whenever they are represented on the screen. Though neurofeedback involves the use of electronic equipment, I believe that it operates along some of the same principles as the Feldenkrais method. Both methods develop increased awareness that can lead to neural changes and neurodifferentiation. (Put differently, when Feldenkrais trained his pupils to refine their sensory awareness of how it felt to perform a movement, he was training them to make more use of the feedback provided by their senses.)

Some introductory books on neurofeedback and a related intervention called low-energy neurofeedback system are listed in the endnotes.

Acknowledgments

WHEN I WAS HALFWAY THROUGH writing this book, my wonderful editor, James H. Silberman, and I found ourselves put to a very personal and unexpected test of its contents.

Jim had a significant stroke that affected both his left arm and leg. As is typical, he was given minimal follow-up on leaving hospital rehab, and when he expressed hope to his neurologist that he might improve, he was told—as people often are—that he must not be fooled by any very minor poststroke improvements he had made: he would very soon plateau, and make no further progress. Jim would have none of it, and decided this was not the neurologist for him. Jim was, after all, one of the first laypeople to recognize the clinical promise of neuroplasticity, when he decided to work on *The Brain That Changes Itself* almost fifteen years ago.

Over the next year and a half, he not only edited this book's remaining chapters, he also energetically applied the techniques described in them (and a few techniques, such as Taub therapy, from the earlier book). Because each chapter addresses a different aspect of neuroplastic healing, there was reason to make use of almost all of them. So Jim not only edited this book, but lived and breathed what is in it. Far from what was predicted for him, he did not plateau, and his process of improvement and brain change did not decelerate; it actually accelerated. In the course of our completing this book, Jim restored most of his lost functions, and no sooner did he finish the editing than he was able to take his first steps unassisted.

So, as the title page says, this is a James H. Silberman book. His care, craft, wise counsel, and deep consideration of the reader's needs and interests are reflected on every page. With his unique combination of relentlessness and patience, he pored over this manuscript many times to sharpen its clarity and accessibility, without simplifying the science or robbing me of my voice. He did not change, in the slightest, his professional approach to the task after the stroke. I soon saw that all that he had learned had indeed made him the ideal neuroplastic pupil, and with the exercise and brain stimulation he now was doing he was as intellectually robust and as sharp as, or even sharper than, he had been before the stroke. When we began this book, I was the resident expert on plasticity, and his role was to help me put what I knew into words. Before we were done, he, by virtue of having practiced what I preached, was the experiential expert, and I was often his interpreter. Both of us, of course, wish this stroke never happened, and yet both of us are aware, given that it did, that there was a strange moral beauty about the fact that we found ourselves in the position to make the best of it, and have done so.

As Hippocrates says in the epigraph to this book, recoveries require not only the physician and the patient but, literally, the people alongside the patient to assist, and in this case, that was Selma Shapiro, Jim's wife. Without Selma's amazingly helpful attitude and indispensable support of Jim, this book would not yet have appeared. Exemplifying the inventiveness and dedication to helping others that I have tried to capture in this book, Edward Taub and physiotherapist Jean Crago at the Taub Clinic, Feldenkrais practitioner Rebecca Gardiner, and laser therapists Fred Kahn and Joanna Malinowska greatly accelerated Jim's neuroplastic recovery.

I THANK ALL THE NEUROPLASTICIANS, as well as their colleagues, research subjects, pupils, and above all their patients and their patients' families, for sharing their stories. Not all of the stories shared could appear in a book this length, but all were essential parts of the research. I thank my own patients, who have taught me so much.

Arthur Fish championed this project from the implausible beginning when I first floated my odd idea that neuroplasticity, energy, and the body had to be linked to better understand how the brain works. He commented brilliantly on portions of the manuscript, and even helped me craft a life that has allowed me to write, research, and think.

Patrick Farrell's impressive passion for the history of science and for literature made him an ideal helper when he began working with me halfway through the long process. He helped as my assistant, with copy editing, with tracking down research, and above all by providing his extremely thoughtful, nuanced reactions to the chapters.

I have been supported by precious companions in serious conversation, who share a rare combination of conscientiousness and intellectual openness, and, fortunately for me, a tenderhearted fondness for each other: Cyril Levitt, Corinne Levitt, Wodek Szemberg, Jacqueline Newell, Waller Newell, Geoffrey Clarfield, Mira Clarfield, Bonnie Fish, Philip Kyriacou, Jordan Peterson, Tammy Peterson, Lyn Rasmussen, Kenneth Hart Green, Sharon Green, Charles Hanly, Margaret Fitzpatrick Hanly, John Moscowitz, Clifford Orwin, Donna Orwin, Thomas Pangle, Lorraine Smith Pangle, Lawrence Solomon, and Patricia Adams. I also thank Kiril Sokoloff and Kate McClure Sokoloff for their enthusiastic support. This largely Canadian group also includes some exemplary physicians: Estera Bekier, Barry Simon, Clare Pain, and Alex Tarnopolsky, who each in his or her way have helped me to think through the great strengths, and limitations, of our current medical paradigm. Dr. Avideh Motmaen-Far, with whom I have had regular conversations about the mind, energy, the body, and fascia, has helped me understand modes of healing I never thought possible. I thank my American physician colleagues Daniel J. Siegel, Meriamne Singer, Mark Sorensen, Eric Marcus, Richard Brown, and Eugene Goldberg. Dr. Ellen Cutler, from whom I have learned immensely about whole-body health, and the body's energy systems, has given me far more than she knows.

Jacqueline Newell, Michael Mazurek, Gerald Owen, Tammy Peterson, and Jordan Peterson commented very helpfully on the manuscript. Jordan and I have had regular conversations on neuroscience and the mind for almost a decade now. I also cherish the ongoing conversations I have had with the American neuroscientists Michael Merzenich, Edward Taub, and Stephen Porges. Conversations with neurosurgeon-neuroscientist Karl Pribram have been few, but very lengthy, over days, intensive and pivotal.

Without even having to use words, Barbara Doidge taught me what a healing presence is, so that it has been easy for me to recognize it in others. All the following have much to teach about influencing the nervous system through the body, wordlessly. Dr. Jayson Grossman, an inimitable teacher, introduced me to the work of the late Dr. George Goodheart, that great clinical genius, who developed applied kinesiology, which combines Chinese energy medicine with Western approaches. I was fortunate enough to be treated in a demonstration by Dr. Goodheart and his colleague David Leaf on one unforgettable day. I thank Judith Neilly, George Roth, David Slabotsky, and Marla Golden for demonstrating the power of osteopathy and other body-based techniques to influence the nervous system. Sifu Philip Mo has shown me how tai chi can reset the brain and nervous system, and the role of energy in that practice.

The following people were helpful, each in his or her own way, in teaching me about mind-body medicine: Ernest Rossi, William O'Hanlon, Claire Frederick, Eric Barnhill, Robert Kidd, David Grand, Marion Harris (for introducing me to the work of Feldenkrais), David Zemach-Bersin, Judith Dack, Joaquin Farias, Robert Harris, Morana Petrofski, Lesley Gates, Heike Raschl, Francine Shapiro, Neil Sharp, John Ratey, Eileen Bach-y-Rita, and Fred Gallo. Also helpful were Leon Sloman, Ates Tanin, Brian Schwartz, Mark Walsh, and Annette Goodman.

Though I did not write about neurofeedback in detail, I trained in it, and learned an immense amount about changing the brain from these neurofeedback scientists and clinicians, in supervision, in courses or through their writings: John Finnick, Moshe Perl, Sebern Fisher, Ed Hamlin, Lynda Thompson, Michael Thompson, Len Ochs, and Jaclyn Gisburne. For their inspiring writing and research that opened my eyes to new topics, I thank Iain McGilchrist, Jaak Panksepp, Oliver Sacks, Robert Schleip, Evan Thompson, Alva Noë, Allan N. Schore, Leonard F. Koziol, Deborah Ely Budding, Thomas Rau, and Elkhonon Goldberg.

On the publishing side, I thank my literary agents at Sterling Lord Literistic for their enthusiastic help, from Chris Calhoun, who helped me talk through and negotiate this project at the beginning, to Flip Brophy, who saw it through, and Ira Silverberg, and now Szilvia Molnar for handling foreign rights. Once the book arrived at Viking, Wendy Wolf championed it and took an extremely helpful bird's-eye view of the book, with her many editorial comments. I thank Janet Biehl for her full immersion in it and astute copy editing, and the patient, always helpful, extremely knowledgeable Bruce Giffords in editorial production. Proofreaders Maureen Clark and Donald Homolka amazed me with their thoroughness, as did Gina Anderson. Henry Rosenbloom, at Scribe, and Helen Conford, at Penguin UK, have been ideal allies.

A number of agencies gave me grants and awards over the years that allowed me to further my scientific development and writing, including the National Institute of Mental Health, in Washington, DC, and the National Health Research and Development Program of Health Canada.

Closer to home, Joshua Doidge helped with research, and has, I believe, done more neuroplastic learning programs than anyone else on planet Earth, showing me what they can do. Brauna Doidge, who has a gift for avoiding inessentials—to safeguard the essentials, of course—helped me in the painful task of cutting down the manuscript.

No book can be written endlessly and do good; the time spent attempting to perfect this one has passed. It no doubt contains errors based upon the limits of my intellectual range and concepts—the errors that I cannot see—alongside errors of fact that I might have caught, had I, as the poet Marvell wrote, "but world enough and time." For both kinds I apologize to you, the reader, and to all the people mentioned above, who have been so generous.

Finally, Karen Lipton-Doidge, my wife and first reader, always intellectually stimulating, kind, and good-humored, has been alongside me throughout this process: on most trips to visit neuroplasticians, training with me in new techniques, helping with research, making prescient comments on the writing, blessing me with all manner of emotional support. First readers see the writing at its worst; this offering, the best that I can do, is for her.

Notes and References

A Note to the Reader About These Notes

All notes are preceded by the page number and a phrase from the text to which they refer. Nestled among these references, the reader will find comments about interesting details, exceptions, historical notes, and more scholarly matters. These comments are preceded by a black dot (•).

Epigraphs

viii **Chasidic saying:** C. Stern, ed., *Gates of Repentance: The New Union Prayerbook for the Days of Awe* (New York: Central Conference of American Rabbis, 1978), p. 3.

viii **"Life is short, and Art long":** Translated by my colleague and friend Waller R. Newell.

Preface

xviii **military metaphors . . . in everyday medical practice . . . Abraham Fuks:** A. Fuks, "The Military Metaphors of Modern Medicine," in Z. Li and T. L. Long, eds., *The Meaning Management Challenge* (Oxford, UK: Inter-Disciplinary Press, 2010), pp. 57–68.

xix • **"battle" against disease:** In the mid-1600s Thomas Sydenham, the "English Hippocrates," wrote of illness, "I attack the enemy within by means of cathartics and refrigerants, and by means of a diet"; and "a murderous array of disease has to be fought against, and the battle is not a battle for the sluggard"; and "I steadily investigate the disease, I comprehend its character, and I proceed straight ahead, and in full confidence, towards its annihilation." *The Works of Thomas Sydenham,* trans. R. G. Latham (London: Sydenham Society, 1848–50), 1:267, 1:33, 2:43.

Chapter 1. Physician Hurt, Then Heal Thyself

5 **most important article in the history of pain:** R. Melzack and P. Wall, "Pain Mechanisms: A New Theory," *Science* 150, no. 3699 (1965): 971–79.

6 **• the German physiologist Manfred Zimmermann:** This was at the Second World Congress on Pain in Montreal in 1978. M. Zimmermann and T. Herdegen, "Plasticity of the Nervous System at the Systemic, Cellular and Molecular Levels: A Mechanism of Chronic Pain and Hyperalgesia," in G. Carli and M. Zimmermann, eds., *Towards the Neurobiology of Chronic Pain* (Amsterdam: Elsevier, 1996), pp. 233–59, 233.

10 **"Central Influences on Pain":** M. H. Moskowitz, "Central Influences on Pain," in C. W. Slipman et al., eds., *Interventional Spine: An Algorithmic Approach* (Philadelphia: Saunders Elsevier, 2008), pp. 39–52.

10 **"Once chronicity sets in . . . difficult to treat":** Ibid., p. 40.

10 **expectations play a major role in the level of pain we will feel:** G. L. Moseley, "A Pain Neuromatrix Approach to Patients with Chronic Pain," *Manual Therapy* 8, no. 3 (2003): 130–40; G. L. Moseley, "Reconceptualising Pain According to Modern Pain Science," *Physical Therapy Reviews* 12 (2007): 169–78, 172.

10 **"an output of the central nervous system":** Moseley, "Reconceptualising Pain," 172.

11 **"The brain . . . mounts a counteroffensive":** Moskowitz, "Central Influences," p. 44.

23 **an ingenious study of people with chronic hand pain:** G. L. Moseley et al., "Visual Distortion of a Limb Modulates the Pain and Swelling Evoked by Movement," *Current Biology* 18, no. 22 (2008): R1047–48.

24 **Preston:** C. Preston and R. Newport, "Analgesic Effects of Multi-Sensory Illusions in Osteoarthritis," *Rheumatology* (Oxford) 50, no. 12 (2011): 2314–15.

26 **patients . . . placebo . . . mostly psychologically unstable . . . untrue:** A. K. Shapiro and E. Shapiro, *The Powerful Placebo: From Ancient Priest to Modern Physician* (Baltimore: Johns Hopkins University Press, 1997), p. 39.

26 **• Tor Wager:** T. D. Wager et al., "Placebo-Induced Changes in fMRI in the Anticipation and Experience of Pain," *Science* 303 (2004): 1162–67; T. D. Wager et al., "Placebo Effects in Human Opioid Activity During Pain," *Proceedings of the National Academy of Sciences* 104, no. 26 (2007): 11056–61; T. D. Wager, "The Neural Bases of Placebo Effects in Pain," *Current Directions in Psychological Science* 14, no. 4 (2005): 175–79. Tor Wager's personal story is recounted in I. Kirsch, *The Emperor's New Drugs: Exploding the Antidepressant Myth* (New York: Basic Books, 2010).

27 **If a response is very rapid . . . placebo:** F. M. Quitkin et al., "Heterogeneity of Clinical Response During Placebo Treatment," *American Journal of Psychiatry* 148, no. 2 (1991): 193–96.

27 **placebo responders were more likely to suffer a relapse:** F. M. Quitkin et al., "Different Types of Placebo Response in Patients Receiving Antidepressants," *American Journal of Psychiatry* 148, no. 2 (1991): 197–203; F. M. Quitkin et al.,

"Placebo Run-In Period in Studies of Depressive Disorders," *British Journal of Psychiatry* 173 (1998): 242–48.

27 **the placebo effect can last for weeks:** T. J. Kaptchuk et al., "Components of Placebo Effect: Randomized Controlled Trial in Patients with Irritable Bowel Syndrome," *British Medical Journal* 336, no. 7651 (2008): 999–1003.

28 **Guy Montgomery:** G. Montgomery and I. Kirsch, "Mechanisms of Placebo Pain Reduction: An Empirical Investigation," *Psychological Science* 7, no. 3 (1996): 174–76.

Chapter 2. A Man Walks Off His Parkinsonian Symptoms

36 **glial cells . . . helping . . . rewire the brain:** R. D. Fields, *The Other Brain* (New York: Simon & Schuster, 2009), p. 24.

37 **Frank Collins and his colleagues discovered GDNF:** L-F. H. Lin et al., "GDNF: A Glial Line–Derived Neurotrophic Factor for Midbrain Dopaminergic Neurons," *Science* 260, no. 5111 (1993): 1130–32; Fields, *Other Brain*, p. 180.

37 **exercise in lab animals had been found to increase GDNF:** M. J. Zigmond et al., "Triggering Endogenous Neuroprotective Processes Through Exercise in Models of Dopamine Deficiency," *Parkinsonism and Related Disorders* 15, supp. 3 (2009): S42–45.

37 **• without medication, most lose the ability to walk:** W. Poewe, "The Natural History of Parkinson's Disease," *Journal of Neurology* 253, supp. 7 (2006): vii2–vii16. Since the advent of drugs, which are used for almost all patients, it has been hard to know what "unmedicated" Parkinson's might look like. Poewe found control drug studies where patients were either on medication or off it because they took a placebo instead. By extrapolating from their rates of decline, he determined that without medication, Parkinson's would lead to a severe disability "after less than 10 years." He found this estimate matched physicians' accounts of decline from the nineteenth century and first half of the twentieth.

37 **drug's effects begin to wane:** E. R. Kandel et al., eds., *Principles of Neural Science*, 4th ed. (New York: McGraw-Hill, 2000), p. 862.

38 **a six-times-normal risk of dementia:** Poewe, "Natural History of Parkinson's."

38 **Margaret Hoehn and Melvin Yahr:** M. M. Hoehn and M. D. Yahr, "Parkinsonism: Onset, Progression and Mortality," *Neurology* 17 (1967): 427–42.

38 **• the substantia nigra:** The substantia nigra is a part of a group of structures called the basal ganglia, usually said to include the caudate, putamen, globus pallidus, substantia nigra, and the subthalamic nucleus. The basal ganglia are involved in processing voluntary motor control and routine behaviors and habits. It can function like a brake and inhibit motor actions. When this "brake" is released, the motor systems become active. Basal ganglia activation also switches from one behavior to the next. Patients with Parkinson's often "freeze" when they try switching to a new activity. A man with the disease may, while walking along, see a line or small obstacle on the pavement and get "stuck in his tracks," unable to step over it because that would require changing his stride.

38 **80 percent of our brain's dopamine is concentrated in . . . the basal ganglia:** Kandel et al., *Principles of Neural Science*, p. 862.

40 • **medication-induced dyskinesias are a result of . . . neuroplastic changes:** B. Picconi et al., "Loss of Bidirectional Striatal Synaptic Plasticity in L-DOPA–Induced Dyskinesia," *Nature Neuroscience* 6, no. 5 (2003): 501–6. The authors gave Parkinsonian rats long-term treatment with L-dopa. Rats that developed dyskinesias had "an altered form of synaptic plasticity," "abnormal information storage in corticostriatal synapses," and chemical aberrations. A healthy brain must be able to both strengthen and weaken its synapses. Weakening may be necessary for forgetting, or erasing connections that are no longer required, possibly allowing that network to do something new. One type of weakening is called synaptic depotentiation. The authors observed that "dyskinetic cases showed no capacity for depotentiation. Such a loss of bidirectional plasticity at corticostriatal synapses may cause a pathological storage of nonessential motor information that would normally be erased, leading to the development and/or the expression of abnormal motor patterns" (p. 504).

40 **"no treatment has yet been identified":** Poewe, "Natural History of Parkinson's."

41 **"jams" the abnormally firing circuits:** J. Bugaysen et al., "The Impact of Stimulation Induced Short-Term Synaptic Plasticity on Firing Patterns in the Globus Pallidus of the Rat," *Frontiers in Systems Neuroscience* 5 (article 16) (2011): 1–8.

42 **Huntington's . . . fast walking . . . onset was significantly delayed:** T. Y. C. Pang et al., "Differential Effects of Voluntary Physical Exercise on Behavioral and BDNF Expression Deficits in Huntington's Disease Transgenic Mice," *Neuroscience* 141, no. 2 (2006): 569–84.

42 **Pepper's small self-published book:** J. Pepper, *There Is Life After Being Diagnosed with Parkinson's Disease* (South Africa: John Pepper and Associates CC, 2003). He later renamed the book *Reverse Parkinson's Disease* (Pittsburgh: Rose Dog Books, 2011).

47 **the four cardinal symptoms:** Almost all neurology textbooks refer to Parkinson's as having four cardinal symptoms, though they often disagree as to which symptoms to include in the four. It seems it is easier to honor the tradition that there must be four than to agree what they are, which points to the fact that it has been hard to sort out what constitutes the core of PD.

47 **"the Parkinsonian features":** I. Litvan, "Parkinsonian Features: When Are They Parkinson Disease," *Journal of the American Medical Association* 280, no. 19 (1998): 1654–55.

47 **two groups of people who get Parkinsonian syndromes:** Ibid.

56 • **It took him three months to . . . support his body weight:** Physiotherapy texts of that era sometimes argued that it was important to analyze a patient's gait. But even the most forward-looking texts today, such as *Neurorehabilitation in Parkinson's Disease,* don't anticipate that physio might reverse motor decline. "The goal of therapy has been largely to help people to maintain what motor capability they have for as long as possible and to help them adjust as their functional levels inevitably decline." M. Trail et al., *Neurorehabilitation in Parkinson's Disease: An Evidence-Based Treatment Model* (Thorofare, NJ: Slack, 2008), p. 24.

59 **The basal ganglia . . . knit together complex sequences of movements and thoughts:** L. F. Koziol and D. E. Budding, *Subcortical Structures and Cognition: Implications for Neuropsychological Assessment* (New York: Springer, 2008), p. 99.

59   **When ... basal ganglia doesn't work ... difficult to learn new cognitive sequences:** O. Nagy et al., "Dopaminergic Contribution to Cognitive Sequence Learning," *Journal of Neural Transmission* 114, no. 5 (2007): 607–12.

60   **substantia nigra ... is responsible for initiating automated sequences of behaviors:** Koziol and Budding, *Subcortical Structures and Cognition*, p. 43.

60   **English footballer with Parkinson's:** O. Sacks, *Awakenings* (New York: Vintage Books, 1999; repr. of 1990 edition; originally published 1973), p. 10.

61   **"The central problem in all Parkinsonian disorders ... is *passivity*":** Ibid., p. 345.

62   **Zigmond's group ... less likelihood of ... Parkinson's ... exercised:** Zigmond et al., "Triggering Endogenous Neuroprotective Processes."

71   **antipsychotic medications ... Usually these Parkinsonian symptoms are reversed:** "One study reported that 16% of cases went on to be confirmed to have idiopathic Parkinson's disease. These people were probably going to develop Parkinson's at some stage in the future in any event but the offending drug 'unmasked' an underlying dopamine deficiency." *Drug-Induced Parkinsonism information sheet,* Parkinson's Disease Society of the United Kingdom, http://www.parkinsons.org.uk/sites/default/files/publications/download/english/fs38_druginducedparkinsonism.pdf.

71   **majority of which are reversible:** K. Ray Chaudhuri and J. Nott, "Drug-Induced Parkinsonism," in K. D. Sethi, ed., *Drug-Induced Movement Disorders* (New York: Marcel Dekker, 2004), 61–75.

77   **exercise was not recommended for ... Parkinson's:** M. A. Hirsch and B. G. Farely, "Exercise and Neuroplasticity in Persons Living with Parkinson's Disease," *European Journal of Physical and Rehabilitation Medicine* 45, no. 2 (2009): 215–29.

77   **only 12 to 15 percent are referred to physiotherapy:** Ibid., 219.

77   **the exercise might actually worsen:** Ibid., 215–29.

78   **Female mice with the human ALS gene ... got worse:** N. C. Stam et al., "Sex-specific Behavioural Effects of Environmental Enrichment in a Transgenic Mouse Model of Amyotrophic Lateral Sclerosis," *European Journal of Neuroscience* 28, no. 4 (2008): 717–23.

79   **roam freely ... they performed better on problem-solving:** D. O. Hebb, "The Effects of Early Experience on Problem Solving at Maturity," *American Psychologist* 2 (1947): 306–7.

79   **van Praag ... use of a running wheel:** H. van Praag et al., "Running Increases Cell Proliferation and Neurogenesis in the Adult Mouse Dentate Gyrus," *Nature Neuroscience* 2, no. 3 (1999): 266–70.

80   **van Dellen, Hannan ... Huntington's ... delay the onset:** A. van Dellen et al., "Delaying the Onset of Huntington's in Mice," *Nature* 404 (2000): 721–22.

81   **running wheel ... delay of Huntington's:** T. Y. C. Pang et al., "Differential Effects of Voluntary Physical Exercise on Behavioral and BDNF Expression Deficits in Huntington's Disease Transgenic Mice," *Neuroscience* 141, no. 2 (2006): 569–84.

81   **"particularly adept at processing novel information":** E. Goldberg, *The New Executive Brain* (New York: Oxford University Press, 2009), pp. 254–55.

81   **can delay onset ... Parkinson's, Alzheimer's, epilepsy:** J. Nithianantharajah and A. J. Hannan, "Enriched Environments, Experience-Dependent Plasticity and Disorders of the Nervous System," *Nature Review: Neuroscience* 7, no. 9 (2006): 697–709; J. Nithianantharajah and A. J. Hannan, "The Neurobiology of Brain and

Cognitive Reserve: Mental and Physical Activity as Modulators of Brain Disorders," *Progress in Neurobiology* 89, no. 4 (2009): 369–82. The following primary research article describes how dementia in HD is delayed by environmental enrichment: J. Nithianantharajah et al., "Gene-Environment Interactions Modulating Cognitive Function and Molecular Correlates of Synaptic Plasticity in Huntington's Disease Transgenic Mice," *Neurobiology of Disease* 29, no. 3 (2008): 490–504.

81 **exercise is as effective as fluoxetine:** T. Renoir et al., "Treatment of Depressive-Like Behaviour in Huntington's Disease Mice by Chronic Sertraline and Exercise," *British Journal of Pharmacology* 165, no. 5 (2012): 1375–89; J. J. Ratey and E. Hagerman, *Spark: The Revolutionary New Science of Exercise and the Brain* (New York: Little Brown, 2008).

82 **Rett's syndrome:** M. Kondo et al., "Environmental Enrichment Ameliorates a Motor Coordination Deficit in a Mouse Model of Rett Syndrome—*Mecp2* Gene Dosage Effects and BDNF Expression," *European Journal of Neuroscience* 27, no. 12 (2008): 3341–50.

82 **schizophrenic-like mice . . . effect is as great as seen with the antipsychotic medication:** C. E. McOmish et al., "Phospholipase C-b1 Knockout Mice Exhibit Endophenotypes Modeling Schizophrenia Which Are Rescued by Environmental Enrichment and Clozapine Administration," *Molecular Psychiatry* 13, no. 7 (2008): 661–72.

82 **proper exercise and cognitive stimulation . . . helps to compensate for . . . genetic predisposition to a neurodegenerative illness:** Nithianantharajah and Hannan, "Neurobiology of Brain and Cognitive Reserve."

82 **exercise . . . the 1950s . . . people with PD . . . benefit from it:** D. S. Bilowit, "Establishing Physical Objectives in the Rehabilitation of Patients with Parkinson's Disease (Gymnasium Activities)," *Physical Therapy Review* 36, no. 3 (1956): 176–78.

83 **• 6-OHDA . . . present in humans beings with Parkinson's disease:** K. Jellinger et al., "Chemical Evidence for 6-Hydroxydopamine to Be an Endogenous Toxic Factor in the Pathogenesis of Parkinson's Disease," *Journal of Neural Transmission Supplement* 46 (1995): 297–314. These animal models of PD are not perfect replicas of the disease, because these drugs cause a onetime loss of dopamine, and PD is progressive. 6-OHDA resembles chemicals the brain uses to pass signals between neurons. It causes cell death in the brain—including death of the dopamine-producing cells—when it oxidizes. A. D. Smith and M. J. Zigmond, "Can the Brain Be Protected Through Exercise? Lessons from an Animal Model of Parkinsonism," *Experimental Neurology* 184, no. 1 (2003): 31–39.

83 **• Parkinson's disease–like animals . . . have complete recoveries:** J. L. Tillerson et al., "Exercise Induces Behavioral Recovery and Attenuates Neurochemical Deficits in Rodent Models of Parkinson's Disease," *Neuroscience* 119, no. 3 (2003): 899–911. These animals ran 15 meters/minute, which is about 0.6 miles per hour. They ran 450 meters a day. Running sessions were separated by 3 hours. In her wonderful review of neuroplasticity and Parkinson's, Sheila Mun-Bryce summarizes the above study this way: "Behavioral recovery was complete in both the 6-OHDA and MPTP groups when exercise was made part of the treatment regime. In comparison, sedentary dopamine depleted animals showed persistent behavioral deficits. Physically active PD animals continued to show no behavioral deficits as long as the twice a day exercise period was maintained."

S. Mun-Bryce, "Neuroplasticity: Implications for Parkinson's Disease," in Trail et al., *Neurorehabilitation in Parkinson's Disease*, p. 46.

83 **"running as well as environmental enrichment greatly reduces the loss of DA [dopamine] cells":** Zigmond et al., "Triggering Endogenous Neuroprotective Processes, S42–45, S43.

84 **exercise . . . nerve growth factors . . . protect the brain . . . Parkinson's:** Ibid.

84 **GDNF is lowered in the substantia nigra:** N. B. Chauhan et al., "Depletion of Glial Cell Line–Derived Neurotrophic Factor in Substantia Nigra Neurons of Parkinson's Disease Brain," *Journal of Chemical Neuroanatomy* 21, no. 4 (2001): 277–88.

84 **BDNF also protects neurons from degenerating:** H. S. Oliff et al., "Exercise-Induced Regulation of Brain-Derived Neurotrophic Factor (BDNF) Transcripts in the Rat Hippocampus," *Molecular Brain Research* 61, no. 1–2 (1998): 147–53.

84 **Rats unable to run produce less BDNF:** J. Widenfalk et al., "Deprived of Habitual Running, Rats Downregulate BDNF and TrkB Messages in the Brain," *Neuroscience Research* 34 (1999): 125–32.

85 **mice that exercise voluntarily . . . increase their BDNF:** Oliff et al., "Exercise-Induced Regulation."

85 **BDNF can also protect neurons:** C. W. Cotman and N. C. Berchtold, "Exercise: A Behavioral Intervention to Enhance Brain Health and Plasticity," *Trends in Neurosciences* 25, no. 6 (2002): 295–301, 296 box 1.

85 **BDNF . . . increase with exercise:** L. Marais et al., "Exercise Increases BDNF Levels in the Striatum and Decreases Depressive-Like Behavior in Chronically Stressed Rats," *Metabolic Brain Disease* 24, no. 4 (2009): 587–97.

85 **exercise can enhance an animal's ability to learn:** S. Vaynman et al., "Hippocampal BDNF Mediates the Efficacy of Exercise on Synaptic Plasticity and Cognition," *European Journal of Neuroscience* 20, no. 10 (2004): 2580–90.

85 **a sedentary lifestyle is a significant risk factor:** S. Vaynman and F. Gomez-Pinilla, "License to Run: Exercise Impacts Functional Plasticity in the Intact and Injured Central Nervous System by Using Neurotrophins," *Neurorehabilitation and Neural Repair* 19, no. 4 (2005): 283–95, 290.

86 **• diaschisis:** The term, from the Greek for "split throughout," is used by clinicians to mean "shocked throughout," and was coined by Constantin von Monakow, a Russian-Swiss neuropathologist, in 1914. He argued that brain damage was not nearly as localized as most believed.

86 **after an injury the brain undergoes an "energy crisis":** C. C. Giza and D. A. Hovda, "The Neurometabolic Cascade of Concussion," *Journal of Athletic Training* 36, no. 3 (2001): 228–35, 232.

86 **an injured brain is especially vulnerable because its energy . . . is so low:** Ibid., 232.

87 **learned nonuse plays a major role in Parkinson's:** J. L. Tillerson and G. W. Miller, "Forced Limb-Use and Recovery Following Brain Injury," *Neuroscientist* 8, no. 6 (2002): 574–85.

88 **cast on the Parkinson's limb . . . movement gains were all lost:** J. L. Tillerson et al., "Forced Limb-Use Effects on the Behavioral and Neurochemical Effects of 6-Hydroxydopamine," *Journal of Neuroscience* 21, no. 12 (2001): 4427–35.

88 **• "decreased physical activity not only is a symptom of PD but also may act to potentiate the underlying degeneration":** J. L. Tillerson et al., "Forced Nonuse in Unilateral Parkinsonian Rats Exacerbates Injury," *Journal of Neuroscience* 22, no. 15

(2002): 6790–99. Tillerson, Zigmond, and Miller demonstrated this by injecting rats with a low dose of 6-OHDA into a single hemisphere of the brain, so that the animals lost 20 percent of their dopamine, which is not enough for the animal to have symptoms. Then some of the animals had a cast put on their nonaffected limb—i.e., their good limb. When the cast was removed after seven days, something strange happened: the 20 percent loss of dopamine in the injected hemisphere was radically increased to a 60 percent loss. In short, that brief deprivation of activity greatly increased the speed of onset of the illness. Dopamine production is very dynamic.

89 **leaped from his wheelchair to save a drowning man:** Sacks, *Awakenings,* p. 10.

89 **On a bike, he appears to be perfectly normal:** A. H. Snijders and B. R. Bloem, "Images in Clinical Medicine: Cycling for Freezing of Gait," *New England Journal of Medicine* 1, no. 362 (2010): e46. For a film of the man riding, see doi: 10.1056/NEJMicm0810287.

89 • **Exercises for balance:** Dr. David Blatt, now fifty-four, an anesthesiologist from Corvallis, Oregon, who was diagnosed with PD in his forties, shows few signs of the illness, and still skis expert-level runs. He attributes the benign course of illness to his exercise program, which challenges his balance system. He thinks his program works by triggering neurotrophic growth factors. He exercises standing on one leg and bending, or balancing himself and juggling while standing on a "Bosu ball," a soft unstable, inflated ball, used in gyms to develop balance. D. Blatt, "Physician, Heal Thyself: A Corvallis Doctor with Parkinson's Disease Finds Help in Exercise—for Himself and His Patients," *Corvallis Gazette Times,* July 10, 2010.

90 **The greater the value of that outcome, the faster people move:** R. Shadmerh and S. Mussa-Ivaldi, *Biological Learning and Control: How the Brain Builds Representation, Predicts Events, and Makes Decisions* (Cambridge, MA: MIT Press, 2012), pp. 291–93.

90 **Parkinson's patients are capable of making motor movements:** P. Mazzoni et al., "Why Don't We Move Faster? Parkinson's Disease, Movement Vigor, and Implicit Motivation," *Journal of Neuroscience* 27, no. 27 (2007): 7105–16, 7115.

91 **"opportunity cost":** Y. Niv and M. Rivlin-Etzion, "Parkinson's Disease: Fighting the Will?" *Journal of Neuroscience* 27, no. 44 (2007): 11777–79.

91 **"The motor system has its own motivation circuit":** Mazzoni et al., "Why Don't We Move Faster?," 7115.

92 • **his conscious walking technique got around this circuit:** Y. Niv et al., "A Normative Perspective on Motivation," *Trends in Cognitive Sciences* 10, no. 8 (2006): 375–81, 377. Niv, Joel, and Dayan point out that habitual movements (such as normal walking) are processed in the lateral part of the striatum and the dopamine-dependent neurons that feed it. Nonhabitual, goal-directed movements are processed by a different circuit, which includes the frontal lobes and the medial part of the striatum. Nonhabitual, goal-directed movement is, I believe, what John Pepper resorted to, in his conscious walking technique, when he paid close attention to each movement and its purpose.

93 • **"Festination . . . hurried against their will":** Sacks, *Awakenings,* p. 6.

94 • **"people find themselves embattled, and even immobilized":** Ibid., pp. 7–8. Sacks points out that bradykinetic patients have a slowed, sticky stream of thought when thinking, termed bradyphrenia (p. 8). Yet even these slowed patients, who appear rigid to an outside observer, are not simply passive; rather, they might better be

described, Sacks writes, as "embattled." He observes, "The appearance of passivity or inertia is deceiving: an obstructive akinesia of this sort is in no sense an idle or restful state, but (to paraphrase de Quincey) '... no product of inertia, but ... resulting from mighty and equal antagonisms, infinite activities, infinite repose.'" Sacks goes on to argue that William James's notion that human beings have two kinds of will, an "obstructive" will and an "explosive" will, applies to the Parkinsonian mental experience: "when the former holds sway, the performance of normal actions is rendered difficult or impossible; if the latter is dominant, abnormal actions are irrepressible. Although James uses these terms with reference to neurotic perversions of the will, they are equally applicable to what we must term Parkinsonian perversions of the will" (p. 7n). I wondered whether John, at times, had a more explosive will than most Parkinson's patients, which allowed him to act and invent his walking intervention. John, according to family reports, has always been a remarkably active person, and it would be very difficult to disentangle, in a man who had Parkinson's for so many decades, whether his active nature was related to his illness.

94 **"vigorous exercise should be accorded a central place":** J. E. Ahlskog, "Does Vigorous Exercise Have a Neuroprotective Effect in Parkinson's?" *Neurology* 77, no. 3 (2011): 288–94.

94 **the lower-intensity exercise, at a walking pace:** L. M. Shulman et al., "Randomized Clinical Trial of 3 Types of Physical Exercise for Patients with Parkinson Disease," *Journal of the American Medical Association: Neurology* (formerly *Archives of Neurology*), 70, no. 2 (2013): 183–90.

94 **Uc ... walking ... led to improvements in the patients' Parkinsonian movement:** Ergun Y. Uc et al., "Phase I/II Randomized Trial of Aerobic Exercise in Parkinson Disease in a Community Setting," *Neurology* 83 (2014): published online.

96 **reduced the risk of dementia ... breakthrough study ... Elwood:** P. Elwood et al., "Healthy Lifestyles Reduce the Incidence of Chronic Disease and Dementia: Evidence from the Caerphilly Cohort Study," *PLoS ONE* 8, no. 12 (2013).

96 • **Cardiff study ... overcame study design problems ... (discussed in the endnotes):** Other studies found that exercise protects against dementia, but this study was a breakthrough because it overcame a problem in many previous studies of dementia. Dementia can start in the brain long before a person qualifies as having a clinical case of it. When a study shows that a person who never exercises, drinks too much, and doesn't watch his weight gets dementia, how can scientists be certain that those "bad behaviors" caused the dementia? Perhaps he already had a low level of dementia, which was why he made bad choices. In science this is called the problem of reverse causality. The scientist thinks that bad behavior causes the disease, but perhaps it could be the reverse, and those with very early dementia—too early to be picked up by their physician—are those who were disinclined to exercise or eat well. It is easy to make this mistake in a short study, one that takes only a snapshot of subjects or follows them only briefly. Before the Cardiff study, ten of eleven studies showed that exercise in midlife correlated with reduced dementia, but they were not long-term studies. But because the Cardiff study followed patients for thirty years, this was not a problem. Dementia is exceedingly rare in the age that the men were at the beginning of the study, and the study took account of the level of cognitive function using exacting tests of each man at the commencement of the study. Thus, the Cardiff

researchers knew that if a person didn't exercise or follow any of the other healthy behaviors, it was not because he already had dementia.

97   **"Only a very small percentage . . . carry . . . inheritance of Alzheimer's":** T. Chow, *The Memory Clinic* (Toronto: Penguin, 2013), p. 69.

97   **"interact with . . . genetic makeup":** Ibid., p. 70.

97   **"is not sufficient to produce Alzheimer's Disease":** Ibid., p. 72.

97   **Another crucial review, in 2011:** J. Ahlskog et al., "Physical Exercise as a Preventive or Disease-Modifying Treatment of Dementia and Brain Aging," *Mayo Clinic Proceedings* 86, no. 9 (2011): 876–84.

98   **significant hippocampal enlargement:** K. I. Erickson et al., "Exercise Training Increases Size of Hippocampus and Improves Memory," *Proceedings of the National Academy of Sciences* 108, no. 7 (2011): 3017–22.

98   **hippocampal enlargement nine years after:** K. I. Erickson et al., "Aerobic Fitness Is Associated with Hippocampal Volume in Elderly Humans," *Hippocampus* 19 (2009): 1030–39.

98   **15 percent of people over seventy have some dementia:** M. D. Hurd et al., "Monetary Costs of Dementia in the United States," *New England Journal of Medicine* 368, no. 14 (2013): 1326–34.

98   **"Ninety Plus" . . . the majority do not have dementia:** M. M. Corrada et al., "Prevalence of Dementia After Age 90: Results from the 90+ Study," *Neurology* 71, no. 5 (2008): 337–43.

Chapter 3. The Stages of Neuroplastic Healing

104   **stroke . . . still living . . . can show signs of atrophy:** L. V. Gauthier et al., "Atrophy of Spared Gray Matter Tissue Predicts Poorer Motor Recovery and Rehabilitation Response in Chronic Stroke," *Stroke* 43, no. 2 (2012): 453–57.

107   **Karl Pribram:** K. H. Pribram, *The Form Within: My Point of View* (Westport, CT: Prospecta Press, 2013).

109   **The brain . . . has no lymphatic system . . . vessels:** R. D. Fields, *The Other Brain* (New York: Simon & Schuster, 2009), p. 42.

110   **Constraint-Induced Therapy . . . increased gray matter in the brain:** L. V. Gauthier et al., "Remodeling the Brain: Plastic Structural Brain Changes Produced by Different Motor Therapies After Stroke," *Stroke* 39, no. 5 (2008): 1520–25.

111   **promote growth, conserve energy:** R. M. Sapolsky, *Why Zebras Don't Get Ulcers*, 3rd ed. (New York: St. Martin's Griffin, 2004), p. 23.

111   **turning off the sympathetic system appears to improve:** M. E. Hasselmo et al., "Noradrenergic Suppression of Synaptic Transmission May Influence Cortical Signal-to-Noise Ratio," *Journal of Neurophysiology* 77, no. 6 (1997): 3326–39.

112   **in sleep the glia open up special channels:** L. Xie et al., "Sleep Drives Metabolite Clearance from the Adult Brain," *Science* 342, no. 6156 (2013): 373–77.

Chapter 4. Rewiring a Brain with Light

114   **Florence Nightingale:** F. Nightingale, *Notes on Nursing: What It Is and Is Not* (London: Harrison, 1860).

115 **Francis Crick . . . turn on certain neurons:** F. H. Crick, "Thinking About the Brain," *Scientific American* 241 (1979): 219–32. See also G. Stix, "A Light in the Brain," *Scientific American* 302 (2010): 18–20.

116 • **Karl Deisseroth . . . optogenetics . . . not . . . useful on patients:** Deisseroth stated recently that he was not advocating "the direct therapeutic application of putting the optics into people." Inserting optic fibers involved "putting in foreign proteins, so who knows what immune reactions there might be. The therapeutic impact would be dwarfed by the basic science impact." Presentation at Mount Sinai Hospital, Department of Psychiatry, University of Toronto, January 11, 2013.

117 **Ward's infants began to improve:** R. H. Dobbs and R. J. Cremer, "Phototherapy," *Archives of Disease in Childhood* 50, no. 11 (1975): 833–36; R. J. Cremer et al., "Influence of Light on the Hyperbilirubinaemia," *Lancet* 1, no. 7030 (1958): 1094–97.

118 **The Romans even had right-to-light laws:** R. Hobday, *The Light Revolution: Health, Architecture and the Sun* (Findhorn, Scotland: Findhorn Press, 2006).

118 • **photosynthesis:** Carbon dioxide + water + light energy —> glucose (sugar) + oxygen. The actual equation is 6 molecules of CO_2 + 6 molecules of H_2O + light energy = $C_6H_{12}O_6$ + 6 molecules of O_2.

119 **Egyptian . . . exposing them to the sun to obtain medical benefits:** H. Györy, "Medicine in Ancient Egypt," in H. Selin, ed., *Encyclopedia of the History of Science, Technology, and Medicine in Non-Western Cultures,* 2nd ed. (New York: Springer, 2008), pp. 1508–18, 1513.

119 **recovering from surgery in a sunlit room:** J. M. Walch et al., "The Effect of Sunlight on Postoperative Analgesic Medication Use: A Prospective Study of Patients Undergoing Surgery," *Psychosomatic Medicine* 67 (2005): 157–63.

119 **Aretaeus . . . "the disease is gloom":** Aretaeus, "On the Therapeutics of Acute Diseases," in F. Adams, ed., *The Extant Works of Aretaeus, the Cappadocian* (London: Sydenham Society, 1856), p. 387.

119 **other light-sensitive cells were found:** D. M. Berson et al., "Phototransduction by Retinal Ganglion Cells That Set the Circadian Clock," *Science* 295, no. 5557 (2002): 1070–73; S. Hattar et al., "Melanopsin-Containing Retinal Ganglion Cells: Architecture, Projections, and Intrinsic Photosensitivity," *Science* 295, no. 5557 (2002): 1065–70.

120 **the SCN, in turn, sends that message to our pineal gland:** Y. Isobe and H. Nishino, "Signal Transmission from the Suprachiasmatic Nucleus to the Pineal Gland Via the Paraventricular Nucleus: Analysed from Arg-Vasopressin Peptide, rPer2 mRNA and AVP mRNA Changes and Pineal AA-NAT mRNA After the Melatonin Injection During Light and Dark Periods," *Brain Research* 1013 (2004): 204–11.

120 *Halobacterium,* **which lives in salt marshes:** J. Spudich, "Color-Sensing in the Archaea: A Eukaryotic-Like Receptor Coupled to a Prokaryotic Transducer," *Journal of Bacteriology* 175 (1993): 7755–61; J. M. Allman, *Evolving Brains* (New York: Scientific American Library, 1999), p. 7.

121 **light-sensitive chemical switches and amplifiers:** K. Martinek and I. V. Berezin, "Artificial Light-Sensitive Enzymatic Systems as Chemical Amplifiers of Weak Light Signals," *Photochemistry and Photobiology* 29 (1979): 637–50.

121 **Szent-Györgyi . . . charge transfer—the molecules often change color:** A. Szent-Györgyi, *Introduction to a Submolecular Biology* (New York: Academic Press,

1960), pp. 54, 80–81; A. Szent-Györgyi, *Bioelectronics: A Study in Cellular Regulations, Defense, and Cancer* (New York: Academic Press, 1968), pp. 19, 26–27, 43.

125 **a particular wavelength will help tissue heal:** T. I. Karu, "Irradiation with He-Ne Laser Increases ATP Level in Cells Cultivated in Vitro," *Journal of Photochemistry and Photobiology B: Biology* 27 (1995): 219–23, 219.

125 **a one-watt laser is thousands of times more intense:** B. B. Laud, *Lasers and Non-Linear Optics* (New Delhi, India: Wiley Eastern, 1991), p. 4.

126 • **wounds so serious that the skin was unable to close over them:** Many such photos can be found in Kahn's three-volume book: F. Kahn, *Low Intensity Laser Therapy in Clinical Practice,* 3 vols. (Toronto: Meditech International, 2008).

127 • **lasers trigger regrowth of normal cartilage:** M. D. C. Cressoni et al., "Effect of GaAIAs Laser Irradiation on the Epiphyseal Cartilage of Rats," *Photomedicine and Laser Surgery* 28, no. 4 (2010): 527–32. Cressoni and colleagues showed that lasers increased the thickness of the cartilage and the number of chondrocytes, or cartilage-producing cells; Y.-S. Lin et al., "Effects of Helium-Neon Laser on the Mucopolysaccharide Induction in Experimental Osteoarthritic Cartilage," *Osteoarthritis and Cartilage* 14, no. 4 (2006): 377–83.

127 **effective in treating osteoarthritis in humans:** P. P. Alfredo et al., "Efficacy of Low Level Laser Therapy Associated with Exercises in Knee Osteoarthritis: A Randomized Double-Blind Study," *Clinical Rehabilitation* 26, no. 6 (2011): 523–33; A. Gur et al., "Efficacy of Different Therapy Regimes of Low-Power Laser in Painful Osteoarthritis of the Knee: A Double-Blind and Randomized-Controlled Trial," *Lasers in Medicine and Surgery* 33 (2003): 330–38.

129 **Naeser . . . studies using lasers for stroke:** M. A. Naeser et al., "Acupuncture in the Treatment of Paralysis in Chronic and Acute Stroke Patients—Improvement Correlated with Specific CT Scan Lesion Sites," *International Journal of Acupuncture and Electrotherapeutics Research* 19 (1994): 227–49; M. A. Naeser et al., "Acupuncture in the Treatment of Hand Paresis in Chronic and Acute Stroke Patients: Improvement Observed in All Cases," *Clinical Rehabilitation* 8 (1994): 127–41; M. A. Naeser et al., "Improved Cognitive Function After Transcranial, Light-Emitting Diode Treatments in Chronic, Traumatic Brain Injury: Two Case Reports," *Photomedicine and Laser Surgery* 29, no. 5 (2010): 351–58; M. A. Naeser and M. R. Hamblin, "Potential for Transcranial Laser or LED Therapy to Treat Stroke, Traumatic Brain Injury, and Neurodegenerative Disease," *Photomedicine and Laser Surgery* 29, no. 7 (2011): 443–46.

130 **when lasers were used to stimulate acupuncture points on the face:** M. A. Naeser et al., "Laser Acupuncture in the Treatment of Paralysis in Stroke Patients: A CT Scan Lesions Site Study," *American Journal of Acupuncture* 23, no. 1 (1995): 13–28.

138 • **The exact frequency of light emitted can be controlled:** The term for this is *coherence,* meaning that the light frequencies coming out of the laser are "a coherent reproduction of the input optical signal." A. E. Siegman, *Lasers* (Mill Valley, CA: University Science Books, 1986), p. 4.

139 **promote the growth of collagen fibers in skin tissues:** S. A. Carney et al., "Effect of the Radiation on Skin Biochemistry," *British Journal of Industrial Medicine* 25, no. 3 (1968): 229–34.

140 • **Laser light triggers ATP production:** The light wavelengths that increase ATP are very specific. As Tiina Karu, the Russian scientist, points out, light at wavelengths of

415, 602, 633, and 650 nanometers enhances ATP production. However, light at 477, 511, and 554 nanometers will not. Karu, "Irradiation with He-Ne Laser."

140 • **Lasers . . . increase the use of oxygen:** A cell, if irradiated by light at wavelengths of 365 or 436 nanometers, will consume more oxygen. Ibid.

141 **the color of a light is a measure of how much energy:** H. Chung et al., "The Nuts and Bolts of Low-Level Laser (Light) Therapy," *Annals of Biomedical Engineering* 40, no. 2 (2012): 516–33.

142 **lasers have a good effect where they are most needed:** J. Tafur and P. J. Mills, "Low-Intensity Light Therapy: Exploring the Role of Redox Mechanisms," *Photomedicine and Laser Surgery* 26, no. 4 (2008): 323–28, 324.

142 • **Human cells in a petri dish will synthesize more DNA:** Human cells synthesize DNA in response to wavelengths of 404, 620, 680, 760, and 830 nanometers of light. *E. coli* grows in response to 404, 454, 570, 620, and 750 nanometers. Yeasts grow in response to 404, 570, 620, 680, and 760 nanometers. T. I. Karu, "Photobiological Fundamentals of Low-Powered Laser Therapy," *IEEE Journal of Quantum Electronics* QE-23, no. 10 (1987): 1703–17.

142 **sunlight . . . serotonin:** G. W. Lambert et al., "Effect of Sunlight and Season on Serotonin Turnover in the Brain," *Lancet* 360, no. 9348 (2002): 1840–42.

143 **"There is an optimal dose of light":** Chung et al., "Nuts and Bolts of Low-Level Laser (Light) Therapy."

151 **low-intensity lasers helped damaged nerves:** S. Rochkind, "Photoengineering of Neural Tissue Repair Processes in Peripheral Nerves and the Spinal Cord: Research Development with Clinical Applications," *Photomedicine and Laser Surgery* 24, no. 2 (2006): 151–57.

151 **a cranial nerve could be healed:** J. J. Anders et al., "Phototherapy Promotes Regeneration and Functional Recovery of Injured Peripheral Nerve," *Neurological Research* 26 (2004): 233–39.

151 **lasering rat brain embryo cells led them to sprout new connections:** S. Rochkind, "Phototherapy in Peripheral Nerve Regeneration: From Basic Science to Clinical Study," *Neurosurgical Focus* 26, no. 2 (2009): 1–6.

152 **lasers can stimulate ATP production:** U. Oron et al., "GaAs (808 nm) Laser Irradiation Enhances ATP Production in Human Neuronal Cells in Culture," *Photomedicine and Laser Surgery* 25, no. 3 (2007): 180–82.

152 **Oron . . . tested this same laser on mice with traumatic brain injuries:** A. Oron et al., "Low-Level Laser Therapy Applied Transcranially to Mice Following Traumatic Brain Injury Significantly Reduces Long-Term Neurological Deficits," *Journal of Neurotrauma* 24 (2007): 651–56.

152 **rats that had had strokes:** A. Oron et al., "Low-Level Laser Therapy Applied Transcranially to Rats After Induction of Stroke Significantly Reduces Long-Term Neurological Deficits," *Stroke* 37 (2006): 2620–24.

152 **reduce scar formation:** U. Oron et al., "Low Energy Laser Irradiation Reduces Formation of Scar Tissue Following Myocardial Infarction in Rats and Dogs," *Circulation* 103 (2001): 296–301.

153 **low-intensity laser irradiation of the blood:** E. N. Meshalkin and V. S. Sergievskii, *Primenenie pryamogo lazernogo izlucheniya v eksperimental'noi i klinicheskoi meditsine* (Application of Direct Laser Radiation in Experimental and Clinical Medicine) (Novosibirsk: Nauka, 1981).

156 **cognitive benefits . . . shown to occur with light:** D. W. Barrett and F. Gonzalez-Lima, "Transcranial Infrared Laser Stimulation Produces Beneficial Cognitive and Emotional Effects in Humans," *Neuroscience* 230 (2014): 13–23.

157 **lowered levels of these proteins using light . . . Alzheimer's:** S. Purushothuman et al., "Photobiomodulation with Near Infrared Light Mitigates Alzheimer's Disease–Related Pathology in Cerebral Cortex—Evidence from Two Transgenic Mouse Models," *Alzheimer's Research and Therapy* 6, no. 1 (2014): 1–13.

157 **retinal damage:** B. T. Ivansic and T. Ivandic, "Low-Level Laser Therapy Improves Vision in a Patient with Retinitis Pigmentosa," *Photomedicine and Laser Surgery* 32, no. 3 (2014): 1–4.

157 **light therapy improves damaged connections:** C. Meng et al., "Low-Level Laser Therapy Rescues Dendrite Atrophy via Upregulating BDNF Expression: Implications for Alzheimer's Disease," *Journal of Neuroscience* 33, no. 33 (2013): 13505–17.

Chapter 5. Moshe Feldenkrais: Physicist, Black Belt, and Healer

160 • **In June 1940 a young Jew escaped:** My principal sources for Feldenkrais's personal history are interviews and conversations with his close friend Avraham Baniel (now in his nineties) and his students and followers Anat Baniel, Marion Harris, and David Zemach-Bersin. Also helpful was Garet Newell, "A Biographical Moshe Feldenkrais," *Feldenkrais Journal*, no. 7 (Winter 1992). Mark Reese's superb, all too brief "A Biography of Moshe Feldenkrais" has been expanded into his masterful biography, *Moshe Feldenkrais: A Life in Movement* (San Rafael, CA: Feldenkrais Press, 2015). The story about Feldenkrais's smuggling secrets in the suitcases is told in this book. As well, Feldenkrais's own curriculum vitae; his autobiographical remarks in his book *The Elusive Obvious;* his books on judo, especially *Higher Judo: Groundwork;* his taped conversations with Karl Pribram; Carl Ginsburg's "Berstein and Feldenkrais: The Fathers of Movement Science," *Feldenkrais Journal*, no. 12 (1997–98); and Dennis Leri, "Feldenkrais and Judo," Newsletter of the Feldenkrais Guild, *In Touch*, 2004. My favorite overall introduction to Feldenkrais's theory is *Embodied Wisdom: The Collected Papers of Moshe Feldenkrais,* ed. E. Beringer (Berkeley, CA: North Atlantic Books, 2010).

160 **contained French scientific secrets and materials:** M. Reese, *Moshe Feldenkrais: A Life in Movement.* See Chapter 3.

165 **"Is there any likelihood that the operation":** M. Feldenkrais, "Image, Movement, and Actor: Restoration of Potentiality: A Discussion of the Feldenkrais Method and Acting, Self-Expression and the Theater" (1966), in Feldenkrais, *Embodied Wisdom,* pp. 93–111, 95.

165 **"I thought I was going insane":** M. Feldenkrais, *The Elusive Obvious, or Basic Feldenkrais* (Capitola, CA: Meta Publications, 1981), p. 45.

166 **"connections between all parts of himself":** M. Reese, "Moshe Feldenkrais's Work with Movement: A Parallel Approach to Milton Erickson's Hypnotherapy," in Jeffrey K. Zeig, ed., *Ericksonian Psychotherapy,* vol. 1, *Structures* (New York: Brunner/Mazel, 1985), p. 415.

166 **"No part of the body can be moved without all the others":** M. Feldenkrais, *Body and Mature Behavior: A Study of Anxiety, Sex, Gravitation and Learning* (1949; reprinted Berkeley, CA: Frog Ltd., 2005), p. 76.

167 **"I was far more absorbed in observing":** Feldenkrais, *Elusive Obvious,* p. 90.

167 **"I believe . . . that the unity of mind and body":** M. Feldenkrais, "Mind and Body" (1964), in *Embodied Wisdom,* p. 28.

167 **"The idea of two lives, somatic and psychic, has . . . outlived its usefulness":** Feldenkrais, *Body and Mature Behavior,* p. 191.

168 **"He could have got a Nobel Prize":** Anat Baniel, interview by author.

169 **"longest apprenticeship":** Feldenkrais, *Elusive Obvious,* p. 24.

169 **"Homo sapiens":** M. Feldenkrais, *Body Awareness as Healing Therapy: The Case of Nora* (Berkeley, CA: Somatic Resources and Frog, 1977), p. 63.

169 **"The mind . . . program the functioning of the brain":** Feldenkrais, *Elusive Obvious,* p. 26.

169 **"the neural substance . . . organizes itself":** Ibid., p. 25.

169 **"My fundamental contention":** Feldenkrais, *Embodied Wisdom,* p. 94.

171 **animals performed tasks . . . without paying attention:** N. Doidge, *The Brain That Changes Itself* (New York: Viking, 2007), pp. 68, 337.

172 **"If I raise an iron bar":** M. Feldenkrais, *Awareness Through Movement: Health Exercises for Personal Growth* (1972; reprinted New York: HarperCollins, 1990), p. 59.

172 **tilt their heads very subtly up and down:** Feldenkrais, *Embodied Wisdom,* p. 7.

172 **"The delay between thought and action":** Feldenkrais, *Awareness Through Movement,* p. 45.

174 **"Do not be serious, eager":** Feldenkrais, *Elusive Obvious,* p. 94.

174 **"Don't *you* decide how to do the movement":** Reese, "Feldenkrais's Work with Movement," p. 418.

175 **Dr. Esther Thelen:** E. Thelen and L. B. Smith, *A Dynamic Systems Approach to the Development of Cognition and Action* (Cambridge, MA: MIT Press, 1994).

175 **"totally awed":** Esther Thelen, "A Dynamic Systems Approach and the Feldenkrais Method," 2012, http://www.youtube.com/watch?v=Le_tFDMB7ds&feature=c4-overview-vl&list=PLrCtcgNcNdtbGbmu6soNs2Toohod3Kox3.

175 **the great judo masters are . . . better "organized":** M. Feldenkrais, *Higher Judo: Groundwork* (1952; reprinted Berkeley, CA: Blue Snake Books, 2010), pp. 32–36.

176 **"As a teacher I can accelerate your learning":** M. Feldenkrais, *Body Awareness as Healing Therapy,* p. xiv.

177 **"It is not a question of eliminating the error":** M. Feldenkrais and H. von Foerster, "A Conversation," *Feldenkrais Journal* 8 (1993): 17–30, 18.

179 **"I have no stereotyped technique":** Feldenkrais, *Body Awareness as Healing Therapy,* p. 9.

180 **"When a skill cannot be performed as before":** Ibid., p. 71.

182 **"I was annoyed with myself":** Ibid., p. 30.

182 **"I was exhilarated":** Ibid., p. 31.

183 **"It was a kind of symbiosis of the two bodies":** Ibid., p. 45.

183 **"a new ensemble":** Feldenkrais, *Elusive Obvious,* pp. 3–4.

183 **resembling a dance:** Ibid., p. 9.

184 **"Recovery is not the right word":** Feldenkrais, *Body Awareness as Healing Therapy,* p. 48.

185 **"'Improvement'" . . . "is a gradual bettering":** Ibid., p. 37.

187 **"Feldenkrais's understanding of habit":** C. Ginsburg, introductory comments to M. Feldenkrais, *The Master Moves* (Cupertino, CA: Meta Publications, 1984), p. 7.

187 **"See how much easier it is":** A. Rosenfeld, "Teaching the Body How to Program the Brain Is Moshe's 'Miracle,'" *Smithsonian* 1, no. 10 (1981): 52–58, 54.

187 **Awareness Through Movement classes can also lengthen muscles:** J. Stephens et al., "Lengthening the Hamstring Muscles Without Stretching Using 'Awareness Through Movement,'" *Physical Therapy* 86 (2006): 1641–50.

188 **80 percent of the brain's neurons:** S. Herculano-Houzel, "Coordinated Scaling of Cortical and Cerebellar Numbers of Neurons," *Frontiers in Neuroanatomy* 4, no. 12 (2010): 1–8, 5.

189 **persistent deficits, and it was believed the cerebellum shows limited plasticity:** L. F. Koziol and D. E. Budding, *Subcortical Structures and Cognition* (New York: Springer, 2009); D. Riva and C. Giorgi, "The Contribution of the Cerebellum to Mental and Social Functions in Developmental Age," *Fiziologiia Cheloveka* 26, no. 1 (2000): 27–31.

194 **"children learn their experience":** A. Baniel, *Kids Beyond Limits: The Anat Baniel Method for Awakening the Brain and Transforming the Life of Your Child with Special Needs* (New York: Perigee, 2012), p. 25.

195 **the throw looked "completely fake":** Feldenkrais, *Embodied Wisdom*, p. 154.

196 **"It is bad in Judo to . . . not to be able to change":** Feldenkrais, *Higher Judo*, p. 94.

196 **"one should always remember . . . fixity . . . do not exist":** Ibid., p. 55.

196 **• Feldenkrais was . . . dying when Avraham Baniel:** The story of Feldenkrais's dying was told to me by Avraham Baniel, in a personal communication.

Chapter 6. A Blind Man Learns to See

197 **• The eye standeth not still:** M. Andreas Laurentius, *A Discourse of the Preservation of the Sight: Of Melancholike Diseases; of Rheumes, and of Old Age*, trans. R. Surphlet, Shakespeare Association Facsimiles no. 15 (1599; London: Humphrey Milford/ Oxford University Press, 1938). Laurentius was physician to France's Henri IV.

201 **many common eye problems:** W. H. Bates, *The Bates Method for Better Eyesight Without Glasses* (New York: Henry Holt, 1981); T. R. Quackenbush, ed., *Better Eyesight: The Complete Magazines of William H. Bates* (Berkeley, CA: North Atlantic Books, 2001); L. Angart. *Improve Your Eyesight Naturally* (Carmarthen, Wales, and Bethel, CT: Crown House Publishing, 2012); A. Huxley, *The Art of Seeing* (Toronto: Macmillan of Canada, 1943).

202 **• lenses were removed . . . could still adjust their focus:** W. H. Bates, *Perfect Sight Without Glasses* (New York: Press of Thos B. Brooks, 1920). For an extended discussion of this controversy, see T. R. Quackenbush, *Relearning to See* (Berkeley, CA: North Atlantic Books, 1997), pp. 50–56.

203 **• Darwin's father, Robert, discovered . . . the eye . . . moves:** R. W. Darwin and E. Darwin, "New Experiments on the Ocular Spectra of Light and Colours," *Philosophical Transactions of the Royal Society* 76 (January 1786): 313–48. For an excellent review of the history of microsaccades, see M. Rolfs, "Microsaccades: Small Steps on a Long Way," *Vision Research* 49, no. 20 (2009): 2415–41, 2416.

203 **When microsaccades are inhibited:** J. K. Stevens et al., "Paralysis of the Awake Human: Visual Perceptions," *Vision Research* 16, no. 1 (1976): 93–98.

203 **retina...information...start to fade:** S. Martinez-Conde et al., "Microsaccades: A Neurophysiological Analysis," *Trends in Neurosciences* 32, no. 9 (2009): 463–75.

205 **70 percent of Asians are now myopic:** K. Rose et al., "The Increasing Prevalence of Myopia: Implications for Australia," *Clinical and Experimental Ophthalmology* 29, no. 3 (2001): 116–20.

205 **severe nearsightedness is associated with:** T. L. Young, "The Molecular Genetics of Human Myopia: An Update," *Optometry and Vision Science* 86, no. 1 (2009): E8–22.

214 **when an animal doesn't use a body part:** N. Doidge, *The Brain That Changes Itself* (New York: Viking, 2007), pp. 58–59.

214 **when people close their eyes and visualize a simple object:** Ibid., pp. 203, 268.

219 **seven sessions with Ginsburg:** D. Webber, "What Does It Mean to See Clearly: The Inside View," *Feldenkrais Journal*, no. 23 (2009): 23.

222 **limit car accidents:** K. K. Ball et al., "Cognitive Training Decreases Motor Vehicle Collision Involvement of Older Drivers," *Journal of the American Geriatrics Society* 58, no. 11 (2010): 2107–13; J. D. Edwards et al., "Cognitive Speed of Processing Training Delays Driving Cessation," *Journals of Gerontology, Series A, Biological Sciences and Medical Sciences* 64, no. 12 (2009): 1262–67.

222 **computer-based exercises can reexpand the visual fields:** I. Mueller et al., "Recovery of Visual Field Defects: A Large Clinical Observational Study Using Vision Restoration Therapy," *Restorative Neurology and Neuroscience* 25 (2007): 563–72; J. G. Romano et al., "Visual Field Changes After a Rehabilitation Intervention: Vision Restoration Therapy," *Journal of the Neurological Sciences* 273 (2008): 70–74.

222 **Susan Barry...*Fixing My Gaze*:** S. R. Barry, *Fixing My Gaze: A Scientist's Journey into Seeing in Three Dimensions* (New York: Basic Books, 2009). See also O. Sacks, "Stereo Sue," *New Yorker,* June 19, 2006; O. Sacks, *The Mind's Eye* (New York: Alfred A. Knopf, 2010).

223 **the retina sends a protein called Otx2:** S. Sugiyama et al., "Experience-Dependent Transfer of Otx2 Homeoprotein into the Visual Cortex Activates Postnatal Plasticity," *Cell* 134 (2008): 508–20.

223 **"The eye is telling the brain when to become plastic":** T. Hensch, "Interview: Trigger for Brain Plasticity Identified: Signal Comes, Surprisingly, from Outside the Brain," Children's Hospital Boston news release, August 7, 2008; reposted in *ScienceDaily,* August 9, 2008.

Chapter 7. A Device That Resets the Brain

231 **• a firing pattern...approximate...being touched:** Currently they divide the 144 electrodes into 16 sectors of 3 by 3 electrodes. At the first moment of firing, the top left of each of the 16 sectors is active, after which the wave goes to the right.

231 **But why stimulate the tongue?:** J. C. Wildenberg et al., "Sustained Cortical and Subcortical Neuromodulation Induced by Electrical Tongue Stimulation," *Brain Imaging and Behavior* 4 (2010): 199–211; Y. Danilov et al., "New Approach to Neurorehabilitation: Cranial Nerve Noninvasive Neuromodulation (CN-NINM) Technology," *Proceedings of SPIE* 9112 (2014): 91120L-1-91120L-10.

232 • **15,000 to 50,000 nerve fibers on the tip of the tongue:** Several nerves supply the tongue. According to Yuri, each lingual nerve (one on each side of the tongue) has 10,000 to 33,000 tactile fibers (for a total of 20,000 to 66,000 fibers). The majority are focused on the tip of the tongue. Another nerve, the chorda tympani (a branch of the facial nerve), deals with taste and pain sensation. There are 3,000 to 5,000 fibers in it (for a total of 6,000 to 10,000 fibers on both sides). So in total the tongue has 26,000 to 76,000 fibers, if we include both sides. The PoNS stimulates only *the front* of the tongue, in a one-inch-square area, not all the fibers. Yuri estimates that the device stimulates from 15,000 to 50,000 fibers. By comparison, the auditory nerve has 30,000 fibers. A. T. Rasmussen, "Studies of the Eighth Cranial Nerve of Man," *Laryngoscope* 50 (1940): 67–83.

232 • **the lingual nerve:** It is a branch of the trigeminal nerve.

233 **Two of these key meridians:** B. Frantzis, *Opening the Energy Gates of Your Body: Qigong for Lifelong Health* (Berkeley, CA: North Atlantic Books, 2006), p. 100.

233 **These tongue points are now being used:** J. G. Sun et al., "Randomized Control Trial of Tongue Acupuncture Versus Sham Acupuncture in Improving Functional Outcome in Cerebral Palsy," *Journal of Neurology, Neurosurgery and Psychiatry* 75, no. 7 (2004): 1054–57; V. C. N. Wong et al., "Pilot Study of Positron Emission Tomography (PET) Brain Glucose Metabolism to Assess the Efficacy of Tongue and Body Acupuncture in Cerebral Palsy," *Journal of Child Neurology* 21, no. 6 (2006): 455–61; V. C. N. Wong et al., "Pilot Study of Efficacy of Tongue and Body Acupuncture in Children with Visual Impairment," *Journal of Child Neurology* 21, no. 6 (2006): 455–61.

236 **a condom for paraplegics with spinal cord injuries:** F. Borisoff et al., "The Development of a Sensory Substitution System for the Sexual Rehabilitation of Men with Chronic Spinal Cord Injury," *Journal of Sexual Medicine* 7, no. 11 (2010): 3647–58.

236 • **some wave patterns will put people to sleep:** Waves can be produced in the array of electrodes by timing when the electrodes fire. Say they have 150 electrodes on the device. They divide them into 6 groups of 25 electrodes, made up of 5 rows of 5 electrodes, and time the firing of each individual electrode. One sequence can have the electrode at the center of the 25 fire first, and then those in the rows around it fire next, and so on, to make an expanding wave, from the center electrode outward. Or they can have the firing begin on the outside rows and move inward to the center one.

239 • **Their first patient was Cheryl:** Y. P. Danilov et al., "Efficacy of Electrotactile Vestibular Substitution in Patients with Peripheral and Central Vestibular Loss," *Journal of Vestibular Research* 17 (2007): 119–30; B. S. Robinson et al., "Use of an Electrotactile Vestibular Substitution System to Facilitate Balance and Gait of an Individual with Gentamicin-Induced Bilateral Vestibular Hypofunction and Bilateral Transtibial Amputation," *Journal of Neurologic Physical Therapy* 33, no. 3 (2009): 150–59; Y. Danilov and M. Tyler, "Brainport: An Alternative Input to the Brain," *Journal of Integrative Neuroscience* 4, no. 4 (2005): 537–50. For the vision device, see, P. Bach-y-Rita et al., "Vision Substitution by Tactile Image Projection," *Nature* 221, no. 5184 (1969): 963–64.

240 **"Is It Possible to Restore Function with Two-Percent":** P. Bach-y-Rita, "Is It Possible to Restore Function with Two-Percent Surviving Neural Tissue?" *Journal of Integrative Neuroscience* 3, no. 1 (2004): 3–6.

242   • **Russian sleep machines, when they cured insomnia:** Electric sleep machines were widely used in Russia for insomnia instead of sleeping pills. In Russia, Yuri's friend and colleague Valery P. Lebedev was a pioneer in sleep machine science. The machines induce sleep using a frequency of 5 to 25 Hz; they use a peak frequency of 75 to 78 Hz to induce anesthesia. Lebedev's work is in Russian. See V. P. Lebedev, *Transcranial Electrical Stimulation, Experimental and Clinical Research: A Collection of Articles* (St. Petersburg: Russian Academy, Pavlov Institute of Physiology, 2005), vol. 2. A number of cranial electrotherapy stimulation (CES) devices, such as the Fisher Wallace stimulator, are available in North America and grew out of the Russian technology. CES devices are about to be FDA approved for insomnia, depression, and anxiety.

253   **Most . . . mild TBI recover . . . within three months:** M. A. McCrea, *Mild Traumatic Brain Injury and Post-Concussion Syndrome: The New Evidence Base of Diagnosis and Treatment* (New York: Oxford University Press, 2008), p. ix.

253   **TBI . . . leading cause of disability and death in young people:** Ibid., p. 3.

253   • **concussions . . . a nineteen-fold increase in . . . Alzheimer's:** A. Schwartz, "Dementia Risk Seen in Players in N.F.L. Study," *New York Times,* September 29, 2009; K. M. Guskiewicz et al., "Association Between Recurrent Concussion and Late-Life Cognitive Impairment in Retired Professional Football Players," *Neurosurgery* 57, no. 4 (2005): 719–26. For a picture of these brains, see "Images of Brain Injuries in Athletes," *New York Times,* December 3, 2012, http://www.nytimes.com/interactive/2012/12/03/sports/images-of-brain-injuries-in-athletes.html?ref=sports.

253   **recovery, only to deteriorate . . . because of a degenerative brain process:** C. Till et al., "Postrecovery Cognitive Decline in Adults with Traumatic Brain Injury," *Archives of Physical Medicine and Rehabilitation* 89, no. 12, supp. (2008): S25–34.

263   • **They put her in an fMRI machine:** J. C. Wildenberg et al., "High-Resolution fMRI Detects Neuromodulation of Individual Brainstem Nuclei by Electrical Tongue Stimulation in Balance-Impaired Individuals," *NeuroImage* 56, no. 4 (2011): 2129–37.

266   **Interneurons . . . signals . . . come at the optimal time:** G. Buzsáki, *Rhythms of the Brain* (New York: Oxford University Press, 2006), p. 77.

266   • **photoreceptors . . . didn't evolve to process that wide a range, but with . . . interneurons, they can:** Visual neuroscientists, according to Yuri, consider the light range we process as a spread of eleven logarithmic units. But each human photoreceptor evolved to process a logarithmic range of only two logarithmic units. Our interneurons allow us to detect signals over the entire eleven-unit range, because a subset of homeostatic interneurons can either excite or inhibit other neurons to which they are connected in an extremely dynamic way, to optimize the range of the visual network to adapt to an average visual environment. See J. Walraven et al., "The Control of Visual Sensitivity: Receptoral and Postreceptoral Processes," in L. Spillman and J. S. Werner, eds., *Visual Perception: The Neurophysiological Foundations* (Toronto: Academic Press, 1977), pp. 81–82, 88–90; O. Marín, "Interneuron Dysfunction in Psychiatric Disorders," *Nature Reviews Neuroscience* 13 (2012): 107–20; A. Maffei and A. Fontanini, "Network Homeostasis: A Matter of Coordination," *Current Opinion in Neurobiology* 19, no. 2 (2009): 168–73.

266   **• Interneurons also help make signals sharper and clearer:** They do so by inhibiting signals from spreading too widely in the network. Through a process called lateral inhibition, they prevent a neuron's signal from becoming diffuse, or having an undue influence on nearby neurons and thus disturbing their signals. An interneuron can also, through feedback, turn off its neuron just after it has sent a signal, so that it doesn't keep bombarding the other neurons it is connected to. (If that didn't happen, the images we see would persist too long, or we would hear sounds longer than they actually occurred.) This function, says Yuri, is the brain's way of providing punctuation, or a full stop, at the end of a sequence of spikes.

276   **Mailer . . . "Every moment . . . one is growing into more":** N. Mailer, *Advertisements for Myself* (New York: Berkley, 1959), p. 355.

277   **published their pilot study of MS:** M. Tyler et al., "Non-invasive Neuromodulation to Improve Gait in Chronic Multiple Sclerosis: A Randomized Double Blind Controlled Pilot Trial," *Journal of Neuroengineering and Rehabilitation* 11 (2014): 79.

278   **• The details of the neuroinflammatory reflex:** The neuroinflammatory reflex was recently discovered by the neurosurgeon and scientist Kevin Tracey, M.D., and Ulf Andersson, M.D., Ph.D., who used electrical stimulation of the vagus nerve to quickly cure a man who had disabling rheumatoid arthritis. The patient, who lived in Mostar, Bosnia, had had years of incapacitating pain in his hands, wrists, elbows, and legs. A small pacemaker-like device was surgically implanted into him that, like the PoNS, injected spikes into the vagus. A wire with an electrode from the pacemaker was inserted directly into the vagus. When the team turned on the electrical stimulation, he went into a clinical remission. The device was able to accomplish what his immune-system-suppressing drugs, all of which have major side effects, could not.

   The vagus nerve has that name because it wanders, like a vagabond, so widely throughout the body, from the brain stem across the chest and into the abdomen. It regulates many bodily functions, including digestion, heart rate, and bladder control, among other things. Its left branch receives sensation from major organs and also distributes signals from the brain to the major organs. It also regulates the recently discovered neuroinflammatory reflex.

   Inflammation triggers the production of molecules called cytokines, which help ward off infection; but when inflammation becomes chronic, these same cytokines become toxic to the tissues. Rheumatoid arthritis, like MS, is an autoimmune disease caused when a person's immune system creates inflammation and attacks the body's cells as though they were foreign invaders. Cytokines accumulate in the cartilage and joints, causing pain and tissue destruction.

   Kevin J. Tracey, Mauricio Rosas-Ballina, and colleagues have described how the neuroinflammatory reflex (and its neural and immunological components) is housed in the vagus nerve. Incoming signals to this reflex sense the inflammation levels, and if they are too high, outgoing signals can turn it off. The mechanism is the following. The vagus nerve sends signals to T-cells (immune system cells that float around in the blood) to make a neurotransmitter called acetylcholine (a chemical usually used to send signals in the brain) to stop the production of cytokines, molecules that foster inflammation.

   The discovery that the brain influences the immune system through this neuroinflammatory reflex has important implications, because brain disorders as diverse as MS, TBI, dementia, autism, depression, and some learning disorders (as well as inflammatory bowel disease, many forms of heart disease, atherosclerosis, cancer, diabetes, and all the autoimmune diseases) have huge inflammatory components. Unfortunately, the drugs that we have that suppress inflammation and the immune system can be dangerous, even causing death, and frequently fail.

Stimulation from the PoNS on the tongue goes to a group of cells in the brain stem called the nucleus tractus solitarius—the same area to which the vagus sends its incoming input. There are many signs that the PoNS helps the vagus regulate the body. For instance, if a patient's blood pressure is too low, the PoNS brings it up to normal. If blood pressure is too high, it lowers itself, homeostatically, toward normal. One man noted that whenever he used the device, he could feel his intestines start to move—a sign the device was regulating his gastrointestinal system, likely through the vagus. MS patients sometimes find their bladder control improves with it.

The discovery of the neuroinflammatory reflex is a major breakthrough. It may be that forms of mind-body medicine, such as meditation, hypnosis, qigong, and yogic breathing, neuroplastically use the mind to train the neuroinflammatory reflex to heal some kinds of inflammatory illness. See M. Rosas-Ballina and K. J. Tracey, "The Neurology of the Immune System: Neural Reflexes Regulate Immunity," *Neuron* 64 (2009): 28–32; U. Andersson and K. J. Tracey, "A New Approach to Rheumatoid Arthritis: Treating Inflammation with Computerized Nerve Stimulation," *Cerebrum,* Dana Foundation, March 21, 2012, http://www.dana.org/news/cerebrum/detail.aspx?id=36272.

Chapter 8. A Bridge of Sound

280   **Plato:** Plato, *The Republic,* trans. Benjamin Jowett (New York: C. Scribner's Sons, 1871), bk. 3, 401d.

286   **"I have an unshakable intuition":** A. A. Tomatis, *The Conscious Ear: My Life of Transformation Through Listening* (Barrytown, NY: Station Hill Press, 1991), p. 2.

287   **"My arrival in the world":** Ibid., pp. 1–2.

287   **"squeeze machine":** T. Grandin, "Calming Effects of Deep Touch Pressure in Patients with Autistic Disorder, College Students, and Animals," *Journal of Child and Adolescent Psychopharmacology* 2, no. 1 (1992): 63–72; J. Anderson, "Sensory Intervention with the Preterm Infant in the Neonatal Intensive Care Unit," *American Journal of Occupational Therapy* 40, no. 1 (1986): 9–26; T. M. Field et al., "Tactile-Kinesthetic Stimulation Effects on Preterm Neonates," *Pediatrics* 77, no. 5 (1986): 654–58; S. A. Leib et al., "Effects of Early Intervention and Stimulation on the Preterm Infant," *Pediatrics* 66, no. 1 (1980): 83–89.

288   **"never easy":** Tomatis, *Conscious Ear,* p. 4.

288   **"I have thought this over carefully":** Ibid., p. 12.

291   • **he could hear only in his new singing range:** Tomatis later confirmed this hypothesis when three of Caruso's friends told him that they walked on Caruso's left because his hearing in his right ear had been damaged by his operation. When Tomatis analyzed a second great operatic singer, Beniamino Gigli, he found he had the same restricted range.

291   **"It was as if Caruso"** ... **"had benefited":** Tomatis, *Conscious Ear,* p. 53.

292   • **"the ear is simply an external attribute of the cerebral cortex":** A. A. Toma-
      tis, "Music, and Its Neuro-Psycho-Physiological Effects. Appendix: 'The Three
      Integrators,'" translated by Terri Brown, presentation to the thirteenth Confer-
      ence of the International Society for Music Education, London, Ontario, August
      17, 1978. The "three integrators" theory appeared in A. A. Tomatis, *La Nuit
      Uterine* (Paris: Stock, 1981), pp. 108–34.

292   **"all, without exception, felt ... well-being":** Tomatis, *Conscious Ear,* p. 55.

294   **a child screaming ... loud as a passing train:** K. Barthel, "The Neurobiology of
      Sound and Its Effect on Arousal and Regulation," presentation to the Integrated
      Listening Systems conference, Denver, CO, September 21, 2011, p. 9.

294   **muscles of the middle ear ... regulated by the brain:** S. W. Porges, *The Polyva-
      gal Theory: Neurophysiological Foundations of Emotions, Attachment, Commu-
      nication, Self-Regulation* (New York: W. W. Norton, 2011), p. 220.

294   **brain map areas for those frequencies ... grow:** J. Fritz et al., "Rapid Task-
      Related Plasticity of Spectrotemporal Receptive Fields in Primary Auditory Cor-
      tex," *Nature Neuroscience* 6, no. 11 (2003): 1216–23; J. C. Middlebrooks, "The
      Acquisitive Auditory Cortex," *Nature Neuroscience* 6, no. 11 (2003): 1122–23.

296   • **had to pass from his left ear to his right hemisphere:** One reason the right
      hearing pathway is shorter has to do with the nerve that enervates the larynx,
      which the right ear monitors, called the recurrent laryngeal nerve. That nerve is
      longer on the left side than the right, because our heart is on the left side of the
      body, and so the left laryngeal nerve has to detour around major vessels attached
      to the heart. P. Madaule, *When Listening Comes Alive: A Guide to Effective
      Learning and Communication* (Norval, ON: Moulin, 1994), p. 42.

296   • **delay, up to 0.4 second:** Tomatis, *Conscious Ear,* pp. 50–51.

297   **the right ear ... hear ... higher speech frequencies:** Ibid., p. 52.

299   **"Everything" ... "easy, even ... English":** Madaule, *When Listening Comes Alive,*
      p. 11.

308   **"It is as if the filtered sound of the mother's voice":** Ibid., p. 73.

309   **D. W. Winnicott:** D. W. Winnicott, "Birth Memories, Birth Trauma and Anxi-
      ety" (1949), in *Through Paediatrics to Psycho-Analysis: Collected Papers* (New
      York: Basic Books, 1975), pp. 174–93.

309   **"the only voice ... in the fetal stage":** Tomatis, *Conscious Ear,* p. 127.

309   **"My own experience as a premature baby":** Ibid.

310   • **inner bones of the ear ... *adult size*:** This had been known since 1670. G. B. El-
      liott and K. A. Elliott, "Some Pathological, Radiological and Clinical Implica-
      tions of the Precocious Development of the Human Ear," *Laryngoscope* 74
      (1964): 1160–71.

310   **played a recording of each mother's voice:** B. S. Kisilevsky et al., "Effects of
      Experience on Fetal Voice Recognition," *Psychological Science* 14, no. 3 (2003):
      220–24.

310   **newborns prefer their mother's voice:** A. J. DeCasper et al., "Of Human Bonding:
      Newborns Prefer Their Mothers' Voices," *Science* 208, no. 4448 (1980): 1174–76.

310   **newborns ... prefer stories ... read ... in ... pregnancy:** A. J. DeCasper and
      M. J. Spence, "Prenatal Maternal Speech Influences Newborns' Perception of
      Speech Sounds," *Infant Behavior and Development* 9, no. 2 (1986): 133–50.

310 • **newborns can distinguish the "mother tongue":** Moon, Lagercrantz, and Kuhl, experts in neonatal language and plasticity, have shown that being exposed to a language in the womb will affect one's ability to perceive it. C. Moon et al., "Language Experienced *in Utero* Affects Vowel Perception After Birth: A Two-Country Study," *Acta Paediatrica* 102, no. 2 (2012): 156–60.

310 **newborns have neural networks sensitive to native speech:** B. S. Kisilevsky et al., "Fetal Sensitivity to Properties of Maternal Speech and Language," *Infant Behavior and Development* 32, no. 1 (2009): 59–71.

310 **"Language, too, possesses a physical dimension":** Tomatis, *Conscious Ear,* p. 137.

311 **"We can imagine the unborn child":** Madaule, *When Listening Comes Alive,* pp. 82–83.

313 **fetal lambs … does not necessarily kill all brain cells … fewer dendritic branches:** J. M. Dean et al., "Prenatal Cerebral Ischemia Disrupts MRI-Defined Cortical Microstructure Through Disturbances in Neuronal Arborization," *Science Translational Medicine* 5, no. 168 (2013): 1–11(168ra7).

313 **"Our findings question current assumptions":** Ibid.

315 • **postrotary nystagmus:** On the phenomenon that "when the rotation is suddenly stopped, nystagmus [occurs] in the opposite direction," see A. Fisher et al., *Sensory Integration: Theory and Practice* (Philadelphia: F. A. Davis, 1991), p. 81.

319 **as the cortex evolved and increased in size, the subcortical structures grew:** S. Herculano-Houzel, "Coordinated Scaling of Cortical and Cerebellar Numbers of Neurons," *Frontiers in Neuroanatomy* 4, no. 12 (2010): 1–8.

320 • **He was enraged, unmanageable, and inconsolable:** You can see Jordan's tantrums, and Paul working with him. Go to the Listening Centre's Web site (note the Canadian spelling of *Centre*) at http://listeningcentre.com/ and click the link at the bottom of the page, to the video *The Child That You Do Have.*

320 **hypersensitive to incoming sensation, most often sound:** E. Gomes et al., "Auditory Hypersensitivity in Autistic Spectrum Disorder," *Pro Fono* 20, no. 4 (2008): 279–84.

323 **"For decades, most doctors told parents that autism was … genetic":** M. Herbert and K. Weintraub, *The Autism Revolution* (New York: Ballantine Books, 2012), p. 5. See also M. R. Herbert, "Translational Implications of a Whole-Body Approach to Brain Health in Autism: How Transduction Between Metabolism and Electrophysiology Points to Mechanisms for Neuroplasticity," in V. W. Hu, ed., *Frontiers in Autism Research: New Horizons for Diagnosis and Treatment* (Hackensack, NJ: World Scientific, 2014).

323 • **"Hundreds of genes":** M. Herbert, "Autism Revolution," presentation at Autism Research Institute Conference, Fall 2012, with slides. See the presentation on http://www.youtube.com/watch?v=LuMUE5E22AE, at the twenty-three-minute mark. See also Herbert and Weintraub, *Autism Revolution,* p. 31.

324 **Many autistic children have immune system abnormalities:** P. Goines and J. Van de Water, "The Immune System's Role in the Biology of Autism," *Current Opinion in Neurology* 23, no. 2 (2010): 111–17, 115.

324 • **They have high rates of gastrointestinal infections:** H. M. R. T. Parracho et al., "Differences Between the Gut Microflora of Children with Autistic Spectrum Disorders and That of Healthy Children," *Journal of Medical Microbiology* 54, no. 10 (2005): 987–91. Seventy percent of autistic children have a history of GI

symptoms, twice the rate of children with normal development. M. Valicenti-McDermott et al., "Frequency of Gastrointestinal Symptoms in Children with Autistic Spectrum Disorders and Association with Family History of Auto-immune Disease," *Developmental and Behavioral Pediatrics* 27, no. 2 (2006): S128–36.

324 • **two hundred major toxic chemicals in their umbilical cord blood:** Many people who care for autistic children report improvements when exposures to toxic chemicals are minimized. Herbert and Weintraub, *Autism Revolution,* pp. 35, 42, 125. Thousands of new artificial chemicals go into the environment each year, and most are untested for long-term health effects. Toxins are known to have a negative impact on the immune system. See P. Grandjean et al., "Serum Vaccine Antibody Concentrations in Children Exposed to Perfluorinated Compounds," *Journal of the American Medical Association* 307, no. 4 (2012): 391–97. See also S. Goodman, "Tests Find More Than 200 Chemicals in Newborn Umbilical Cord Blood," *Scientific American* (2009).

324 **inflammation was "particularly striking in the cerebellum":** D. L. Vargas et al., "Neurological Activation and Neuroinflammation in the Brain of Patients with Autism," *Annals of Neurology* 57, no. 1 (2005): 67–81, 77.

325 **antibodies coming from their mothers:** The studies are reviewed in Goines and Van de Water, "Immune System's Role."

325 **23 percent of mothers . . . had such antibodies:** D. Braunschweig et al., "Autism-specific Maternal Autoantibodies Recognize Critical Proteins in Developing Brain," *Translational Psychiatry* 3 (2013): e277, doi:10.1038/tp.2013.50.

325 **monkeys . . . behaviors similar to those of autistic children:** M. D. Bauman et al., "Maternal Antibodies from Mothers of Children with Autism Alter Brain Growth and Social Behavior Development in the Rhesus Monkey," *Translational Psychiatry* 3 (2013): e278, doi:10.1038/tp.2013/47.

325 **high levels of antibodies:** A. Enstrom et al., "Increased IgG4 Levels in Children with Autism Disorder," *Brain, Behavior, and Immunity* 23, no. 3 (2009): 389–95.

325 • **vaccinations . . . in a** *subgroup* **of children is controversial:** We often hear in the media that all medical experts think that vaccinations offer no risk, are safe, and *couldn't possibly* harm a child. The mainstream medical position is far more nuanced. The Centers for Disease Control publish a thirty-four-page "Guide to Vaccine Contraindications and Precautions." *Contraindications* is a medical term for situations in which an intervention should *not* be used *or its use should be altered,* such as for people who have had significant or life-threatening reactions to the vaccine or to a component of it; for people who have abnormal immune systems or certain infections; or for those who have had adverse reactions before, among other situations. The general medical consensus is that vaccines are sometimes harmful for some individuals, and some have been taken off the market for this reason. The key question for autism is, might some potentially autistic children qualify for precautions or contraindications, and have these children specifically been studied? Herbert describes what these children look like in *Autism Revolution.* Some experts say that this subgroup has not been studied in relation to vaccinations. Dr. David Amaral, director of research at the University of California, Davis, MIND Institute, one of the world's leading research institutes on autism and inflammation, said (in a recent PBS special) of children

at risk for autism, "Vaccinations for those children actually may be the environmental factor that tips them over the edge of autism. And I think it is incredibly important still, to try and figure out what, if any, vulnerabilities in a small subset of children might make them at risk for having certain vaccinations." The new science of vaccinomics, which aims to develop personalized vaccines tailored to a person's genetic profile and individual medical history, acknowledges that our current one-size-fits-all approach to vaccines is less than optimal, and that for some people, some current vaccines may be ineffective, and for other people some may be harmful. See M. W. Moyer, "Vaccinomics: Scientists Are Devising Your Personal Vaccine," *Scientific American* (June 24, 2010), http://www.scientificamerican.com/article/vaccinomics-personal-vaccine/. Jordan Rosen and "Timothy," discussed earlier in this chapter, both had an autistic regression within one week of receiving a vaccination at eighteen months.

325   **Chronic inflammation disturbs developing neuronal circuits:** R. H. Lee et al., "Neurodevelopmental Effects of Chronic Exposure to Elevated Levels of Pro-Inflammatory Cytokines in a Developing Visual System," *Neural Development* 5, no. 2 (2010): 1–18.

325   **"underconnected":** M. A. Just et al., "Cortical Activation and Synchronization During Sentence Comprehension in High-Functioning Autism: Evidence of Underconnectivity," *Brain: A Journal of Neurology* 127, no. 8 (2004): 1811–21.

325   **neurons at the front of the brain . . . poorly connected:** S. E. Schipul et al., "Inter-regional Brain Communication and Its Disturbance in Autism," *Frontiers in Systems Neuroscience* 5, no. 10 (2011), doi: 10.3389/fnsys.2011.00010.

325   **Other brain areas show "overconnectivity":** R. Coben and T. E. Myers, "Connectivity Theory of Autism: Use of Connectivity Measures in Assessing and Treating Autistic Disorders," *Journal of Neurotherapy* 12, no. 2 (2008): 161–79.

326   **Abrams . . . autistic children . . . voice is underconnected to . . . reward center:** D. A. Abrams et al., "Underconnectivity Between Voice-Selective Cortex and Reward Circuitry in Children with Autism," *Proceedings of the National Academy of Sciences* 110, no. 29 (2013): 12060–65.

326   **"did not register any change of expression":** L. Kanner, "Autistic Disturbances of Affective Contact," *Nervous Child* 2 (1943): 217–50, 231.

326   **mother's voice, oxytocin is secreted in his brain:** L. J. Seltzer et al., "Social Vocalizations Can Release Oxytocin in Humans," *Proceedings of the Royal Society: Biology* 227, no. 1694 (2010): 2661–66.

327   **oxytocin levels are significantly lower in people with autism:** C. Modahl et al., "Plasma Oxytocin Levels in Autistic Children," *Biological Psychiatry* 43, no. 4 (1998): 270–77.

327   • **"social engagement system":** S. W. Porges et al., "Reducing Auditory Hypersensitivities in Autistic Spectrum Disorders: Preliminary Findings Evaluating the Listening Project Protocol," *Frontiers in Pediatrics* (in press). The intervention exercised the brain's regulation of the middle ear muscles. Autistic children listening to the filtered music began to show more facial expression and stopped averting their gaze in the presence of people; half had their sound sensitivities reduced, and 22 percent showed improved emotional regulation, whereas only 1 percent in the control group did. Clearly, the social engagement system was being turned on. Porges's program is not yet available to consumers. Music works because, as

Porges points out, it "duplicates the frequency band of the human voice." Porges, *The Polyvagal Theory: Neurophysiological Foundations of Emotions*, p. 250. See pp. 26–27 and 250–53 for his theory of how the middle ear developed.

330 **"In the eyes of many, dyslexia"**: P. Madaule, "The Dyslexified World," originally presented at the "Listening and Learning" conference, Toronto, 1978; published in T. M. Gilmour, P. Madaule, and B. Thompson, eds., *About the Tomatis Method* (Toronto: Listening Centre Press, 1989), p. 46; a slightly different version is online at http://www.listening centre.com/pdf/01dyslexie.pdf.

334 **"flew in the face of all my clinical experience"**: Ron Minson, "A Sonic Birth," in D. W. Campbell, ed., *Music and Miracles* (Wheaton, IL: Quest Books, 1992).

335 **good auditory "attention span"**: Madaule, *When Listening Comes Alive*, p. 113.

335 **"the ability to cut out parasitic information"**: Ibid.

336 **Ritalin given to very young animals**: W. A. Carlezon et al., "Enduring Behavioral Effects of Early Exposure to Methylphenidate in Rats," *Biological Psychiatry* 54, no. 12 (2003): 1330–37.

336 **"The movement triggers dopamine, which is key for motivation and attention"**: N. Doidge, *The Brain That Changes Itself* (New York: Viking, 2007), pp. 106–7; J. Ratey, *Spark: The Revolutionary New Science of Exercise and the Brain* (New York: Little, Brown, 2008), p. 136.

336 **very-high-sugar foods**: B. S. Lennerz et al., "Effects of Dietary Glycemic Index on Brain Regions Related to Reward and Craving in Men," *American Journal of Clinical Nutrition* 98, no. 3 (2013): 641–47; M. R. Lyon, *Healing the Hyperactive Brain: Through the New Science of Functional Medicine* (Calgary, AB: Focused Publishing, 2000).

337 **• people with ADHD also have decreased brain volume in the cerebellum**: "Anatomical MRI studies have found reduced volumes, mainly supporting the idea that a distributed circuit that includes the right prefrontal cortex, the caudate nucleus, the cerebellar hemispheres and a subregion of the cerebellar vermis, underlies ADHD." F. X. Castellanos and R. Tannock, "Neuroscience of Attention-Deficit/Hyperactivity Disorder: The Search for Endophenotypes," *Nature Reviews* 3, no. 8 (2002): 617–28, 620. The caudate is part of the basal ganglia. See also Russell Barkley, who, reviewing the brain scan data, observes that people with ADHD have less brain volume in the right frontal cortex, the basal ganglia, and the cerebellum. R. A. Barkley, *Attention-Deficit Hyperactivity Disorder*, 3rd ed. (New York: Guilford Press, 2006), pp. 222–23.

337 **As patients get better . . . the cerebellum increases**: S. Mackie et al., "Cerebellar Development and Clinical Outcome in Attention Deficit Hyperactivity Disorder," *American Journal of Psychiatry* 164, no. 4 (2007): 647–55.

338 **music . . . positive reward . . . Menon . . . Levitin . . . fMRI scans**: V. Menon and D. Levitin, "The Rewards of Music Listening: Response and Physiological Connectivity of the Mesolimbic System," *NeuroImage* 28 (2005): 175–84.

338 **• People with ADHD have smaller basal ganglia**: "When an organism attends to one perception, it inhibits attention to other input. For example, when the organism switches focus or selects a motor response, the other possible selections are inhibited. . . . The frontal cortices, which are an essential participant in the 'looped' architecture of the basal ganglia, clearly play an important role in inhibitory control. . . . However, the first region in which massive inhibitory

control mechanisms can be found is within the basal ganglia. . . . Cortico-basal ganglia 'loops' modulate attention and behavior. Inhibitory output from the basal ganglia to the various target nuclei . . . gate the focus of attention and action depending upon the organism's purpose.

"This elevates the basal ganglia as a major player in cognition and executive control. The inhibitory mechanisms of the basal ganglia challenge the view of cortical supremacy in cognition. The basal ganglia very likely comprised the brain's first executive system, and they continue to heavily contribute to cognitive and behavioral control." L. F. Koziol and D. E. Budding, *Subcortical Structures and Cognition: Implications for Neuropsychological Assessment* (New York: Springer, 2008), p. 20. See also p. 197. See P. C. Berquin et al., "Cerebellum in Attention-Deficit Hyperactivity Disorder: A Morphometric MRI Study," *Neurology* 50, no. 4 (1998): 1087–93.

338 **inhibiting . . . anything unrelated to the main task:** Koziol and Budding, *Subcortical Structures,* pp. 194–97.

339 **leap before they look:** D. G. Amen, *Healing ADD* (New York: Berkley, 2001), pp. 90–92.

339 **Sound therapy . . . Minson and Pointer . . . the vagus nerve:** R. Minson and A. W. Pointer, "Integrated Listening Systems: A Multisensory Approach to Auditory Processing Disorders," in D. Geffner and D. Ross-Swain, eds., *Auditory Processing Disorders: Assessment, Management, and Treatment,* 2nd ed. (San Diego: Plural, 2012), pp. 757–71.

341 **"sensations as 'food for the brain'":** J. Ayres, *Sensory Integration and the Child,* 25th anniversary ed. (Los Angeles: Western Psychological Services, 2005), p. 6.

343 **"slumping in their cells like wet dishrags":** Tim Wilson, "A l'Ecoute de l'Univers: An Interview with Dr. Alfred Tomatis," in T. M. Gilmor, P. Madaule, and B. Thompson, eds., *About the Tomatis Method* (Toronto: Listening Centre Press, 1989), p. 211.

344 **"had been chanting in order to 'charge' themselves":** Ibid.

344 **four hours a night:** Ibid., p. 223.

345 • **Kraus . . . sound waves . . . Mozart . . . brain's waves:** The recordings are taken from the person's brain stem, one of the first areas to receive the incoming signals from the ear. The technique is called auditory brain stem response (ABR). N. Kraus, "Listening in on the Listening Brain," *Physics Today* 64 (2011): 40–45; also N. Kraus and B. Chandrasekaran, "Music Training for the Development of Auditory Skills," *Nature Reviews Science* 11 (2010): 599–605; E. Skoe and N. Kraus, "Auditory Brain Stem Response to Complex Sounds: A Tutorial," *Ear and Hearing* 31, no. 3 (2010): 1–23; N. Kraus, "Atypical Brain Oscillations: A Biological Basis for Dyslexia?" *Trends in Cognitive Science* 16, no. 1 (2011): 12–13.

346 **listen to a waltz rhythm:** S. Nozaradan et al., "Tagging the Neuronal Entrainment to Beat and Meter," *Journal of Neuroscience* 31, no. 28 (2011): 10234–40.

346 **hooked nine pairs of guitarists up to EEGs:** U. Lindenberger et al., "Brains Swinging in Concert: Cortical Phase Synchronization While Playing Guitar," *BMC Neuroscience* 10, no. 1 (2009): 22. A video can be seen at http://www.biomedcentral.com/imedia/2965745562100252/supp2.mpg.

347 **subcortical brain areas . . . once thought to lack plasticity, are . . . neuroplastic:** E. Skoe et al., "Human Brainstem Plasticity: The Interaction of Stimulus Probability and Auditory Learning," *Neurobiology of Learning and Memory* 109, no. 2014 (2013): 82–93.

348 **Levitin ... "dopamine ... improving people's moods":** D. J. Levitin, *This Is Your Brain on Music: The Science of Human Obsession* (Toronto: Dutton, 2006), p. 187.

349 **"A few weeks after the music":** A. A. Tomatis, *La libération d'oedipe, ou de la communication intra-utérine au langage humain* (Paris: Les éditions ESF, 1972), pp. 100–102. This translation is by Paul Madaule.

Afterword to the Paperback Edition

354 **knows what the world is like ... basic commitments:** T. S. Kuhn, *The Structure of Scientific Revolutions* (1962; reprinted, enlarged Chicago: University of Chicago Press, 1970), p. 5.

354 ***Where Medicine Went Wrong:*** B. J. West, *Where Medicine Went Wrong: Rediscovering the Path to Complexity* (Toh Tuck Link, Singapore: World Scientific Publishing Co., 2006), p. 124–26.

357 **Oliver Sacks ... "all sorts of generalizations":** O. Sacks, *On the Move: A Life* (Toronto: Knopf, 2015), p. 173.

358 **"Imagine I cart a pig ..." Ramachandran explains: "I think it's fair to say":** Both Ramachandran quotes from, V. S. Ramachandran and S. Blakeslee, *Phantoms in the Brain* (New York: William Morrow and Company, Inc., 1998), p. xiii.

359 **John Ioannidis, M.D. ... 35 percent ... RCTs cannot be replicated:** S. Ebrahim et al., "Reanalyses of Randomized Clinical Trial Data," *Journal of the American Medical Association* 312, no. 10 (2014): 1024–32, 1027; J. P. A. Ioannidis, "Why Most Published Research Findings Are False," *PLoS Medicine* 2, no. 8 (2005): 696–701.

363 **He has developed many techniques ... Web site:** See http://www.fariastechnique.com.

367 **multicenter study ... BrainHQ ... improvements:** G. W. Rebok et al., "Ten-Year Effects of the Advanced Cognitive Training for Independent and Vital Elderly Cognitive Training Trial on Cognition and Everyday Functioning in Older Adults," *Journal of the American Geriatrics Society* 62, no. 1 (2014): 16–24.

368 **The retina not only has two kinds of photosensitive cells:** D. Zelinsky, "Neuro-optometric Diagnosis, Treatment and Rehabilitation Following Traumatic Brain Injuries: A Brief Overview," *Physical Medicine and Rehabilitation Clinics of North America* 18 (2007): 87–107.

369 **brain does in fact have a lymphatic system:** K. Alitalo et al., "A Dural Lymphatic Vascular System That Drains Brain Interstitial Fluid and Macromolecules," *Journal of Experimental Medicine* 212, no. 7 (2015): 991–99.

Appendix 1. A General Approach to TBI and Brain Problems

371 **a combination of cognitive stimulation and physical and social stimulation reduces post-TBI brain shrinkage:** L. S. Miller et al., "Environmental Enrichment May Protect Against Hippocampal Atrophy in the Chronic Stages of Traumatic Brain Injury," *Frontiers in Human Neuroscience* 7 (2013): 506.

Appendix 2. Matrix Repatterning for TBI

373 **Shock waves from a bomb blast:** Y. Chen et al., "Concepts and Strategies for Clinical Management of Blast-Induced Traumatic Brain Injury and Posttraumatic Stress Disorder," *Journal of Neuropsychiatry and Clinical Neurosciences* 25 (2013): 103–10.

Appendix 3. Neurofeedback for ADD, ADHD, Epilepsy, Anxiety, and TBI

378 **Some introductory books on neurofeedback:** J. Robbins, *A Symphony in the Brain: The Evolution of the New Brain Wave Biofeedback* (New York: Grove Press, 2000); M. Thompson and L. Thompson, *The Neurofeedback Book: An Introduction to Basic Concepts in Applied Psychophysiology* (Wheat Ridge, CO: Association for Applied Psychophysiology and Biofeedback, 2003); S. Larsen, *The Healing Power of Neurofeedback: The Revolutionary LENS Technique for Restoring Optimal Brain Function* (Rochester, VT: Healing Arts Press, 2006); S. Larsen, *The Neurofeedback Solution: How to Treat Autism, ADHD, Anxiety, Brain Injury, Stroke, PTSD, and More* (Toronto: Healing Arts Press, 2012).

Index

David Wootton, *The Invention of Science: A New History of the Scientific Revolution*

Christopher Tyerman, *How to Plan a Crusade: Reason and Religious War in the Middle Ages*

Andy Beckett, *Promised You A Miracle: UK 80–82*

Carl Watkins, *Stephen: The Reign of Anarchy*

Anne Curry, *Henry V: From Playboy Prince to Warrior King*

John Gillingham, *William II: The Red King*

Roger Knight, *William IV: A King at Sea*

Douglas Hurd, *Elizabeth II: The Steadfast*

Richard Nisbett, *Mindware: Tools for Smart Thinking*

Jochen Bleicken, *Augustus: The Biography*

Paul Mason, *PostCapitalism: A Guide to Our Future*

Frank Wilczek, *A Beautiful Question: Finding Nature's Deep Design*

Roberto Saviano, *Zero Zero Zero*

Owen Hatherley, *Landscapes of Communism: A History Through Buildings*

César Hidalgo, *Why Information Grows: The Evolution of Order, from Atoms to Economies*

Aziz Ansari and Eric Klinenberg, *Modern Romance: An Investigation*

Sudhir Hazareesingh, *How the French Think: An Affectionate Portrait of an Intellectual People*

Steven D. Levitt and Stephen J. Dubner, *When to Rob a Bank: A Rogue Economist's Guide to the World*

Leonard Mlodinow, *The Upright Thinkers: The Human Journey from Living in Trees to Understanding the Cosmos*

Hans Ulrich Obrist, *Lives of the Artists, Lives of the Architects*

ALLEN LANE
an imprint of
PENGUIN BOOKS

Recently Published